Blaber's Foundations for Paramedic Practice

Blaber's Foundations for Paramedic Practice
A theoretical perspective

Fourth edition

Edited by Amanda Y. Blaber

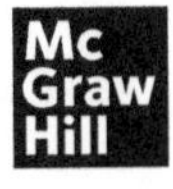

Open University Press

Open University Press
McGraw Hill
Unit 4
Foundation Park
Roxborough Way
Maidenhead
SL6 3UD

email: emea_uk_ireland@mheducation.com
world wide web: www.mheducation.co.uk

First edition published 2008
Second edition published 2012
Third edition published 2019
First published in this fourth edition 2025

Executive Editor: Sam Crowe
Editorial Assistant: Hannah Jones
Content Product Manager: Graham Jones

A catalogue record of this book is available from the British Library

ISBN-13: 9780335252732
ISBN-10: 0335252737
eISBN-13: 9780335252749

Typeset by Transforma Pvt. Ltd., Chennai, India

Praise for this book

"The work that paramedics do is so much more than clinical skills. Patient care is delivered in a complex environment that includes patient perspectives, legal and ethical frameworks, an evolving research base and so much more. Blaber's Foundations for Paramedic Practice provides an excellent overview of these elements in one place. It is both a useful resource for experienced paramedics and essential reading for those just starting out on their journey to registration."

Dr Matt Capsey, PhD, MSc, PgCLTHE, FHEA, MCPara;
Senior Lecturer in Paramedic Practice, University of Cumbria, UK

"This text provides a thorough and insightful exploration of the contemporary aspects that are part of modern paramedic practice, appealing not only to paramedics and paramedic students, but many others working alongside them as well.

New and updated chapters reflect the everchanging nature of the UK paramedic profession, in terms of an ever-expanding scope of practice and increasing professional responsibilities. The many chapter contributors, with their specialist interests and expertise, add significant weight to the quality and value of the book, the content of which is written in a comprehensive, authoritative yet accessible style that will greatly benefit the reader."

Aidan Ward, Senior Lecturer in Paramedic Science,
University of Northampton, UK

"The fourth edition of Blaber's Foundations for Paramedic Practice has been constructed by an incredible wealth of knowledgeable health Care practitioners, who have captured the true essence for being an operation paramedic on today's front-line service. For me the key theme throughout the text is the undertone of how important mental awareness (the hidden psychology) is for today practitioners. Students often come into this profession blinkered by the highly published 'hero paramedic'. This book embeds 'solid foundations' for any aspiring paramedic and is certainly of high value to

Contents

List of contributors

Amanda Blaber has many years of experience in several higher education institutions, lecturing both nurses and paramedics in healthcare subjects, on both undergraduate and postgraduate courses. Amanda is a freelance academic writer and editor. Clinically, Amanda's background is in emergency care, but more recently she has contributed to the COVID-19 vaccination campaigns and now does some work in primary care. Amanda has contributed to national education paramedic forums and curriculum design workshops. She has extensive knowledge and experience in curriculum design and validation processes, and undertakes occasional consultancy work for the College of Paramedics. Amanda is an Honorary Fellow of the College of Paramedics. She is the author/co-editor of *Student Paramedic Survival Guide*; *Assessment Skills for Paramedics*; *Clinical Leadership for Paramedics*; *Independent Prescribing for Paramedics* and the theoretical textbook *Foundations.* Amanda is extremely proud of the contribution she and her colleagues have made to the education of paramedics in the UK.

Mike Brady Dip He, BSc (Hons), PG Dip (ACP), PhD, Consultant Paramedic, Assistant Clinical Director of Remote Clinical Welsh Ambulance Services University NHS Trust. Mike is a consultant paramedic and a clinical academic focusing on emergency, urgent and unscheduled care. He has a specialist interest in digital care, remote consultations and clinical decision support systems. His published research interests include telephone triage, remote clinical decision-making, digital care, end-of-life care, child safeguarding and using patient experience as evidence to improve services. Mike began his career as a rapid response paramedic with the Great Western Ambulance Service after graduating with a diploma in paramedic science from the first undergraduate university paramedic science course in Wales. He completed his BSc Honours degree and started his PhD in 2012, focusing on the paramedic's role in child safeguarding. Mike has completed a postgraduate diploma in advanced clinical practice and still spends time in clinical practice. Mike has been a lecturer in emergency and unscheduled care, an academic author and a clinical leader to a range of nurses and allied health professions, predominantly in 999 and 111 contact centres, where most of his recent research has been focused and where he has overseen and directly coordinated various large-scale programmes of digital clinical change. He is currently the Assistant Clinical Director of Remote Clinical Care at Welsh Ambulance Services University NHS Trust. This role involves leading, influencing and setting clinical direction for remote clinical decision-making and triage for the organisation. It involves interpreting national policy and new legislation, understanding its impact on the organisation and the profession, and influencing how it is implemented.

James Brogan is Principal Lecturer for the Paramedic Practice course at Robert Gordon University (RGU), Aberdeen. In this role, James leads all paramedic provision at RGU and is also responsible for areas across other disciplines and streams of work within the School. James has significant experience in paramedicine and the education of medical and non-medical pre-hospital practitioners. He has worked at several institutions, providing education and leadership, and teaching pre- and post-registration practitioners across medical and non-medical programmes in the UK and internationally. James is a member of the Scottish Collaboration of Paramedic Educators (SCoPE) and the Scottish Government Overarching Steering Group on Paramedic Education.

Vince Clarke BSc (Hons), PGCE, MA, EdD, FHEA, MCPara, Associate Professor (Learning and Teaching). Vince is Programme Lead for the BSc Honours in Paramedic Science at the University of Hertfordshire, Hatfield, where he has been employed since 2016. He joined the London Ambulance Service in 1996, qualified as paramedic in 1998 and entered the Education and Development Department in 2001. He worked as part of the higher education team and developed in-house paramedic programmes in addition to working closely with higher education partner institutions. A Health and Care Professions Council partner since 2006, Vince has been involved in the regulatory approval of a wide range of paramedic educational programmes across the UK as well as assessing continuing professional development submissions and sitting on the Conduct and Competence Fitness to Practise panel hearings. Vince has served as Trustee for Education for the College of Paramedics, the UK's professional body for paramedics, having also held the position of Head of Endorsements. He maintains clinical currency and works for the London Ambulance Service as a bank paramedic. Vince also works as an independent paramedic expert witness for the courts and prepares reports on breach of duty for both claimants and defendants. Vince's professional doctorate in education focused on the theory–practice relationship in paramedic undergraduate education. This work informed the development of university-accredited ambulance service paramedic Practice Educator courses and forms the basis for the College of Paramedics' approach to practice-based learning.

Madeleine Cole BSc (Hons) Paramedic Practice. After finishing university, Maddi spent four years working for the Ambulance Service from 2018 to 2022. During this time, she worked on the frontline throughout the COVID-19 pandemic, as a clinical advisor in the ambulance control centre and within the practice education department. Her interest in frailty and long-term condition management led her to move into primary care where she is due to start her advanced clinical practitioner training. Alongside this, she also spent a year working as a lecturer practitioner at the University of Brighton on the paramedic science degree programme. Maddi has always had a keen interest in public health and health promotion to support people to live well for longer. Maddi believes that encouraging patients to have autonomy over their care and allowing space for clinicians to *open up* conversations about health and wellbeing provides opportunity for holistic, patient-centred care. She hopes her contribution will help others understand the complex nature of public health and how health inequalities can impact the accessibility and uptake of services and public health promotions.

Steve Cowland is Senior Lecturer in the Department of Paramedic Science, City St George's, University of London. Before joining City St George's in 2015, Steve worked for the London Ambulance Service for over 30 years where, as a paramedic training officer and course director, he developed, with higher education institutions, both Foundation and BSc paramedic degree courses. Now working at City St George's, Steve continues to mentor paramedic students and develop practice placement provision for them as well as seeking opportunities for further placement experiences. As the paramedic profession is becoming more expansive in nature and the need for more varied and inter-professional placements is becoming an essential requirement of course content, Steve continues with the team at City St Georges to develop these opportunities so that they become an intrinsic part of the student paramedic experience.

Professor Bob Fellows OBE, FCPara, BSc, PGCE, MSc. Bob is a paramedic consultant and educationalist of many years' service in paramedic education, specific to pre-hospital and out-of-hospital care, with a focus on pre-registration curriculum design. With a career spanning over 40 years in the NHS ambulance service and higher and further education, Bob has been a specialist visitor for the regulator in education and continuing professional development (CPD), and both a pioneer of the professional body and an employee, including head of education for six years. He has published several texts and, together with Graham Harris, is co-author of a *History of the Paramedic Profession – A Modern Success.* Inspired by his own father, who worked for the London Ambulance Service in the 1950s, Bob encouraged his son to become an enhanced paramedic for London and South Central. Bob's mother was also a nurse and his daughter is a doctor working in cardiology. Now retired clinically, Bob maintains his association with paramedicine through educational links to the College of Paramedics and assessing CPD with the Health and Care Professions Council.

Professor Rachael Fothergill PhD, BSc (Hons), Head of Clinical Audit and Research, London Ambulance Service. Rachael joined the London Ambulance Service in 2000 and has been their head of clinical audit and research for the last 24 years. She has a wealth of experience in pre-hospital research supported by her background as a health scientist. Rachael is an Honorary Professor at Warwick University's Medical School and a Visiting Professor of Kingston University's Faculty of Health, Social Care and Education. She is the chair and a founding member of the UK's National Ambulance Research Steering Group and sits on numerous trial steering groups and project management committees for academic and charitable organisations. She has published widely on pre-hospital research, including in the *New England Journal of Medicine* and *The Lancet.* Her involvement in research and clinical audit, both within the UK and internationally, has influenced pre-hospital clinical guidelines, leading to changes in clinical practice and patient care.

Ann French qualified as a registered nurse in 1988 and worked as a staff nurse in the Division of Neurosciences. When Teesside Hospice opened in 1994, Ann was a sister in the in-patient unit, providing specialist palliative care for patients with life-limiting illnesses, after which she became a Macmillan clinical nurse specialist working in the community. Ann is now acting Dean in the School of Health and Life Sciences at Teesside University and is involved in a variety of palliative care modules. She completed her PhD in palliative care at the International Observatory on End of Life Care, Lancaster University, her research focusing on how people with a life-threatening illness cope at the end of life.

Georgina Gill HCPC Paramedic, BSc (Hons). After qualifying as a paramedic, Georgina worked in an NHS ambulance service where she developed a special interest in the care of older adults and frailty. She later moved to East Surrey Hospital to work as a Teaching Fellow in geriatric medicine. During this time, she contributed to Series 11 and 12 of the MDTea Podcast (https://thehearingaidpodcasts.org.uk/mdtea-podcast/) in addition to working within an emergency department-based frailty service. She then worked as a community frailty practitioner, completing comprehensive geriatric assessments and advanced care plans. Georgina has recently returned to the ambulance service and hopes to complete her masters to become an advanced clinical practitioner. When not at work, she is most often found being active, whether that's walking, cycling, swimming or in the gym.

Vicky Gooch BSc, DipHE, PG Cert, MSC, HEA Fellow. Vicky is an advanced practitioner currently working in primary care. She worked as a senior lecturer/assistant professor at two different universities between 2016 and 2023, where she contributed to the Paramedic BSc programmes. Vicky believes that using a patient-centred approach is essential in clinical practice: treating each person as an individual regardless of their diagnosis. She hopes that increasing awareness of the challenges faced by people living with dementia will result in improved care for all.

Liam Hamilton MSc, BSc (Hons). Liam is currently Clinical Simulation Fellow in the Faculty of Education, Health and Human Sciences, University of Greenwich. Liam trained as a paramedic in London before moving to Kent. His career as a paramedic in the ambulance service saw him working on frontline ambulances, fast response cars and the Special Operations Response Team (SORT), before becoming an operational team leader and operational commander. He sat on a professional practice group and contributed to and led on local and trust-wide initiatives. He has mentored and developed students and staff throughout his career, leading him to pursue a career in higher education. Serving through the COVID-19 pandemic changed the way Liam looked at his decision-making and how it changed paramedic practice. Identifying the need to bridge the gap between traditional paramedic training and practice, he joined the University of Greenwich as a Clinical Simulation Fellow, specialising in Human Factors and decision-making in pre-hospital care. He works in a multidisciplinary team to design and develop new concepts, and deliver clinical simulation scenarios for paramedics and other registered healthcare professionals. Liam also volunteers for a charity who deliver basic life support and bleed control sessions for young people at risk or involved with gang violence. With a keen interest in the forensic and legal aspects of pre-hospital care, he undertakes occasional shifts as a paramedic within the prison service.

Graham Harris FCPara, BSc, PGCE, MSc. Graham is a paramedic educationalist of long standing in healthcare education, specific to pre-hospital care, with a focus on paramedic practice and experience in developing and leading paramedic degree programmes within the university sector. His career to date spans over 50 years across the military, NHS ambulance service, higher education and the professional body. He is a prolific contributor to educational texts dealing with paramedic practice, including the acclaimed *Assessment Skills for Paramedics* and *Clinical Leadership for Paramedics* – he co-authored chapters in all four editions. He is a co-author of the *History of the Paramedic Profession – A Modern Success.* He has been instrumental in the development of numerous College of Paramedics publications and acted as the College representative on several of the sub-committees that implemented the findings of the Paramedic Evidence-based Education Project (PEEP) report, being the prime link between the UK College of Paramedics and Health Education England (HEE) in the development and implementation of key strategic documents, including chairing the Quality Assurance Agency Paramedic Subject Benchmark Statement (2016). He has held the Alternate and Elected representative London Region, Assistant Director, Director of Professional Standards and National Education Lead posts for the College of Paramedics. He has also been a member and chair of the Education Advisory Committee.

Nikki Harvey RGN has a masters in child protection and until recently was the Head of Safeguarding for the Welsh Ambulance Services University NHS Trust (WAST), a position she held since 2017. Nikki has over 20 years' experience working collaboratively within the safeguarding and public protection arena in a variety of health service settings. On behalf of WAST, Nikki has been instrumental in the development and implementation of a digital safeguarding reporting system which is now in use across Wales. She has been influential in strategic safeguarding, chairing the National Ambulance Safeguarding Assurance Group (NASAG) for several years. Having recently retired early, part of Nikki's legacy will be the impact of her revolutionising safeguarding reporting in WAST.

Kath Jennings SFHEA, MA, PGCert HE, BA (Hons) MCPARA. Kath is a Senior Lecturer, School of Health Sciences, University of Greenwich. Kath has worked as a paramedic academic since 2010 in two higher education institutions and has held roles as academic section lead, programme leader, module leader, personal tutor and in curriculum development. As well as teaching paramedic science, Kath teaches across inter-professional modules teaching adult and children's nursing and midwifery students. Kath has written about leadership in this book because, in addition to having held various leadership roles in her academic career, she currently leads on a leadership and clinical decision-making module within the BSc Hons Paramedic Science degree programme at the University of Greenwich. Kath's clinical experience was gained while working for the London Ambulance Service NHS Trust as an emergency medical technician and a paramedic. She is currently undertaking doctoral studies in the field of paramedics and knife crime. Her other research interests include end-of-life care for paramedics, paramedic students' understanding of emotional labour in paramedic practice, inter-professional education and paramedics' management of traumatic injuries.

Gwenan Jones-Parry MSc, BSc (Hons), DipHE Paramedic Science, Senior Safeguarding Specialist, Welsh Ambulance Service University NHS Trust (WAST). Gwenan is a registered paramedic who worked on an ambulance and rapid response vehicle in South Wales before specialising and joining the safeguarding team. Contributing to strategic and operational safeguarding, providing safeguarding advice to colleagues, attending multi-agency safeguarding forums and developing safeguarding training all are part of her daily role. Gwenan has played a key part in the work to digitalise the safeguarding reporting process, making safeguarding reports more accessible to colleagues and the reporting process more efficient. Having been through the newly qualified paramedic process and become a practice educator herself, supporting paramedic students while on placement, Gwenan understands the importance of combining theory, knowledge and practical application. Gwenan is pleased to have had the opportunity to author and co-author the safeguarding chapters of this book. All paramedics will face complex safeguarding matters during their career, so it is essential that they are equipped to recognise and report these concerns appropriately. Gwenan hopes that these safeguarding chapters support paramedics, in any role and at all points within their career, to *Think Safeguarding!*

John Krohne Dip He Nursing (Mental Health), BSc, PG Cert, MSc, HEA Fellow. John is the joint course leader for Mental Health Nursing at the University of Brighton. He has clinical experience in a variety of mental health settings, including psychiatric intensive care and working age/ older adult in-patient services. Between 2003 and 2016, John worked in education roles supporting nurse mentors and students in clinical practice across adult, child and mental health fields. This included the role of Education Lead for a Community NHS Trust providing adult/child services before joining the University of Brighton as a senior lecturer in 2016. In this role, John contributes both to pre-registration nursing, paramedic, radiography and midwifery programmes and post-registration modules teaching dementia, ethics and leadership. John has a passion for dementia teaching and believes it is important for healthcare professionals to use the lived experience of the person with dementia to inform their practice, moving beyond the diagnosis and focusing on the individual.

Carol Lloyd NNEB, BEd Hons, Dip C, MA, PhD. Carol is Senior Lecturer in Humanistic Counselling and Childhood Studies, University of Chichester, and a UKCP-accredited psychotherapist. Carol first trained as a nursery nurse. In her early vocational journey, she made the decision to train as an early years teacher, specialising in the 3–8-year age group. Carol's career and experience with supporting children focused on education. However, while undertaking her teacher training, she experienced a life-changing event and embarked on the counselling route to help with trauma. Moving in a parallel path vocationally to education, she began her counselling training. Carol progressed to teach an MA in Transpersonal Arts and Practice (Somatic art psychotherapy) in 2009 researching cancer and trauma. Carol continues to be involved in training counsellors to degree level and private practise counselling adults and children as an accredited expressive arts psychotherapist. In 2014, Carol undertook her PhD into researching a potential for integrating the sharing of children's sleep dreams within an educational context, aiming to merge two disciplines. Her research is underpinned by the psychoanalytical work of Carl Jung and was completed in 2020. In summary, Carol has over 30 years' experience working in the disciplines of delivering mental health teaching in higher education settings and her private practise as a psychotherapist with adults and children. Carol's contribution to the chapters in this book is aimed at the integration of the psychological theory of the personality, concepts of the development of the unconscious towards consciousness and the unique diversity of a human personality. By reading her contributions, it is hoped paramedics will be be inspired to study and perceive the sum of all the parts of a child's psyche and the complexities of neurodiversity. Carol hopes readers will become wiser in their professional knowledge and feel more skilled in their professional approach to trauma or emergency situations.

Christopher Matthews is a Critical Care Paramedic Manager and a Senior Lecturer on a BSc (Hons) Paramedic Science degree course. He is also a Fellow of the Higher Education Academy. Chris commenced his ambulance career after leaving the Royal Marine Commandos as a commissioned officer, following an exciting and varied career. Using his previous valuable experiences, Chris quickly progressed to become a critical care paramedic, due to his keen interest in the management of high acuity patients. He believes that expert pre-hospital critical care must become an integral component within all Ambulance Trusts. His time in the military and as a critical care paramedic has enabled him to see the importance of human factors within paramedicine. He developed one of the very first university modules to deliver Human Factors and leadership education to student paramedics and he hopes all paramedic courses and Ambulance Trusts will embrace teaching in this field. Chris has achieved many awards during his ambulance career, including one from the Royal Humane Society for bravery, and he is about to complete his MSc in Advanced Clinical Practice.

Ptolemy Neoptolemos joined the North East Ambulance Service in 2004, becoming a registered paramedic in 2007, spending time working as a team leader. In 2015, he joined Teesside University as a Senior Lecturer in Paramedic Practice and was also Representative Trustee for the North East with the College of Paramedics during this time. Currently, Ptolemy is acting Head of Department for Nursing and Midwifery in the School of Health and Life Science at Teesside University, and contributes to higher education provision across the School. He is currently studying for his PhD, focusing on the coping mechanisms used by student paramedics in dealing with occupational stress with a particular focus on maladaptive coping strategies.

Alison Robinson qualified as a registered general nurse in 1991 and has spent all of her career within oncology, palliative care and nurse education. For most of her career, Alison has held cancer nurse specialist roles, primarily head/neck cancer and lung cancer. She also managed and led a Macmillan Cancer Information Centre before moving into an educational role within an NHS Trust. In 2014, Alison joined Teesside University as a senior lecturer to pursue her interest in nurse education and workforce development. Alison is currently a Principal Lecturer in Learning and Teaching in the School of Health and Life Science at Teesside University, supporting the development of programmes within nursing and midwifery. Following the completion of her MSc in 2013, her particular interests are in service improvement and leadership.

Joanna Shaw MRes, BSc (Hons). Joanna is Clinical Audit Manager, London Ambulance Service NHS Trust. Since joining the Trust, Joanna has had responsibility for managing the service's clinical audit programme, producing changes to the Trust's clinical practice and improving the care delivered to patients. She monitors clinical audit activities across the Trust, supporting and facilitating other staff undertaking clinical audit, both internally and externally, by providing individual tuition and running clinical audit training sessions. Joanna has accreditations in Advanced Clinical Audit, Trainer in Clinical Audit and Significant Event Audit. Joanna also has a history supporting health research projects in the voluntary sector with a BSc (Hons) in Biology and Statistics from Keele University and an MRes in Health and Social Care from the University of Manchester. Joanna has published her work in several peer-reviewed research journals and has presented at numerous national and international conferences.

Lucy Shaw BSc (Hons) Paramedic Practice. After finishing university, Lucy worked as a paramedic for the ambulance service from 2018 to 2023, working on the frontline throughout the COVID-19 pandemic. After a short career break, Lucy plans to start working as an urgent community response paramedic helping people within the community to avoid hospital admission. Lucy is interested in communication theory as it is not only crucial to providing effective and compassionate care but is also essential to our everyday lives and relationships. She believes that our communication skills are something we should all continue to improve.

Chris Storey is a HCPC Paramedic and Senior Lecturer. Chris started working for the University of Brighton as a Senior Lecturer on the BSc (Hons) Paramedic Science course in 2015. He balanced this with working 'on the road' as an ambulance paramedic with South East Coast Ambulance Service. Now full time at the university, he teaches anatomy and physiology and patient physical assessment, as well as being the admissions tutor for the course. He has retained his paramedic registration and does voluntary work for the ambulance service in his spare time.

Claire Tinker MSc, PGCert HE, BSc (Hons). Claire is a registered paramedic and currently a Senior Lecturer in the School of Education, Health and Human Sciences, University of Greenwich. Claire started her paramedic journey in 1996 and worked for the London Ambulance Service NHS Trust in a variety of roles, including cycle response paramedic, London's Air Ambulance flight paramedic and clinical tutor. She completed an MSc in Advanced Practice at the University of Greenwich before leaving the NHS for the University of Cumbria to launch the Paramedic Degree Apprenticeship Programme in London.

Jackie Whitnell works within the NHS and has done so for more than 30 years. Her career spans theatre and intensive care nursing, sick children's nursing and health visiting. Jackie has an MA in Sociology of Health and a BSc (Hons) in Psychology. Jackie has also worked as a senior lecturer in several universities across South East England, teaching all aspects of child health, including atypical and developmental psychology to students studying paramedic science, nursing, midwifery and childhood studies. Jackie returned to nurse practice during the COVID-19 pandemic to aid the vaccination programme and continues to work at her local GP practice.

Professor Julia Williams PhD, FC Para, FHEA, Professor of Paramedic Science. As Head of Research for the College of Paramedics, Julia is committed to increasing the capacity and capability of paramedics within paramedic research, and she takes every opportunity to inform other agencies about the rich talent that exists within the paramedic profession in relation to clinical research, highlighting the positive contribution paramedics can make to the health and care research agenda. Over the years, she has been involved in a variety of qualitative, quantitative and mixed methods research studies related to different aspects of paramedic practice; unscheduled emergency and urgent healthcare provision; paramedic education; and the health and wellbeing of the paramedic workforce.

Acknowledgements

Since my initial involvement with paramedic education many years ago, when there was only one higher education institute in the UK running undergraduate and postgraduate courses, there has been an exponential increase in the number of education programmes being offered. The College of Paramedics has, and continues to be, instrumental in guiding the education of future paramedics. I was fortunate to be involved in the early stages of this development and, as a nurse educator (at that point), was privileged that my paramedic colleagues were so welcoming, keen, receptive and willing to listen, learn and work collaboratively to develop the first curriculum guidance document. Obviously, the paramedic profession has so much expertise and in so many fields now, that it is self-governing and only occasionally requires input from colleagues from other professions. That is the way it should be.

The four (Blaber's) *Foundations* texts have followed a similar evolutionary path: now, having many of the chapters being written by paramedics or collaborations of education teams from various institutions and/or ambulance services. My thanks to everyone, past and present, who has contributed to the education of student paramedics. Paramedicine has meant that I have had the pleasure of getting to know and working with many people across the UK that I would not otherwise have done. It has also been very special and a source of pride for me to follow the career paths of many of my ex-students, some of whom have contributed to this and previous texts. The paramedic network is most definitely alive and well.

Special thanks to the contributors who have been *in this from the beginning*: Steve, Bob, Rachael, Graham and Jackie. You have been consistent, enthusiastic, committed and have always delivered 100 per cent. To all at OU Press for their assistance, commitment and expertise, especially Sam and Hannah.

To my long enduring family and friends who have *lived* all four editions with me – thank you for your ideas, thoughts, proofreading, patience, care and love during the process, which I know can at times be arduous, time-consuming and hard work. But, I love it!

Finally, to Jackie, without whose encouragement and support, *Foundations* would not exist. It was your enthusiasm, we-can-do-this attitude, drive, commitment, expertise and wholehearted belief in me that got us to this point today. Thank you!

Introduction

Amanda Y. Blaber

There is always a starting point, whether that be, for example, your decision to make paramedicine your career or what educational path to take into the profession… similarly, this book acts as a starting point for you. It is hoped that it will ignite your curiosity and passion to learn more and educate you to the point where you will be the best paramedic you can be. If that is the case, *Foundations* will have served its purpose.

This book (and previous editions of it) was never intended to be a 'one-stop' shop for paramedic education, but a springboard to help you on your education journey. You also need to conduct your own further reading, investigations and research.

If you look through the chapter content of each of the four (Blaber's) *Foundations for Paramedic Practice* texts (2008, 2012, 2019, 2024), some chapters will have been removed, some updated and many replaced. Together with the first, second and third editions, this text reflects a historical journey of the paramedic role in the UK. It is also important to recognise that politics will affect the National Health Service, in addition to society at large and societal expectations. All of these factors (and more) affect clinicians' roles, working conditions, opportunities and the care given to patients. It is hoped that this text helps you to see how inextricably linked many of these subjects are and how changes in one area can affect many others. The complexities of care are many and varied.

Hints to help you use this book effectively

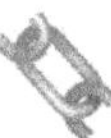 Throughout the chapters, the symbol to the left serves as a prompt to readers to **'link to'** other chapters, where you can read more on a specific subject or subjects.

 **Reflection: points to consider**

You will also find '**Reflection: points to consider**' boxes, where you are invited to consider what you have just read and apply it to your own life experience and/or practice.

There are many **case studies** sprinkled throughout the text. We invite you to read these and then link theory to practice, addressing the questions posed. It is hoped that these features bring the book to life for the reader and help make links to practice more explicit and encourage critical thinking.

Interpersonal communication: a foundation of practice

Lucy Shaw

> **In this chapter:**
> - Introduction
> - Why is this relevant?
> - The basics of communication
> - Verbal features of communication
> - Non-verbal communication
> - Communicating with patients: exploring the case study
> - Inter-professional communication tools
> - Conclusion
> - Chapter key points
> - References and suggested reading

INTRODUCTION

Communication is one of the most fundamental elements of human existence and is integral to our lives from birth. It involves the transfer of information between people and it is difficult to think of any situation when a person is not communicating in some way or other, because even when you are not speaking, your body is constantly presenting a stream of non-verbal messages to those around you (Gamble and Gamble, 2017, 2023). Outwardly, communication appears normal and straightforward, whereas in fact it is complex and open to many influences, which can lead to being misunderstood, if the meaning within the communication is not clear and consistent in all the forms that the information is being sent, received and understood (Pavord and Donnelly, 2015).

WHY IS THIS RELEVANT?

In health care, being able to communicate effectively is vital (Vermier et al., 2015). Communication is one of the '6 Cs of Care' (NHS Professionals,

2023), a set of fundamental values that healthcare staff must demonstrate to provide a high standard of patient care. Arguably, communication is one of the most important skills required by paramedics (O'Toole, 2023). Without interpersonal communication, paramedics would not be able to talk to patients, know the location of their next call, hand over a patient to the staff in an emergency department, or undertake most of their clinical skills safely. Hence, the ability to communicate with patients, relatives, colleagues and the public is seen as an essential skill for ambulance clinicians and all healthcare practitioners (Pavord and Donnelly, 2015; HCPC, 2024). Despite the importance of communication, it has often been seen as a soft skill and not as important as the technical skills, such as cannulation and intubation. However, Lucas et al. (2015) are critical of this view, suggesting communication should be considered alongside, and equal to, those technical skills, because communication is integral to their performance. Despite communication being such a fundamental part of professional practice, 22 per cent of written complaints received by the National Health Service are concerned with communication issues alone, either from staff to patient, staff to staff, or patient to staff (O'Hara et al., 2019). It is clear, then, that all clinicians should be constantly aware of 'what and how they communicate', because it could have either a positive or negative effect on every aspect of their relationships with patients, relatives and colleagues. So, communication warrants a place at the heart of practice.

THE BASICS OF COMMUNICATION

Communication is a two-way process that includes the exchange of information, thoughts and feelings by speaking, body language, or writing of some sort, according to *The Oxford English Dictionary* (2024). It has been established for some time that only 7 per cent of communication is attributed to the words used, while 38 per cent is derived from the tone of voice used and a further 55 per cent from non-verbal cues (Mehrabian, 1981).

The most common model of interpersonal communication proposes that one person is 'the sender' who formulates a message and sends it verbally, non-verbally, or in a combination of the two, to another person, 'the receiver'. Once a message has been sent, the receiver uses his or her senses (hearing, sight, etc.) to receive it. The receiver then interprets that message and responds verbally, non-verbally or both, with what they think is appropriate feedback to the sender, based on the receiver's interpretation. The original sender, then, in turn, interprets that feedback and responds, based on what they think the feedback was (Shannon and Weaver, 1949). If the message contains conflicting verbal and non-verbal cues, known as a 'mixed message', it may be misunderstood and thus misinterpreted. Hence, all clinicians need to send clear messages – where there is consistency between the verbal and non-verbal features – so as to minimise any potential misunderstandings.

However, communication is open to a range of factors that influence the way we formulate and send messages (encoding) and interpret messages (decoding). Both the sender and receiver encode and decode the meaning of the message through the verbal and non-verbal features of communication alongside their senses (Argyle, 1988). This process is influenced by many other factors associated with each of us – our social identity, personality, values, beliefs, gender, culture, status, to name just a few (Hartley, 1999) (see Figure 1.1). So all clinicians should consider how these factors influence what they communicate and how the patient's sociocultural factors influence how that communication is interpreted, particularly within multicultural societies, where differences in values, beliefs and behaviours need to be respected to enable paramedics to provide good quality care to a diverse patient group and prevent offence being caused inadvertently (Pavord and Donnelly, 2015; HCPC, 2024). In addition, the social situation in which communication occurs can positively or negatively influence the effectiveness of that communication (see Figure 1.1). If a situation was time-critical or complex, for example, it would require very clear, direct communication.

VERBAL FEATURES OF COMMUNICATION

Verbal communication is, in essence, a deliberate conscious process, because people select the words from their vocabulary to communicate what they want to say (Gamble and Gamble, 2017). The meaning of the messages we communicate may change depending on the paralinguistic features used to convey them. The paralinguistic features outlined in Figure 1.2 are used to emphasise the meaning of the message the sender wishes to send.

Paramedics are expected to use professional vocabulary with colleagues and other professionals whose understanding of that terminology may vary, yet also be able to translate that communication to meet the needs of patients whose cognitive development and communication abilities will also vary. The optimum level of communication is that which is clear, understandable and appropriate to the situation and people involved.

Clearly, when someone speaks in order to convey a verbal message, it needs to be loud enough for the intended recipient to hear it (Pavord and Donnelly, 2015). The volume used to send a message will vary depending on the situation – for example, two paramedics talking at a busy roadside would need to speak louder than when talking to a patient in their home.

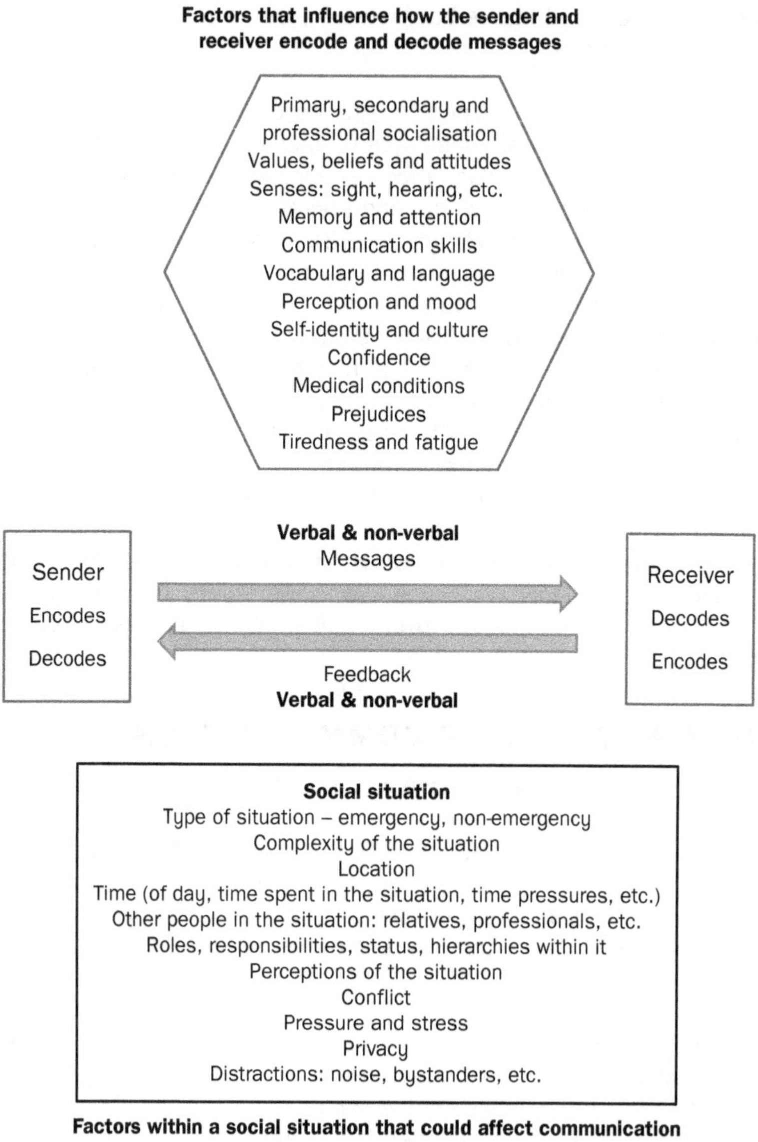

Factors that influence how the sender and receiver encode and decode messages

Primary, secondary and
professional socialisation
Values, beliefs and attitudes
Senses: sight, hearing, etc.
Memory and attention
Communication skills
Vocabulary and language
Perception and mood
Self-identity and culture
Confidence
Medical conditions
Prejudices
Tiredness and fatigue

Sender		Receiver
Encodes	**Verbal & non-verbal** Messages →	Decodes
Decodes	← Feedback **Verbal & non-verbal**	Encodes

Social situation
Type of situation – emergency, non-emergency
Complexity of the situation
Location
Time (of day, time spent in the situation, time pressures, etc.)
Other people in the situation: relatives, professionals, etc.
Roles, responsibilities, status, hierarchies within it
Perceptions of the situation
Conflict
Pressure and stress
Privacy
Distractions: noise, bystanders, etc.

Factors within a social situation that could affect communication

Figure 1.1   A model of communication

Source: Adapted from Shannon and Weaver (1949), Hartley (1999), Pavord and Donnelly (2015).

Furthermore, ensuring an appropriate volume is important in terms of the effectiveness of the communication: too loud and a patient may think you are shouting at them, too soft and they may not hear you at all – both could

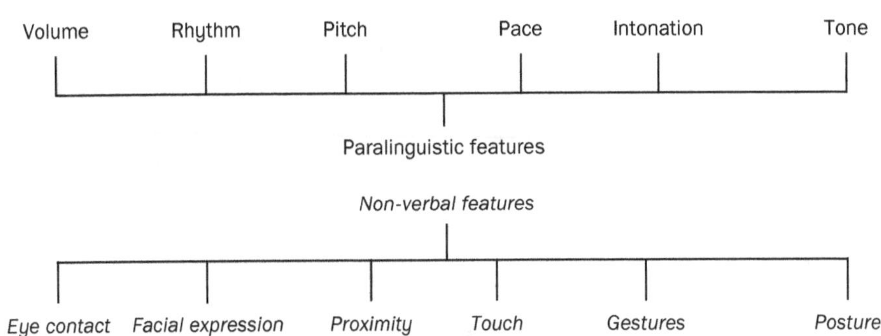

Figure 1.2 Paralinguistic and non-verbal features of communication

limit the patient's ability to interpret the meaning of the message correctly, and potentially leave them with a lasting negative impression of how clinicians communicate.

Closely linked to volume is pitch – usually the higher the volume, the higher the pitch of voice. If these two elements are linked to a fast pace and rhythm of speaking, it could – paralinguistically – communicate a sense of urgency, but it could also be interpreted as a sign of stress or panic. Thus, the possible consequences of clinicians using a raised volume, pitch, pace and rhythm include that the recipients of the message may potentially think the situation is serious, or perhaps that the clinician is unsure of what they are doing. Changes in these aspects of speech may, in part, be due to alterations in the clinician's level of anxiety during a patient interaction, particularly if it is a stressful one. Additionally, the more the clinician feels under pressure, the more these features will be reflected in their voice.

Intonation is the emphasis used to communicate a particular tone or mood and the paralinguistic features are used to do this. Hence, controlling the intonation of the voice by having a calm pace, rhythm and tone at an appropriate volume will likely communicate confidence, caring and trustworthiness. Tonal qualities that infer sarcasm, for example, should be avoided.

Case study 1.1

You attend a care home for an elderly patient who has fallen over. When you arrive, the patient is lying on the floor of the living room with other residents walking around and the TV on very loud. The staff advise you that the patient is hard of hearing. Next, you attend a child who has been generally unwell for a few days and is now having difficulty breathing; the child is sitting with her parents and is crying.

- How can you adapt your verbal communication to suit each patient? Consider the paralinguistic features of speech: volume, rhythm, pitch, pace, intonation and tone.
- How can you adapt your non-verbal communication so that it is appropriate for each patient? Consider the non-verbal features: eye contact, facial expression, proximity, gesture and posture.
- What could you do to make the situation better for communicating with each patient? Consider changes you could make to the environment – for example, switching the TV off/removing distractions, incorporating toys/objects to demonstrate what you'll do, or using communication aids.

Paramedics communicate with patients of all ages, backgrounds and with varying communication needs. It is important to be able to adapt how you communicate to work best for each patient and their needs. Being an effective communicator puts patients and their family members at ease. If a patient has communication needs, ask the patient and their relatives how they communicate best and whether they utilise a particular technique or piece of equipment to aid them.

NON-VERBAL COMMUNICATION

In addition to verbal communication, people instinctively use their bodies to communicate non-verbally. Furthermore, non-verbal communication – in a similar manner to the paralinguistic features of speech – can replace, supplement or contradict the meaning of the verbal message being sent (Gamble and Gamble, 2017). Often, non-verbal cues are unconscious manifestations of thoughts and feelings. Consequently, it is difficult for an individual to have total conscious control over their non-verbal cues and to some degree they will always communicate non-verbal messages they are unaware of, even if they pay close attention to their own body language, which may lead to unintentional miscommunication (Hartley, 1999).

Eye contact

Eye contact is a significant form of non-verbal communication. It is an important way that people initiate and maintain communication and its use by paramedics can show they are interested and care about their patients.

Usually, the receiver will maintain eye contact with the sender for the main part of the message, while the sender will at times look away and return to have eye contact with the receiver. Consequently, if you were not to look at a patient or relative when communicating with them, this could be a sign you are either not listening to them or are not interested in what they have to say. However, if the patient is avoiding eye contact but demonstrating they are listening by giving suitable verbal responses with appropriate paralinguistic features, it may be that in this case it would be culturally insensitive or even rude to maintain eye contact (Pavord and Donnelly, 2015).

Facial expression

Like the eyes, the face is one of the most expressive parts of the human body (Gamble and Gamble, 2017), and feelings such as anger, joy and surprise are often easily identifiable from a person's facial expressions. It is evident that paramedics will encounter situations that they find shocking, fearful or surprising, and there is a strong likelihood that they may display those emotions via their facial expressions. Patients can recognise the emotions and mood states displayed by paramedics when caring for them (O'Toole, 2023). Again, the implications are that clinicians need to have the self-awareness to understand the non-verbal cues they exhibit and the effect they may have on the person they are communicating with (Pavord and Donnelly, 2015; Moss, 2020).

Reflection: points to consider

Consider the importance of reflecting on the reactions that patients and family members have demonstrated or expressed as a result of your facial expressions during certain types of calls.

- Have you observed a colleague make unprofessional and inappropriate facial expressions?
- If so, how did this make you feel?
- How would you address this if it happened again?

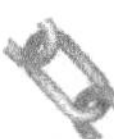

Chapter 6 for more on communication and human factors and **Chapter 18** for discussion on how we make decisions.

Gestures and posture

Together with facial expressions, both gestures and posture can emphasise and clarify the meaning of the spoken message (Gamble and Gamble,
2017). People often use their hands to gesture when they are speaking.
Some gestures like pointing can be problematic, depending on the context
in which they are used; for example, pointing to a piece of equipment can
be appropriate but pointing at a patient is not. Equally, making large gestures may convey enthusiasm, but used extensively in a patient interaction
can move the focus away from the patient to the ambulance clinician, which
may or may not be helpful depending on the situation.

Posture includes the way you stand, sit and position your body. It is generally accepted that, if possible, when talking to patients, paramedics should
maintain an open posture – that is, not crossing one's arms or legs –
because standing with your arms crossed in front of a patient or relative
can be interpreted as confrontational and uncaring. Thus, an open posture
suggests you are willing to communicate with the patient, as does position-
ing yourself at the same level as the patient to maintain direct eye contact.
Clearly, maintaining an open posture would not be possible at the scene of
a road traffic accident, but the principles ought to be applied where appropriate to communicate with patients and relatives.

Both posture and gestures can have a positive effect on establishing and
maintaining good communication, especially if used in combination with
eye contact. If these are used appropriately, it suggests the paramedic is
concerned for the patient, is willing to listen to them, and is paying attention to what they say. But if used unwisely, it might suggest to the patient
or relative that the paramedic is uncaring, unwilling to listen and not compassionate (Pavord and Donnelly, 2015; Moss, 2020).

Proximity

People also communicate by how closely they stand or sit next to another
person. This is referred to as personal space or proximity. Generally during social interactions, people who do not know each other tend to stand
approximately at arm's length from one another. This distance is often
reduced when people know each other, or when one person gives permission directly or indirectly for someone to enter their personal space and
touch them. Being too close can cause discomfort and unease and be perceived as threatening, even if touch is not involved.

Touch is another significant element of non-verbal communication for ambulance clinicians, because much of the care given requires touch, such as

placing a blood pressure cuff, stabilising a C-spine, and so on. Although touch is an instinctive form of communication, it can be misinterpreted, so be sure to touch patients on socially acceptable parts of the body, such as the hands, if that is clinically appropriate, until you have direct or implied consent to touch them elsewhere to undertake a procedure (Clarke et al., 2024).

 **Reflection: points to consider**

Thinking about the above non-verbal cues, how might you be able to identify the following:

- Someone was not listening to you.
- A colleague was interested in what you were saying.
- The person you were talking to was worried.
- A colleague tells you to do something quickly.

Case study I.2

An ambulance was called to an urgent care centre by a doctor who had assessed a 56-year-old patient. The patient had suspected pneumonia and was breathless, with low oxygen saturations, low blood pressure, a raised pulse and pyrexia. Two paramedics arrived at the reception desk. The first paramedic called the patient's name across the crowded waiting room. The patient identified themselves by raising their hand and saying 'yes'. The paramedic did not move from the desk and responded loudly, 'Do you want to do this here or in the back of the ambulance?'

Immediately, the second paramedic established eye contact with the patient, smiled, crossed the waiting room and sat on the chair next to them. The paramedic introduced themselves, and explained that they needed to undertake an assessment and that they could either try to find somewhere in the centre to do it, or they could undertake it in the ambulance. The patient agreed to the latter. This paramedic then asked whether the patient could walk and whether they needed assistance to get to the ambulance. This paramedic walked alongside the patient while reassuring them with touch and calm conversation. Once in the ambulance, the first paramedic sat diagonally across from the patient and asked a range of questions and recorded the answers on their documentation. During this they did not have any eye contact or look at the patient at all and used a very 'matter of fact' tone of voice. In a similar tone, they also asked the second paramedic to undertake a range of clinical observations and administer some oxygen, which they did. While doing this, the second paramedic explained to the patient what was happening, engaged in some conversation, maintained eye contact and used positive non-verbal communication. The second paramedic then left the patient, explaining that they were going to drive them to the local hospital. The first paramedic remained with the patient, in the same seated position, but did not speak or look at the patient during the journey. On arrival, the first paramedic left the ambulance and went into the emergency department, while the second paramedic helped the patient out of the ambulance and into a wheelchair before taking them into the department.

- How appropriate were the features of communication used in this case study?
- What impact might they have on the potential public view of the paramedic profession?
- If you were a patient, which of these paramedics would you like to care for you and why?

COMMUNICATING WITH PATIENTS: EXPLORING THE CASE STUDY

In case study 1.2, different levels of therapeutic communication are evident, some positive and others less so. Effective communication with patients, relatives and the public is an essential and integral part of the role of the paramedic from the very outset of a patient interaction (O'Toole, 2023; HCPC, 2024). The main concern in this case study is that it is the real-life experience of a patient. It demonstrates very different first impressions of the paramedic profession to the patient and the other people in the waiting room.

When encountering a patient, first impressions are important and can significantly influence how that patient interaction unfolds. First impressions consist of both verbal and non-verbal features. So, wearing a clean smart uniform, establishing both eye and verbal contact and introducing yourself are all key elements. According to Turner and Sefika (2016), from the start, effective communication should incorporate:

- beginning with a smile not a bias;
- having self-awareness and respect for others;

- listening, with care, compassion and appreciation;
- answering with understanding and empathy;
- explaining professionally with compassion.

If these are present, then the potential for the development of a compassionate relationship is increased, allowing the clinician and patient to make a personal connection with one another. It is believed that this fosters a deeper level of care and support and makes it more likely that the patient feels they have been cared for with dignity and respect.

In case study 1.2, the second paramedic did demonstrate positive elements of communication, by using both verbal and non-verbal communication to demonstrate the elements proposed by Turner and Sefika (2016). The positive elements of their initial communication style were that they established eye contact, smiled, moved towards the patient, sat at the level as the patient and introduced themselves. In contrast, the first paramedic did none of this; indeed, their communication style perhaps was one of projecting power, or perhaps they were just tired or fatigued. But if the latter were the case, it is questionable whether they should have demonstrated this to the degree they did, and they should at least have tried to appear caring and professional (HCPC, 2024), but this could also demonstrate the level of stress and pressure paramedics face in their role and the emotional demands of their work. It was clear that if the patient wanted care, they would have to go to the first paramedic and not the other way around. If the second paramedic had not approached the patient, the outcome might have been different; the patient might have felt vulnerable and perhaps under pressure to comply with the first paramedic's wishes. This could have resulted in the patient feeling undervalued and pressured, potentially setting the scene for frustration and confrontation or even a complaint at a later point.

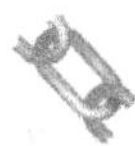

Chapter 4 for ethical considerations, **Chapter 9** for power of the professions and **Chapter 10** for factors affecting patients' decision to access health care.

Reflection: points to consider

Go to the 'hello my name is …' website (www.hellomynameis.org.uk) and find out who started this campaign and why they did so. Play some of the video clips on the site to help you do this.

Throughout case study 1.2, the second paramedic maintained good eye contact, used a supportive tone of voice and listened to the patient. Initially, both paramedics afforded the patient some degree of choice in terms of where they could be examined. The first paramedic addressed the situation in such a way that the patient might have felt they had no option but to go with the paramedic to the ambulance. Or, if the patient wanted to express any concerns, they would have no choice but to have done so across the waiting room, or asked the paramedic to approach them. The patient might not have felt comfortable with either of these options. Therefore, the first impression made by this paramedic was not one of wanting to listen, but one of just wanting to get the 'job done'. By contrast, the second paramedic did show they were listening and respected the patient as an individual. They gave the patient some choice, discussed it in a sensitive manner, and tried to protect the patient's privacy and dignity by discussing it next to them, even though it was in a crowded waiting room. Throughout the interaction the two paramedics maintained very different communication styles, one professional, compassionate and respectful, the other not, thereby demonstrating a contradiction in the standards of conduct and performance recommended for practice (HCPC, 2024).

Effective communication is an essential part of patient-centred care and is essential to professional practice (HCPC, 2024). If used correctly, it can significantly help a patient feel they have been treated and respected as an individual (Turner and Sefika, 2016; Moss, 2020). If effective communication was used by other professionals with paramedics, it would make the paramedics feel valued and respected too. The significance of this is that communication is not just about ensuring people receive the correct information and that the correct information is collected, it is also about making sure that patients and staff feel valued, trusted and respected through the way they are communicated with. The clinical outcome of a situation should be significantly improved because there is an effective exchange of information.

Communication can also affect the way a patient perceives a situation and potentially can make the difference between a positive or negative clinical outcome (Vermier et al., 2015). In case study 1.2, it was fortunate that the clinical outcome was a positive one, but the impact the two paramedics had on the patient was significantly different, one appearing kind, compassionate and caring, the other not; one making the patient feel like a respected individual, with time for the patient, the other not. Hence, all clinicians need to consider which words they use and how they emphasise them to give clear, caring, empathetic and assertive messages to patients and not ones that indicate the clinician's frustrations, attitudes or assumptions. It is certainly clear that in any situation, the elements in the model outlined in Figure 1.1 clearly do contribute to effective communication.

INTER-PROFESSIONAL COMMUNICATION TOOLS

Much of the communication that paramedics are involved in requires information about the specifics of a given situation to be transmitted quickly, accurately and effectively, either at the scene or in a handover situation (O'Toole, 2023). Hence, the need for effective inter-professional communication is a key element of paramedic practice (HCPC, 2024). Standardised handover frameworks provide a systematic way of promoting the effective and comprehensive transfer of key clinical information from one clinician to another, thus reducing the risk of information being forgotten or overlooked within the handover (Rosenberg et al., 2009; Murray et al., 2012; Flynn et al., 2017). In 2010, the NHS published 'Safer Care', advocating the use of the SBAR tool (NHS Institute for Innovation and Improvement, 2010). In 2011, the World Health Organization issued a patient safety curriculum guide document (WHO, 2011), advocating SBAR (in some countries known as ISBAR). With specific reference to emergency care, in 2016 NICE advocated a standard pre-alert for trauma patients (NICE, 2016), which made specific reference to the ATMIST tool, which is now the UK standard pre-alert tool in the UK. These frameworks provide paramedics with a structured format by which to hand over key information about the patient and the situation. But this also means that the clinician receiving the information knows the broad areas of information to expect within the handover, and therefore what to ask for if there appear to be any gaps in the information provided.

The research evaluating these tools suggests they are useful and can enhance communication and handover, although it has also been established that their effectiveness can be influenced by a range of communication factors, such as time, status, busyness, and the relationships of the people involved in the handover (Bost et al., 2012; Flynn et al., 2017). These factors are highlighted in the model of communication outlined in Figure 1.1. Therefore, to use these tools effectively, the aforementioned issues also have to be addressed. For example, the information provided and the way it is communicated by a clinician has to be valued by the other clinicians involved, and issues like status, hierarchy and time have to be overcome to ensure that the relevant information is handed over and clearly understood. Hence, the models of communication and theories that support them directly underpin communication in practice.

All the issues discussed above concerning clear verbal and non-verbal communication are relevant to inter-professional communication, as the information gained through these processes will at some point be recorded in written documentation (Vermier et al., 2015).

Reflection: points to consider

Take a look at Figure 1.3. Think back to when you recently handed over patient information to another clinician or healthcare professional. Write down what you remember you said about the patient and their condition. Now put the information under the headings (SBAR, ATMIST, ASHICE) in each of the frameworks.

- Did you have something in every area for each?
- Would using one of these frameworks help you structure your handovers in future?

CONCLUSION

Interpersonal communication involves the complex exchange of information between people who constantly send and receive messages from one another and is a fundamental element of a paramedic's practice. The way a paramedic encodes and sends messages will affect the way patients and colleagues decode and interpret those message. This may lead to clear accurate communication or miscommunication, depending on the factors which influence the way the paramedic and the patient or colleague are interacting in that situation. It is important to remember, therefore, that both verbal and non-verbal communication are inextricably linked and it is the way a paramedic uses them in combination that impacts on their interactions with their patients and colleagues and can positively or negatively affect the outcome of a situation. It is this combination that allows paramedics to effectively communicate a range of messages from the very subtle to the blatantly obvious. The social situation in which communication occurs will also affect the sending, receiving and interpretation of any particular message, whether given by the paramedic, the patient or colleague, and whether it occurs at an accident scene, in an ambulance, in a patient's home or in an emergency department. It is of vital importance that our communication is effective and sensitive to the situation and the people involved. All clinicians need to be constantly aware not only of what they say, but also how they say it. Our interactions with patients and families require thought (prior to and during our communications) and are deserving

(1) SBAR	(2) ATMIST	(3) ASHICE
(S) Situation • Identify yourself • Identify the patient by name • Give details about the situation, e.g. patient involved in a road traffic collision • Give any details of initial vital signs, oxygen given, level of consciousness, etc. • Describe your concerns **(B) Background** • Give the patient's reason for admission • Explain significant medical history • Current medication and allergies • Procedures you have undertaken • Medications given by you and those normally taken by the patient • Treatments/procedures you have undertaken **(A) Assessment** • Vital signs • Contraction pattern • Clinical impression and concerns **(R) Recommendations** • Explain what you think the patient needs now • Make suggestions • Clarify expectations	**(A) Age** Age and sex of casualty **(T) Time** Estimated time of arrival and time incident occurred **(M) Mechanism of injury** • The gross mechanism of injury, e.g. motor vehicle collision, stab wound to chest • Details of other factors known to be associated with major injuries, e.g. entrapment, vehicle rollover, occupant ejected from vehicle **(I) Injury** What can be seen or suspected **(S) Signs** Vital signs including heart rate, blood pressure, respiratory rate, oxygen saturation, Glasgow Coma Score **(T) Treatment** Treatment given to the patient	**(A) Age** What is the patient's age? **(S) Sex** Is the patient male or female? **(H) History** What happened to the patient, e.g. road traffic collision, etc. **(I) Injuries sustained** Stab wound to the chest, fractured femur, etc. **(C) Condition** Patient's vital signs, including heart rate, blood pressure, respiratory rate, oxygen saturation, Glasgow Coma Score **(E) Estimated time of arrival** Time of arrival at the receiving hospital

Figure 1.3 Examples of frameworks to support handover

Source: Collated and adapted from NHS Institute for Innovation and Improvement (2010), Jeffreys et al. (2021).

of reflection afterwards. Communication is at the forefront of our practice and is an essential fundamental skill that we can strive to improve throughout our careers. Furthermore, when communicating about patients to other healthcare professionals, there is a need to ensure that all information is accurate and, frequently, given quickly. Hence, handover frameworks provide a systematic means to facilitate the effectiveness of communication between ambulance clinicians and other members of the inter-professional team, thus promoting quality care through skilled communication.

Chapter key points:

- We are always in a state of communicating something to someone.
- Communication is a mix of verbal and non-verbal elements – both act as carriers of the messages we send and receive.
- The way we formulate, send, receive and interpret messages is influenced by our values, beliefs, social identity, perceptions and the context in which the communication occurs.
- Communication is a fundamental and vital part of all healthcare professionals' practice, because care and treatment cannot be effective without communication of some kind.
- Communication is a central component in providing compassionate patient-centred care in a multicultural society.
- Communicating patient information to other professionals needs to be accurate and undertaken quickly and effectively, to promote quality care.

REFERENCES AND SUGGESTED READING

Argyle, M. (1988) *Bodily Communication*, 2nd edition. London: Routledge.

Association of Ambulance Chief Executives & Joint Royal Colleges Ambulance Liaison Committee (AACE/JRCALC) (2022) *JRCALC Clinical Guidelines 2022*. Bridgwater: Class Professional Publishing.

Blaber, A. and Harris, G. (eds.) (2014) *Clinical Leadership for Paramedics*. Maidenhead: Open University Press.

Bost, N., Crilly, J., Patterson, E. and Chaboyer, W. (2012) Clinical handover of patients arriving by ambulance to a hospital emergency department: a qualitative study, *International Emergency Nursing*, 20 (3): 133–41.

Clarke, V., Harris, G. and Cowland S. (2024) Ethics and law for the paramedic, in A.Y. Blaber (ed.) *Blaber's Foundations for Paramedic Practice: A Theoretical Perspective*. London: Open University Press.

Eggins, S. and Slade, D. (2015) Communication in clinical handover: improving the safety and quality of the patient experience, *Journal of Public Health Research*, 4 (666): 197–99.

Flynn, D., Francis, S., Robalino, S., Lally, J. et al. (2017) A review of enhanced paramedic roles during and after hospital handover of stroke, myocardial infarction and trauma patients, *BMC Emergency Medicine*, 17 (5): 1–13.

Gamble, T.K. and Gamble, M. (2017) *Nonverbal Messages Tell More: A Practical Guide to Nonverbal Communication.* New York: Routledge.

Gamble, T.K. and Gamble, M. (2023) *The Interpersonal Communication Playbook.* London: Sage.

Gault, I., Shapcott, J., Luthi, A. and Reid, G. (2016) *Communication in Nursing and Healthcare.* Los Angeles, CA: Sage.

Hartley, P. (1999) *Interpersonal Communication*, 2nd edition. London: Routledge.

Health and Care Professions Council (HCPC) (2024) *Standards of Conduct, Performance and Ethics.* Available at: https://www.hcpc-uk.org/standards/standards-of-conduct-performance-and-ethics/.

Hendrickson, S.W. (2008) *SBAR Basics: A Resource Guide for Healthcare Managers.* Marblehead, MA: HCP Pro.

Jeffreys, C., Maxwell, D., Fitzpatrick, D. and Loughrey, J.P. (2021) *Handover; skills to enhancing the PHEM-EM interface*, ed. L. Fraser. Royal College of Emergency Medicine, E-learning platform. Available at: www.rcemlearning.co.uk/reference/handover-skills-to-enhancing-the-phem-em-interface/#163213647806-ae833d2e-e833 (accessed 23 April 2024).

Loseby, J. and Lyon, R. (2013) Clinical handover of the trauma and medical patient: a structured approach, *Journal of Paramedic Practice*, 5 (10): 563–67.

Lucas, P.V., McCall, M., Eccleston, C., Lee, E. et al. (2015) Prioritising the development of paramedic students' interpersonal skills, *Journal of Paramedic Practice*, 7 (5): 242–48.

Mehrabian, A. (1981) *Silent Messages: Implicit Communication of Emotions and Attitudes*, 2nd edition. Belmont, CA: Wadsworth.

Moss, B. (2020) *Communication Skills in Nursing, Healthcare and Social Care*, 5th edition. London: Sage.

Murray, S.L., Crouch, R. and Ainsworth-Smith, M. (2012) Quality of the handover of patient care: a comparison of pre-hospital and emergency department notes, *International Emergency Nursing*, 20 (1): 24–27.

National Institute for Health and Care Excellence (NICE) (2016) *Major trauma: service delivery*, NICE Guideline 40. Available at: https://www.nice.org.uk/guidance/ng40 (accessed 23 April 2014).

NHS Institute for Innovation and Improvement (2010) *Safer care: SBAR.* Available at: https://www.england.nhs.uk/improvement-hub/wp-content/uploads/sites/44/2017/11/SBAR-Implementation-and-Training-Guide.pdf (accessed 9 April 2024).

NHS Professionals (2023) *The 6 Cs of care.* Available at: https://www.nhsprofessionals.nhs.uk/nhs-staffing-pool-hub/working-in-healthcare/the-6-cs-of-care (accessed 9 April 2024).

O'Hara, J.K., Reynolds, C., Moore, S., Armitage, G. et al. (2019) What can patients tell us about the quality and safety of hospital care? Findings from a UK multi-centre survey study, *BMJ Quality and Safety*, 27 (9): 673–82.

O'Toole, G. (2023) *Communication in Paramedic Practice.* London: Elsevier.

Pavord, E. and Donnelly, E. (2015) *Communication and Interpersonal Skills*, 2nd edition. Banbury: Lantern.

Rosenberg, L.A., Leitzsch, J. and Little, B.W. (2009) Systematic review of handoff mnemonics literature, *American Journal of Medical Quality*, 24 (3): 196–204.

Shannon, C.E. and Weaver, W. (1949) *The Mathematical Theory of Communication.* Urbana, IL: University of Illinois Press.

The Oxford English Dictionary (2024) Communication. Oxford: Oxford University Press. Available at: https://www.oxforddictionaries.com/oed (accessed 7 April 2024).

Turner, S.Y. and Sefika, K. (2016) *The Three Fundamental Principles of Effective Communication in Healthcare Settings.* Amazon Media, Kindle edition.

Vermier, P., Vandijck, D., Degroote, S., Peleman, R. et al. (2015) Communication in healthcare: a narrative review of the literature and practical recommendations, *International Journal of Clinical Practice*, 69 (11): 1257–67.

World Health Organization (WHO) (2011) *Patient safety curriculum guide: multi-professional edition.* Available at: https://www.who.int/publications/i/item/9789241501958 (accessed 23 April 2024).

Reflective practice for paramedics

Claire Tinker, with contributions from James Brogan

> **In this chapter:**
>
> - Introduction
> - Why is this relevant?
> - Benefits of reflective practice
> - Defining the terms: critical reflection and reflexivity
> - What should I reflect upon?
> - Approaching reflection
> - Reflective models and frameworks
> - When to reflect
> - Conclusion
> - Chapter key points
> - References and suggested reading

INTRODUCTION

The College of Paramedics (CoP) defines a paramedic as working

> ... *autonomously as a generalist clinician across a range of healthcare settings, usually in emergency, primary or urgent care. They may also specialise in clinical practice, education, leadership or research. (CoP, 2019)*

> *Paramedics have a unique role that intersects healthcare, public health, social care and public safety. The rapidly evolving face of healthcare affords increasing opportunities for paramedics to break down barriers, help to remove inefficiencies and be a key contributor to future models of health and care. (CoP Interactive Career Framework, no date)*

It is clear from the above descriptions that paramedics may find themselves in increasingly varied roles, in many different aspects of the health and care sector. The ability to reflect both personally and professionally is central for any healthcare professional.

WHY IS THIS RELEVANT?

For paramedics, reflective practice is a key component of professional development, involving the evaluation of their experiences and actions to improve future performance. This evaluation process allows the identification of strengths and weaknesses, the opportunity to learn from previous experiences and to make informed decisions in complex and dynamic situations. In addition, reflective practice promotes critical thinking skills, empathy towards patients and effective communication within the healthcare team. By regularly engaging in reflective practice, paramedics can enhance their clinical expertise and provide optimal care to patients. Having a healthy scepticism of your abilities, attitudes and behaviours is key to challenging practice, and the insight provided by reflective practice creates an opportunity to learn from them and improve professional practice.

This chapter will consider the benefits of reflective practice, what to reflect on and when and suggestions for achieving a structured and meaningful approach.

BENEFITS OF REFLECTIVE PRACTICE

It is not the mountains we conquer, but ourselves.

– Sir Edmund Hillary

There are a wide range of benefits to reflective practice that may not be immediately obvious. If done properly and not treated as a tick-box exercise, reflection helps to develop an understanding of challenging situations and supports the professional journey of all paramedics, irrespective of education or experience.

Continuous professional development

It is acknowledged that health and care professionals should engage in reflective practice as a necessary component of their ongoing professional development. A joint statement by the chief executives of the statutory regulators of healthcare professionals in the UK asserts that practising reflection not only improves the individual practitioner but also the team they are part of. It also assures the public that clinicians regularly assess their practice and strive to improve what they do and how they operate (HCPC, 2019). The statement makes it clear that to promote professional growth and strengthen professional dedication, teams should be encouraged to make time for reflection. It is also made clear that registrants will not be asked by their regulator to provide their personal reflective notes to investigate a concern about them.

Understanding reflective practice and the need to record the outcome of reflection to support continuous improvement is a requirement of the Standards of Proficiency (HCPC, 2023), see Box 2.1. Maintaining current knowledge and skills through continuous professional development necessitates the use of reflective practice; consequently, an essential component of paramedics' ongoing professional development is understanding when and how to reflect. The use of reflective practice is necessary to maintain current knowledge and skills; as a result, knowing when and how to reflect is a crucial part of paramedics' ongoing professional development.

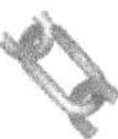 **Chapter 21** for more on continuing professional development for the paramedic.

Box 2.I Reflective practice for paramedics (HCPC, 2023)

Your standards of proficiency require you to:

- Understand the value of reflective practice and the need to record the outcome of such reflection to support continuous improvement (Standard 10.1).
- Recognise the value of multidisciplinary reviews, case conferences and other methods of review (Standard 10.2).
- These methods exist because understanding the value of reflection is important for meeting all of your standards of proficiency.

Clinician mental health and wellbeing

Setting aside time to reflect on situations encountered in practice can seem onerous when workloads are high and healthcare organisations are under pressure, but doing so can help lower levels of anxiety by giving back a sense of control and reducing the risk of burnout. By slowing down and deepening our awareness we can, step by step, contribute to informed, evidence-based practice, and share learning that will benefit future service users exponentially. By understanding what we can – and cannot –

accomplish in practice, we can learn to be compassionate and realistic with ourselves (Bassot, 2020).

Communication and collaboration

Reflective practice facilitates improved communication skills if used to explore interactions with patients, colleagues and interdisciplinary teams, leading to enhanced collaboration and patient-centred care. Reflective practice tends to be viewed as an individual activity but there are benefits from understanding the wider impact of events on the team and organisation. The National Health Service group reflection programme 'Schwartz Rounds' was designed to provide employees across all disciplines a chance to get together and explore the emotional components of their jobs. The outcomes from this initiative have found that staff who attend regularly report feeling less stressed, less isolated, and are better able to care for their patients (The Point of Care Foundation, 2016).

Cultural competence and humility

Cultural development within paramedicine is the integration of cultural competence, sensitivity and awareness into practice. This involves understanding and respecting the cultural backgrounds, beliefs, values and practices of the diverse communities served by paramedics. Having the ability to build rapport in a cross-cultural context is crucial in improving patient outcomes (Ross et al., 2018). Although there is a paucity of research on the use of reflective practice as a tool to develop cultural humility, there is some evidence that experiential learning in combination with reflective writing can be advantageous (Sanchez et al., 2019).

Developing the evidence base

Meeting the Professional Standards for Paramedics (HCPC, 2023) requires an engagement with the evidence base to ensure quality of practice. Reviewing the evidence base as part of the reflective process not only encourages the incorporation of findings into practice but also can identify gaps in the literature that create a symbiotic relationship between reflective practice and the evidence base.

DEFINING THE TERMS: CRITICAL REFLECTION AND REFLEXIVITY

Reflection is a state of mind and a continuous attitude towards life and work; we might look back on life experiences such as a holiday or job interview and consider how they made us feel, what was good or bad about them, and create a plan to avoid or repeat the event. This process when applied to our work can help us understand where we are in our practice and develop rather than repeat our practice year on year (Bolton and Delderfield, 2017; Johns, 2017).

Critical reflection

The opportunity for learning and professional development in this process comes from not just looking back and describing events but from *critically* evaluating them and considering how they relate to the evidence base. These findings are then applied to action plans for future practice, thus ensuring that the level of care provided continues to improve.

To facilitate professional growth, critical reflection improves professional practice by helping you understand what you are doing, why you are doing it, and the consequences of your decisions and actions. This allows you to be better able to approach unknown and unexpected situations in a way that meets your needs as well as those of others. Superficial reflection lacks criticality and can be vulnerable to personal biases and unchallenged assumptions that might be found within organisational cultures. Creating a critical argument with yourself introduces depth to the analysis, reinforcing the importance of critical thinking skills in reflective practice (Collen, 2022). This level of scrutiny can be an uncomfortable process, as using a critical approach to reflection in academic and professional contexts requires shifting our viewpoint, deepening our understanding and strengthening our knowledge in ways that ultimately bring about transformation and change. A critical approach to reflection should provide an unbiased viewpoint on your experience as well as an explanation for your behaviours, emotions, and responses to situations. Since it can be difficult to bring that level of objectivity to personal experiences, it is useful to cross-check your conclusions with your peers or other observers (Cottrell, 2023).

On a superficial level, it may be possible to use pre-existing knowledge to solve routine and familiar problems, but expert practitioners can employ a deeper level of knowledge and understanding and engage in critical reflection. Without engagement in reflective practice, professional development is stalled and the risk of clinical errors increases. The novice may make appropriate clinical decisions in both simple and complex situations by employing logic and reasoning; conversely, an experienced clinician may arrive at an incorrect diagnosis if they fail to appreciate the need for reflection when presented with a complex case or contradictory data (Royce et al., 2019).

Reflexivity

The deliberate, in-depth examination of one's perspective, values and presumptions is known as *reflexivity*. To be reflexive is to examine the limits of our knowledge and to explore how our personal and professional values relate to organisational structures (Bolton and Delderfield, 2017). For the paramedic, this may involve an examination of how the demands of the workplace influence the care provided and our attitude towards patients. Greater empathy between the patient and the practitioner is promoted by this process (Koshy et al., 2017).

Reflexivity also involves thinking from within experiences – working out how our presence at an event influences actions and outcomes. The reflexive practitioner would not just ask what happened and how it can be improved but pose deeper questions about assumptions that were made and what external pressures influenced decision-making (Bolton and Delderfield, 2017). The examination of the boundaries of our knowledge and how our actions affect organisational structures that contradict our own is what it means to be reflexive. Paramedics must be self-aware, and understand themselves, their ideal standard of care and the realities of their practice to genuinely comprehend and respond to the experiences of their patients. Reflection on one's viewpoint, values and presumptions is supported by this focus and is a crucial component of professional development (Cottrell, 2023). Paramedics examining the congruence between their perceived role identity and what they encounter in practice may create cognitive dissonance and frustration which affects mental wellbeing (Collen, 2022; Mausz et al., 2022). Utilising a reflective practice approach to professional identity and the paramedic's place within an organisation may reduce chronic stressors.

To become a reflexive practitioner, we should examine the limits of our knowledge and explore how our personal and professional values relate to organisational structures (Bolton and Delderfield, 2017). For the paramedic, this may involve an examination of how the demands of the workplace influence the care provided and our attitude towards patients. Becoming a paramedic is centred around a need to help people, save lives and be part of an 'exciting' profession (Ross et al., 2016), but the realities of the workplace can be frustrating. This contradiction between professional identity and the reality of the job can lead to frustration with some patient presentations (Collen, 2022; Mausz et al., 2022). Engaging in more sophisticated and varied processes of reflection and reflexivity on this challenge can create greater empathy between the patient and the practitioner (Koshy et al., 2017).

WHAT SHOULD I REFLECT UPON?

Critical incidents

There is an assumption in the literature that paramedics should reflect on things that go wrong – so-called 'critical incidents' – and, of course, this is an important response to errors and mistakes if we wish to avoid their repetition. Critical incidents may be an obvious prompt for reflection but limiting reflective practice to negative experiences risks making it a punitive process. This type of reflection requires openness and honesty without fear of blame and should be balanced with positive outcomes; indeed, there is merit in reflecting on events that went well, which can be more rewarding and help build confidence. The process should leave you feeling positive and hopeful; indeed, reflection on a positive outcome is something to be shared (Koshy et al., 2017; HCPC, 2023).

Feedback

Feedback can be a trigger for reflection on both positive and negative outcomes. Historically, paramedics received little feedback on their clinical performance or health-related outcomes, which has fed the perception that only exceptional and negative incidents initiate reflection. Paramedics have expressed a desire to receive more information about outcomes for emotional and developmental motives (Eaton-Williams et al., 2020). One of the anticipated benefits of receiving meaningful feedback on patient outcomes, especially in complex cases and non-conveyed patients, is a willingness to engage in reflective practice (Eaton-Williams et al., 2020).

APPROACHING REFLECTION

Preparing to reflect requires some consideration of what the focus of the reflection should be and whether the time available is sufficient to do justice to the work. It may be prudent to focus on one aspect of a situation and allow more depth to the reflection. You should also consider who the audience of your reflection will be and how you will structure it. A personal record may be written in an informal style and structure but if you feel that findings from the reflection may benefit other paramedics, consideration should be given to writing for publication or sharing with a group reflection. If you believe that learning from the reflection may help a wider audience, consider how the content might need to be changed to meet the needs of this potential audience (Cottrell, 2023). Taking your reflections to a peer reviewer can be beneficial because they can highlight issues that you might have missed and can serve as a beneficial educational experience for the other clinicians involved (Koshy et al., 2017).

It is particularly important to ensure that confidentiality is maintained throughout the reflection and that no participant is identifiable – this includes both colleagues and patients. In high-profile cases that have been reported by the media, anonymizing names may not be enough to achieve this, as participants may be identifiable by their age, gender, ethnicity or role. It is crucial to gain express consent in writing if you are using identifiable information for reasons not related to care or treatment (HCPC, 2021).

REFLECTIVE MODELS AND FRAMEWORKS

If you are new to reflective practice, it can be helpful to think about the framework within which you will structure your reflection to avoid missing important steps and the chance to develop your professional practice.

A structured approach to reflective practice is supported by a variety of frameworks. Well-known frameworks include Kolb's Learning Cycle (Kolb, 1984), Gibbs' Reflective Cycle (Gibbs, 1998), Rolfe, Freshwater and Jasper's Reflective Model (Rolfe et al., 2001), and Johns' Model of Reflection (Johns, 1994), which are summarised in Table 2.1. These key contributions to reflective practice have been developed further for paramedic practice by Willis (2010) and Wade (2013) in more contemporary frameworks. These contemporary interpretations include specific references to evidence-based practice and, in the case of Willis, the role of ethics and human factors in the evaluation. Developing your clinical decision-making abilities requires a solid grasp of the evidence base, particularly in complex situations, so these contemporary models may be better suited to your professional development as a paramedic.

Unless prescribed by an academic programme or publisher guideline, you are certainly not compelled to use any particular model and you may develop your approach. Box 2.2 lists the commonalities of reflective models which you may adapt to create your process. Ensure you don't skip sections or questions that make you feel uncomfortable – the process of reflection may not always be an easy one. For more detail on all of the models listed in Table 2.1, see the specific texts cited there.

WHEN TO REFLECT

Reflection is a cycle of self-observation and self-evaluation that can occur at different points in a situation. For example, as you administer morphine to a patient and observe the effects and side effects of the drug, you draw on your pre-existing knowledge and past experiences of administering morphine and adapt the administration accordingly. Schön (1983) defines this

Table 2.1 Summary of frameworks

Framework	Components/stages (Wade, 2013)	Suitability
Kolb's Learning Cycle (1984)	• Concrete experience • Reflective observation • Abstract conceptualisation • Active experimentation	A four-stage model supports reflection of a hands-on experience. Promotes testing strategies for future occurrences
Gibbs' Reflective Cycle (1998)	• Description • Feelings • Evaluation • Analysis • Conclusion • Action plan	Builds on Kolb's model to include prompt questions. The cyclical model is well-suited for examining situations that occur regularly
Rolfe, Freshwater and Jasper's Reflective Model (2001)	• What? • So What? • Now what?	This three-stage model appears simple but requires comprehensive reflective questioning
Johns' Model of Reflection (1994)	• Describe the experience. • Reflection • Influencing factors • Could I have dealt with it better? • Learning	A cyclical model developed for nursing – designed to analyse complex decision-making
Willis' Reflective Models (2010)	Model 1 (cyclical): • Description • Areas for investigation • Literature search • Ethical implications for practice • Next time Model 2 (hierarchical): • What happened? • Human factors • Clinical application • Supporting literature • Next time	A more contemporary set of models designed with paramedic practice in mind. A flexible approach that considers ethical issues, human factors and the evidence base

Framework	Components/stages (Wade, 2013)	Suitability
	Model 3 (cyclical): • Discuss • Key issues • Supporting evidence – evidence base • Next time	

Box 2.2 Commonalities of reflective models

Description of the experience: Involves providing a detailed account of the experience, event or situation being reflected upon. It sets the stage for understanding the context and identifying key elements.

Feelings and emotions: An exploration of the emotions and feelings associated with the experience.

Critical analysis (evaluation of actions): An evaluation of the experience including your actions, decisions and responses to events. This should include what went well, what could have been done differently, and identifying factors that influenced the outcomes. This stage may include examining how events relate to the evidence base and the consideration of alternative strategies. The broader context of the experience, including environmental, cultural or organisational factors, can also be considered and provide insight into how external elements may have influenced the situation.

Identification of learning: As reflective practice is centred around learning and growth, this stage is key in identifying lessons learned from the experience and a consideration of how these insights can be applied in the future.

Goal setting or action planning: Involves outlining specific, achievable goals based on the insights gained through reflection. These goals serve as a roadmap for future actions. This step is crucial for translating insights into action.

process as 'reflecting in action' – that is, thinking about what you are doing, reflecting at the time of the event, reviewing your actions, and making judgements based on your knowledge and experiences. You may recognise this process as something that we do in all facets of our daily lives, including reviewing our decisions on situations, such as deciding which route to take to work and adapting the plan when we encounter traffic congestion by drawing on pre-existing knowledge of the route and past experiences of it to make judgements.

Schön (1983) refers to the retrospective perspective as 'reflection on action'. This takes place after the event, critically analysing what you did and why, how it relates to the evidence base, and what changes you might make for future practice. The retrospective process of reflecting on action is a more formal activity involving a deeper review of knowledge by searching the literature to determine how our actions aligned with the evidence base and what could be changed in future iterations of the event.

Collen (2022) introduced the concept of 'The Garden Path Test' for paramedics – the idea that you can challenge your practice and decisions if not directly 'in action', then immediately afterwards. Engaging in reflection at this point provides an opportunity to evaluate clinical decisions and perhaps take an opportunity to liaise with colleagues to discuss those concerns. A benefit of this approach allows you to 'clear your head' and mentally decompress before attending to your next patient. By pausing to reflect in this way, you are allowing 'system two' thinking to dominate, which allows time for considered thought to occur (Kahneman, 2012).

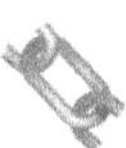 **Chapter 6** for more on human factors in health care.

CONCLUSION

Reflective practice is an integral part of the paramedic's lifelong learning journey from novice to expert. By routinely engaging in reviews of knowledge, skills and behaviours, we deepen self-awareness of our performance. An in-depth examination of personal and professional values and how our involvement in patient interactions influences outcomes encourages scrutiny of both the evidence base and the pressures that influence clinical decision-making and where the boundaries of our knowledge lie.

Critically reflective accounts provide important evidence of professional development and how the standards set by the HCPC are met. Using contemporary frameworks to structure reflection encourages consideration of the ethical issues and human factors affecting practice, and identifying gaps in knowledge informs the trajectory of your professional development.

> ## Chapter key points:
>
> - Reflection is so much more than merely recalling an event.
> - Ensure that you do not only reflect on negative incidents – it is also important to explore positive, well-organised care events.
> - There are a variety of structured reflective frameworks available, so ensure you read widely to select the most suitable framework for your needs.
> - It is important to distinguish between critical reflection and reflexivity.
> - Reflection is a statutory requirement of your registration as a paramedic and forms the basis of your continuing professional development.

REFERENCES AND SUGGESTED READING

Bassot, B. (2020) *The Reflective Journal*, 3rd edition. London: Bloomsbury Academic.

Bolton, G. and Delderfield, R. (2017) *Reflective Practice, Writing and Professional Development*, 4th edition. London: Sage.

College of Paramedics (CoP) (2019) *What is a paramedic?* Bridgwater: College of Paramedics (due for updated release 2024). Available at: https://collegeofparamedics. co.uk/COP/BecomeAParamedic/Become_a_Paramedic.aspx?hkey=f10838de-b67f-44a0-83b7-8140d8cdba83&WebsiteKey=9a9b21e9-7e94-4adf-a89a-ebe1cb57da56 (accessed 3 April 2024).

College of Paramedics (CoP) (no date) *Interactive Career Framework.* Bridgwater: College of Paramedics. Available at: https://collegeofparamedics.co.uk/COP/ ProfessionalDevelopment/Interactive_Career_Framework.aspx (accessed 3 April 2024).

Collen, A. (2022) *Decision Making in Paramedic Practice*, 2nd edition. Bridgwater: Class Professional Publishing.

Cottrell, S. (2023) *Critical Thinking Skills: Effective Analysis, Argument and Reflection*, 4th edition. London: Bloomsbury Academic.

Eaton-Williams, P., Mold, F. and Magnusson C. (2020) Exploring paramedic perceptions of feedback using a phenomenological approach, *British Paramedic Journal*, 5 (1): 7–14.

Gibbs, G. (1998) *Learning by Doing: A Guide to Teaching and Learning Methods.* Oxford: Further Education Unit, Oxford Polytechnic.

Health and Care Professions Council (HCPC) (2019) *HCPC unites with health regulators to issue joint statement in support of reflective practice across healthcare*. Available at: https://www.hcpc-uk.org/news-and-events/news/2019/hcpc-unites-with-health-regulators-to-issue-joint-statement-in-support-reflective-practice-across-healthcare/#:~:text=The%20chief%20executives%20of%20nine%20healthcare%20regulators%2C%20including,of%20good (accessed 7 April 2024).

Health and Care Professions Council (HCPC) (2021) *Key principles of confidentiality*. Available at: https://www.hcpc-uk.org/standards/meeting-our-standards/confidentiality/guidance-on-confidentiality/key-principles-of-confidentiality/ (accessed 7 April 2024).

Health and Care Professions Council (HCPC) (2023) *Standards of Proficiency for Paramedics*. Available at: https://www.hcpc-uk.org/standards/standards-of-proficiency/paramedics/ (accessed 9 April 2024).

Johns, C. (1994) Nuances of reflection, *Journal of Clinical Nursing*, 3 (2): 71–75.

Johns, C. (2017) *Becoming a Reflective Practitioner*. Chichester: Wiley.

Jones, J., Bion, J., Brown, C., Willars, J. et al. (2020) Reflection in practice: how can patient experience feedback trigger staff reflection in hospital acute care settings, *Health Expectations*, 23 (2): 396–404.

Kahneman, D. (2012) *Thinking, Fast and Slow*. New York: Farrar, Straus & Giroux.

Kolb, D. (1984) *Experiential Learning: Experience as the Source of Learning and Development*. Upper Saddle River, NJ: Prentice Hall.

Koshy, K., Limb, C., Gundogan, B., Whitehurst, K. et al. (2017) Reflective practice in health care and how to reflect effectively, *International Journal of Surgical Oncology*, 2: e20. Available at: https://doi.org/10.1097/IJ9.0000000000000020.

Mausz, J., Donnelly, E.A., Moll, S., Harms, S. et al. (2022) Role identity, dissonance, and distress among paramedics, *International Journal of Environmental Research and Public Health*, 19: 2115. Available at: https://doi.org/10.3390/ijerph19042115.

Minnican, C. and O'Toole, G. (2020) Exploring the incidence of culturally responsive communication in Australian healthcare: the first rapid review on this concept, *BMC Health Service Research*, 20: 20. Available at: https://doi.org/10.1186/s12913-019-4859-6.

Rolfe, G., Freshwater, D. and Jasper, M. (2001) *Critical Reflection in Nursing and the Helping Professions: A User's Guide*. Basingstoke: Palgrave Macmillan.

Ross, L., Hannah, J. and Van Huizen, P. (2016) What motivates students to pursue a career in paramedicine?, *Australasian Journal of Paramedicine*, 13 (1): 484. Available at: https://doi.org/10.33151/ajp.13.1.484.

Ross, L., Jennings, P., Gosling, C. and Williams, B. (2018) Experiential education enhancing paramedic perspective and interpersonal communication with older patients: a controlled study, *BMC Medical Education*, 18: 239. Available at: https://doi.org/10.1186/s12909-018-1341-9.

Royce, C., Hayes, M. and Schwartzstein, M. (2019) Teaching critical thinking: a case for instruction in cognitive biases to reduce diagnostic errors and improve patient safety, *Academic Medicine*, 94 (2): 187–94.

Sanchez, N., Norka, A., Corbin, M. and Peters, C. (2019) Use of experiential learning, reflective writing, and metacognition to develop cultural humility among undergraduate students, *Journal of Social Work Education*, 55 (1): 75–88.

Schön, D.A. (1983) *The Reflective Practitioner: How Professionals Think in Action.* New York: Basic Books.

The Point of Care Foundation (2016) *About Schwartz Rounds.* Available at: https://www.pointofcarefoundation.org.uk/our-programmes/staff-experience/about-schwartz-rounds/ (accessed 9 April 2024).

Wade, C. (2013) Planning and writing an evidence-based critical reflection, *Journal of Paramedic Practice*, 3 (4): 190–96.

Willis, S. (2010) Becoming a reflective practitioner: frameworks for the prehospital professional, *Journal of Paramedic Practice*, 2 (5): 211–16.

3 Using clinical audit to improve patient care

Rachael T. Fothergill and Joanna Shaw

In this chapter:

- Introduction
- Why is this relevant?
- Clinical governance
- What is clinical audit?
- Peer review, critical incident analysis, deep dives and quality improvement
- What are the benefits of clinical audit?
- The role of the paramedic in clinical audit
- Conclusion
- Chapter key points
- References and suggested reading
- Useful websites

INTRODUCTION

This chapter is a brief introduction to the concept of using clinical audit as a tool to improve clinical quality and patient care. The process of clinical audit dates back to the mid-nineteenth century, and today, it plays an important role in ensuring that the highest standard of care is delivered to patients across the NHS. This chapter outlines the process and importance of clinical audit, and briefly touches on other approaches to reviewing health care. An understanding of these approaches is the foundation not only of paramedic practice, but all other healthcare provider roles. Some definitions are included and sources of further reading provided.

WHY IS THIS RELEVANT?

Clinical audit has a direct effect on paramedic practice and is something that clinicians are involved with on a daily basis, even though they may not realise it. It can change practice by influencing protocols, policy development and treatments. Everything the paramedic does in practice is subject to the rigours of clinical audit. Clinical audit is reliant upon accurate clinical documentation and, as such, it is important that healthcare practitioners are aware of how their clinical records are used and how this influences future patient care.

CLINICAL GOVERNANCE

Clinical governance provides a mechanism for ensuring that quality is at the heart of the NHS. It is aimed at improving standards of clinical practice and ensuring that decisions are based on the most up-to-date evidence of what is clinically effective. Clinical governance is not simply concerned with achieving and maintaining high standards, but with continuously improving them to create an environment of clinical excellence. It has been defined as 'a mission not just to do well, but to do better' (Donaldson, 2000: 7).

It is generally recognised that before the UK government introduced clinical governance into the NHS in 1997, there was a distinct lack of organisational responsibility for quality. Within a couple of years, the Health Act of June 1999 (Section 18) established a statutory duty of quality requiring NHS Trusts to monitor and improve the care they provide.

It is helpful to view clinical governance as an 'umbrella' beneath which there are a number of key components that combine to make a quality organisation. Essentially, clinical governance is about:

- clear lines of responsibility and accountability for the quality of clinical care;
- a comprehensive programme of quality improvement activities;
- clear policies for managing risks, and procedures for identifying and addressing poor performance.

Clinical audit is one of the principal methods for measuring clinical quality and identifying improvements in health care, and has been described as one of the cornerstones of clinical governance (Oyebode et al., 1999).

WHAT IS CLINICAL AUDIT?

Clinical audit is a quality assurance and improvement tool. There are many definitions of clinical audit, but they generally all have the same key elements: the systematic review of the quality of care against explicit criteria and making improvements where indicated. Box 3.1 provides the Healthcare Quality Improvement Partnership definition of clinical audit.

> ## Box 3.1 Definition of clinical audit
>
> 'A quality improvement cycle that involves measurement of the effectiveness of healthcare against agreed and proven standards for high quality, and taking action to bring practice in line with these standards so as to improve the quality of care and health outcomes' (Healthcare Quality Improvement Partnership, 2011: xi).

The emergence of clinical audit

The work of Florence Nightingale in the 1850s is widely considered to be one of the earliest examples of clinical audit. By monitoring medical practices during the Crimean War, she was able to identify a link between poor sanitation and high mortality rates. Florence and her team of nurses methodically introduced strict sanitation procedures and were able to report a significant decrease in patient deaths.

Clinical audit (or 'medical audit' as it was once known) was not formally introduced into professional practice in the NHS until 1989 when the government published its White Paper *Working for Patients* (DH, 1989). This paper also set out the government's expectation that regular, systematic audit was something in which every doctor would participate. Just a few years later, it became clear that all healthcare professionals, not just hospital doctors, should play an active part in audit, and so medical audit evolved into clinical audit. In 1997, along with the introduction of clinical governance, the government identified clinical audit as important to achieving a high-quality NHS (DH, 1997, 1998). In 2000, clinical audit became further embedded into health care when the *NHS Plan* (DH, 2000) made it a requirement for all NHS organisations and a mandatory obligation for all doctors employed in, or under contract to, the NHS. Ten years later, in 2010, the government began linking NHS payment arrangements to quality measures reported in national clinical audits, solidifying a commitment to clinical audit.

The important role of clinical audit in the NHS has been highlighted by a number of high-profile public inquiries. The 2001 report of the investigation into the deaths of babies following heart surgery during the 1990s at the Bristol Royal Infirmary cited a 'lax approach to safety, secrecy about doctors' performance and a lack of monitoring'. The report recommended that clinical audit 'must be fully supported by Trusts', 'should be compulsory for all healthcare professionals providing clinical care', and the 'requirement to participate in it should be included as part of the contract of employment' (DH, 2002).

The value of clinical audit was further emphasised by the inquiry into the deaths of patients under the care of the general practitioner, Dr Harold Shipman. The government's response to the Shipman Inquiry (DH, 2007) acknowledged the progress to clinical governance that had been made by the NHS since the period covered by the Inquiry but indicated that had such processes been in place at the time, 'it is highly unlikely that the abuses could have continued for such long periods without being detected'. The report reiterated the significance of all clinicians participating in clinical audit 'so that any problems are picked up by them and their peers at the earliest possible stage'. The Morecambe Bay Investigation of serious incidents in maternity services at Furness General Hospital (FGH), which included the deaths of mothers and babies, described clinical governance systems throughout the Trust as inadequate with a failure to present a complete picture of how the maternity unit was operating. The investigation report, the Kirkup Report, identified a range of key issues that comprised a lack of robust clinical governance activity at unit level and specified the need for a continuing audit programme in response to the results of investigations (Kirkup, 2015). More recently, in 2022, the Ockenden Report presented the findings and recommendation of the largest inquiry into a single service in the NHS's history. This review of maternity services at the Shrewsbury and Telford Hospital NHS Trust (Ockenden, 2022) identified concerns that included a lack of planned audits being undertaken, a failure to monitor and a failure to develop robust action plans to effect a change in practice. The review found that the management of maternity audits resulted in 'a significant lost opportunity to improve the quality of maternity care at the Trust throughout the entire period of the maternity review'.

Clinical audit clearly has an important role to play in the NHS, and all healthcare professionals should have a basic understanding of its principles. This position is supported by a number of professional bodies including, but not limited to, the General Medical Council, the Royal College of Emergency Medicine and the Health and Care Professions Council. The latter's *Standards of Proficiency for Paramedics* (HCPC, 2023) specifies that paramedics 'must be able to assure the quality of their practice … engage in evidence-based practice, monitor and systematically evaluate the quality of practice'. All of these elements are an integral part of clinical audit and, as such, every paramedic has a role to play in clinical audit.

The clinical audit process

The clinical audit process consists of an iterative cycle of steps known as the audit cycle (see Figure 3.1). It involves selecting a topic, setting standards for clinical practice and then measuring actual practice to determine

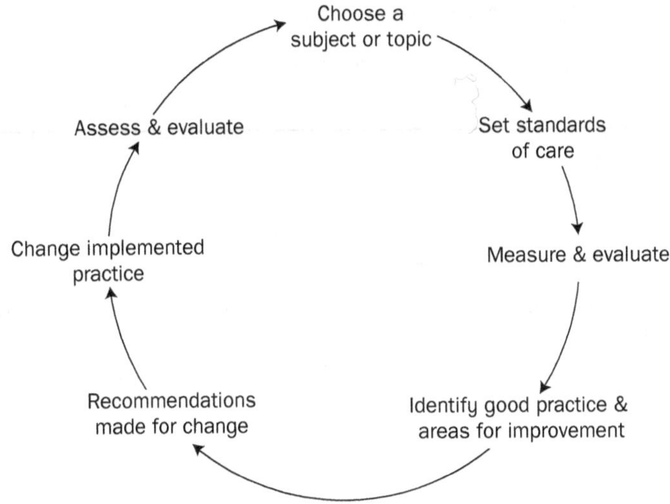

Figure 3.1   The audit cycle

Source: Contains public sector information licensed under the Open Government
Licence v3.0. Adapted from DH (1997), based on information in NICE (2002).

whether the standards are being met. If practice is shown to deviate from
the accepted standard, then reasons must be identified and improvements
made. After a suitable time interval, clinical practice must be reassessed
(re-audited) against the original criteria to confirm an improvement in healthcare delivery. The whole audit process should continue through as many
cycles as necessary until there is evidence that improved standards of care
are being delivered and maintained.

Topic selection

As any audit project will inevitably involve a significant investment of
resources, topic selection needs careful consideration. Practically any area
of clinical care can be selected as a topic for clinical audit, as long as it is
measurable and has the potential to provide assurance or improvements
to services and patient care. Topic selection will largely be determined at a
local level (ideally with input from key stakeholders) and involve a variety of
sources, including complaints, clinical incident reports and feedback from
patient questionnaires or focus groups. The need for a particular clinical
audit can also be triggered by the introduction of new drugs or interventions,
new guidance or new care pathways. It is also common for topics to be specified at a national level through, for example, government-commissioned
programmes and NICE guidance.

Criteria, standards and exceptions

When a topic has been chosen, the criteria, expected standards of care and any exceptions to delivering that care must be established. Criteria are essentially explicit statements that describe the aspects of care being measured (for example, 'adequate analgesia must be given to patients in pain') and are used to assess the quality of care provided.

There are three types of criteria that can be measured:

- **Structure:** what was needed (e.g. the availability of resources and facilities)?
- **Process:** what was done/what action was taken (e.g. the treatment given)?
- **Outcome:** what was the clinical result (e.g. the patient's health status)?

Process criteria are generally considered to be the most sensitive measures of the quality of care, although within the NHS there is growing interest in the use of outcome measures. It is important to use outcome measures with caution as there are often many different factors that contribute to an outcome (such as other treatments and co-existing clinical conditions) and, as such, it is possible that patients who receive a good level of care may experience poor outcomes, and vice versa. Furthermore, some important outcomes occur long after care is provided, so it can be difficult to tease out the direct impact of a particular clinical intervention. This latter limitation is particularly pertinent to ambulance services where patients are frequently handed over to hospitals or other healthcare providers within a relatively short period of time. Outcome measures are also, in practice, often difficult to collect. When examining outcomes as part of ambulance service clinical audit, it is sometimes necessary to collect information not only from ambulance service clinical records, but from the records of other organisations that subsequently cared for the patient. With limited resources and access to external data sources, it is often a challenge for ambulance services to obtain data from other organisations. Ambulance services may find it less problematic and more useful to select, where practical, outcomes that occur within a short period relative to the incident, such as those at the point of patient handover to another healthcare professional or within a few days of such handover.

Another challenge with undertaking an outcomes audit is the proximity to research. While it is possible to utilise observational research methods (such as patient questionnaires and focus groups) to obtain outcome information for clinical audit, these approaches will need to be considered within the UK Framework for Health and Social Care Research (Health Research Authority, 2017), with issues of confidentiality and ethics being key, and the necessary approvals (including organisation research approvals and approvals from the NHS Research Ethics Committee as appropriate) being secured in advance.

Nonetheless, despite the potential limitations, outcome measures can be extremely powerful, particularly when used in conjunction with process measures.

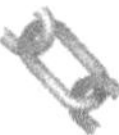 Turn to **Chapter 5** to read about the importance of research within the paramedic profession.

Standards are defined as expected levels of performance – that is, how often it is expected that the care given will comply with the criteria. Standards are usually expressed as percentages (e.g. 100 per cent of patients in pain should receive adequate analgesia or have a clearly documented exception).

Exceptions are valid clinical reasons why the standard of care could not be delivered (e.g. contraindication to analgesia). Exceptions should not include organisational issues, such as lack of equipment or lack of staff, as it is important for any clinical audit to be able to measure and highlight such issues with the ultimate aim of driving change.

Criteria, standards of care and exceptions within UK ambulance services are mainly derived from national ambulance clinical practice guidelines, other guidelines as appropriate (e.g. NICE) and local protocols.

Recommendations and actions

Once the data has been collected and practice measured, areas of care that do or do not meet the set standards are identified. Where care is found to meet the expected standard, it is important to communicate this and congratulate those involved, which may be at an individual, departmental or organisational level. When clinical practice does not meet the expected standard, recommendations for improving practice must be developed and an action plan devised. Once approved by the Trust's relevant executive committees, the recommended changes and actions are implemented in a systematic fashion.

A common criticism of the clinical audit process is that recommended changes are sometimes not fully or effectively implemented. For an audit to succeed in delivering change, it is important that there is strong clinical leadership and 'buy-in' at a senior level within the organisation. It is also crucial that key stakeholders, including relevant clinicians, patients or service users, and staff, whose support is necessary to implement changes, are involved from the outset. Key stakeholder involvement ensures that ownership of the project lies with those who are most likely to be affected by its findings. Their involvement also ensures commitment and increases the likelihood that changes to practice, and thus improvements to patient care, will be achieved.

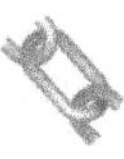 **Chapter 17** for more detail on clinical leadership.

PEER REVIEW, CRITICAL INCIDENT ANALYSIS, DEEP DIVES AND QUALITY IMPROVEMENT

There are a number of common methods of reviewing health care within the NHS that are often mistakenly considered to be clinical audit; these include peer review, critical incident analysis, deep dives and quality improvement projects. Peer review typically involves a group of clinicians randomly selecting a small sample of records for patients who were recently under their care, and considering as a group whether the best care was provided. Critical incident analysis usually involves multidisciplinary teams reviewing cases that have caused concern or where there were unexpected, adverse outcomes. Deep dive reviews are increasingly being used by NHS Trusts to examine known or potential issues or concerning trends, and to provide assurance about the safety and quality of care. Quality improvement is closely aligned with clinical audit, but is not the same. Where clinical audit asks whether we are performing to the acceptable standard and identifies areas for improvement, quality improvement specifically focuses on making continual small changes to improve an existing service. All of these approaches, when used on their own, are very useful, but they can be even more impactful when used alongside clinical audit, or even integrated as a data collection tool during the measuring practice stage of the audit cycle.

WHAT ARE THE BENEFITS OF CLINICAL AUDIT?

Effective clinical audit is vital to the NHS; it brings many benefits to organisations, healthcare professionals, patients and the public. Clinical audit enables organisations and practitioners to demonstrate, to themselves and to others, the effectiveness and quality of their services. It can provide reassurance that patients are receiving the best possible care and increase confidence in the quality of the service as a whole. Where clinical audit identifies areas for improvement, it can aid practitioners and organisations by pinpointing where further education and training are needed, and so can provide opportunities for learning and development. It can also highlight to organisations areas where new investment and resources are needed to support clinical practice. Most importantly, clinical audit can reduce variability in practice and improve standards of clinical care.

Clinical audit can also bring benefits to the participating paramedic, providing valuable, first-hand experience of using evidence as a tool for change, enabling them to be a direct part of that change, and demonstrating their commitment to continued professional development. It can provide a different view of clinical practice, contributing to improved skills and confidence. In addition, by providing insight into how information from clinical records is used, it can enhance the paramedic's own documentation and record-keeping skills.

As clinical audit typically relies on extracting information from patient records, improvements to documentation and the processes for capturing clinical information may occur, even if the standard of documentation itself is not the objective of the audit. By reporting levels of missing information and identifying issues associated with documentation and data capture mechanisms, action may be taken to improve record keeping, data accuracy and accessibility.

Clinical audit can also provide a valuable contribution to the existing medical evidence base. Using clinical audit findings to add to the evidence base is particularly important in the pre-hospital arena where research evidence for many interventions, although accumulating, may be lacking. Indeed, it is now common practice to find the results and recommendations from ambulance service clinical audits being used to inform local protocols and national ambulance clinical practice guidelines.

THE ROLE OF THE PARAMEDIC IN CLINICAL AUDIT

HCPC registrant paramedics are expected to meet specific standards of proficiency (HCPC, 2023) in order to 'be able to assure the quality of their practice':

- 'monitor and systematically evaluate the quality of practice, and maintain an effective quality management and quality assurance process working towards continual improvement' (2023: 11.3);
- 'participate in quality management, including quality control, quality assurance, clinical governance and the use of appropriate outcome measures' (2023: 11.4);
- 'recognise the value of gathering and using data for quality assurance and improvement programmes' (2023: 11.6).

As in other NHS organisations, ambulance service clinical audit is extremely dependent upon the information documented by the practitioner and the importance of high-quality, complete documentation should not be underestimated. Full and accurate documentation allows those reviewing clinical records to gain a more comprehensive picture of the care that was delivered, which, in turn, leads to accurate interpretations and decisions about patient care. Ultimately, without a high standard of documentation, clinical audit cannot accurately assess the real clinical situation and deliver appropriate changes to practice and real improvements for patients. Even if not directly involved in a clinical audit project, the paramedic still has a part to play by ensuring high-quality, full and accurate documentation.

 **Reflection: points to consider**

How often are documentation audits carried out in your NHS Trust? Do you understand the importance of your documentation and the link to clinical audit?

CONCLUSION

This chapter has highlighted some important areas of practice rooted in providing a high-quality service. It is hoped that the various sections have improved your knowledge and understanding of the concepts of clinical audit and quality improvement, and the way in which systematically reviewing clinical practices can inform and improve patient care.

Chapter key points:

- Clinical audit is undertaken across all healthcare environments and the outcome can influence practice and provide real benefits for patients.
- All paramedics have a key role to play in improving the care delivered by their organisation, whether directly or indirectly, and clinical audit is an integral component of this.
- Full and accurate documentation allows the systematic review of practices, which in turn leads to tangible actions to improve care.

REFERENCES AND SUGGESTED READING

Department of Health (DH) (1989) *Working for Patients*, Cm 555. London: HMSO.

Department of Health (DH) (1997) *The New NHS: Modern, Dependable*, Cm 3807. London: HMSO.

Department of Health (DH) (1998) *A first class service: Quality in the NHS*. Available at: webarchive.nationalarchives.gov.uk/+/http://www.dh.gov.uk/en/Publications andstatistics/Publications/PublicationsPolicyAndGuidance/DH_4006902 (accessed 1 April 2024).

Department of Health (DH) (2000) *The NHS Plan: A Plan for Investment, a Plan for Reform*, Cm 4818-I. London: HMSO.

Department of Health (DH) (2002) *Learning from Bristol: The Department of Health's response to the Report of the Public Inquiry into children's heart surgery at the Bristol Royal Infirmary 1984–1995*, Cm 5363. London: TSO. Available at: https://assets.publishing.service.gov.uk/media/5a7c743540f0b62aff6c1c71/5363.pdf (accessed 1 April 2024).

Department of Health (DH) (2007) *Safeguarding patients: The Government's response to the recommendations of the Shipman Inquiry's fifth report and to the recommendations of the Ayling, Neale and Kerr/Haslam Inquiries*. Available at: https://assets.publishing.service.gov.uk/media/5a7c71a940f0b62aff6c1b5a/7015.pdf (accessed 1 April 2024).

Donaldson, L.J. (2000) Clinical governance: a mission to improve, *British Journal of Clinical Governance*, 5 (1): 6–8.

Health and Care Professions Council (HCPC) (2023) *Standards of Proficiency for Paramedics*. Available at: https://www.hcpc-uk.org/standards/standards-of-proficiency/paramedics/ (accessed 1 April 2024).

Health Research Authority (2017) *UK Policy Framework for Health and Social Care Research*. Available at: www.hra.nhs.uk/planning-and-improving-research/policies-standards-legislation/uk-policy-framework-health-social-care-research/uk-policy-framework-health-and-social-care-research (accessed 1 April 2024).

Healthcare Quality Improvement Partnership (2011) *New Principles of Best Practice in Clinical Audit*. Oxford: Radcliffe Publishing.

Kirkup, B. (2015) *The Report of the Morecambe Bay Investigation*. Available at: https://assets.publishing.service.gov.uk/media/5a7f3d7240f0b62305b85efb/47487_MBI_Accessible_v0.1.pdf (accessed 1 April 2024).

National Institute for Clinical Excellence (NICE) (2002) *Principles for Best Practice in Clinical Audit*. London: Radcliffe Medical Press.

Ockenden, D. (2022) *Findings, conclusions and essential actions from the independent review of maternity services at the Shrewsbury and Telford Hospital NHS Trust*. Available at: https://assets.publishing.service.gov.uk/media/62433358d3bf7f32b317e8e5/Final-Ockenden-Report-print-ready.pdf (accessed 7 April 2024).

Oyebode, F., Brown, N. and Parry, E. (1999) Clinical governance: application to psychiatry, *Psychiatric Bulletin*, 23: 7–10.

USEFUL WEBSITES

National Institute for Health and Care Excellence (NICE), Open Athens: https://openathens.nice.org.uk/ (accessed 1 April 2024).
OpenGrey: www.opengrey.eu/ (accessed 1 April 2024).
PubMed: www.ncbi.nlm.nih.gov/pubmed/ (accessed 1 April 2024).

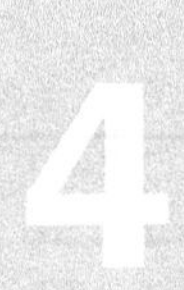

Ethics and law for the paramedic

Vince Clarke, Graham Harris
and Steve Cowland

In this chapter:

- Introduction
- Why is this relevant?
- Ethics
- Law
- Professional regulation
- Accountability and clinical negligence
- Capacity and consent
- Confidentiality and data protection
- Conclusion
- Chapter key points
- References and suggested reading

INTRODUCTION

The role of paramedics has undergone immense development since becoming allied health professional (AHP) registrants in September 2000, with the term 'paramedic' now being synonymous with primary, urgent, community, acute, emergency and critical healthcare arenas. Paramedics are required to work within the legal parameters dictated by legislation, and readers are reminded to refer to the most up-to-date government documents and laws. All areas of paramedic practice – notably, the gaining of consent, drug administration, issues of confidentiality and data protection – must be undertaken within the legal framework of the respective UK nation in which the paramedic practises.

WHY IS THIS RELEVANT?

Paramedics often meet people in extremely difficult and distressing personal circumstances and at critical times in their lives. Patients and families can be vulnerable during these moments, so it is crucial that paramedics understand the key legal and ethical issues that may impact on their decision-making. Without an understanding of the ethical principles, legislation or legal precedents that apply to their practice, paramedics may potentially be at risk of incurring fitness to practise investigations, civil litigation or, in extreme cases, criminal charges. No text can prepare the reader for all eventualities, but a discussion of the key legal and ethical issues is vital for safe, competent and professional practice.

ETHICS

Ethics can be considered a 'moral code' and, as such, can be very subjective. There are many textbooks devoted to ethical principles and theories, including a number that focus specifically on medical ethics. Such texts often contain ethical scenarios for the reader to dissect, discuss and consider. Examples of subject matter for this type of scenario could include termination of pregnancy, resource allocation, assisted suicide, end-of-life issues, organ donation or 'saviour siblings', to name but a few. The difficulty with such ethical dilemmas from the perspective of the paramedic is that they tend to be focused on situations that occur in non-emergency environments within health care and can, therefore, be viewed as less relevant to the paramedic. However, with the expansion of the role of the paramedic to include alternative treatment pathways, and an increasing tendency to be able to treat at the point of contact, or refer patients to areas other than emergency departments (EDs), a deeper understanding of ethical decision-making should be considered 'a must' for paramedics who are now at the front line of 'out-of-hospital' rather than 'pre-hospital' care.

The role of the paramedic often demands rapid decision-making capability where it could be argued that ethical considerations are put aside for clinical decisions to be made. There are generally very clear clinical guidelines for paramedics to follow, but there are also rarely considered ethical decision-making processes that accompany them.

The principles of ethics proposed by Beauchamp and Childress (2019) are a good starting point for the paramedic (see Box 4.1). Their 'four principles' approach provides paramedics with the basic tools that they need to enable them to consider ethics in their practice. By considering each of the four principles, paramedics can weigh up their decisions and ensure that they are in the best interests of the patient while being ethically sound.

The principles proposed by Beauchamp and Childress are just one approach to ethics and even these cannot be covered in great depth in an introductory

> ## Box 4.1 The 'four principles' approach to ethics
>
> 1. *Respect for autonomy – 'self-rule'.* Autonomy is the principle that allows an individual to have control over their being. This means that any decision that they make about their treatment must be respected.
> 2. *Non-maleficence – 'do no harm'.* This principle advocates not causing undue harm to the patient. Such harm may be considered direct physical harm, such as the insertion of an intravenous cannula, or harm brought about by failing to consider foreseeable outcomes of a proposed course of action, such as leaving a vulnerable patient at home when their presentation requires hospitalisation. The negative impact of any harm must be balanced against the potential benefit.
> 3. *Beneficence – 'do good'.* This principle advocates maximising benefits and minimising harm to patients. Beneficence underlies all of the actions of the healthcare professionals and can be allied with the term 'best interests'. It is important to note that a patient's perspective of what is in their best interests may not always be the same as that of the healthcare professionals dealing with them. In these cases, there may appear to the paramedic to be a conflict between beneficence, non-maleficence and autonomy.
> 4. *Justice – 'what is right?'* This principle looks at what is right or fair in any given situation. For example, patients who have mental health problems have the same right to appropriate treatment as those who do not. In the paramedic's world, situations such as availability of resources and time spent on scene with patients could be considered when looking at justice.

text of this type. To give the paramedic an introduction to how these principles may be considered in practice, each of the principles will be discussed alongside the case studies presented later in this chapter.

LAW

Law in the UK comes from several sources, including legislation from Parliament, case law, books of authority, custom and law reform. For aspects of law, the UK is generally divided into three territories: Scotland, Northern Ireland, and England and Wales. The majority of legislation and case law is consistent between the territories, but there may be specific legislative requirements within each area, so the paramedic must be familiar with the peculiarities of the territory in which they practise.

The legal system in place within the UK can be broadly divided into two main branches: criminal law and civil law. Table 4.1 details the differences and similarities between these two areas.

Table 4.1 Criminal law and civil law

	Criminal law	**Civil law**
Purpose	To protect society by maintaining law and order	To uphold the rights of individuals and to settle disputes
Participants	The case is brought by the Crown Prosecution Service on behalf of the State, and is represented as the Crown versus the defendant, e.g. *R vs Shipman*	The case is brought by one individual or organisation against another individual or organisation, e.g. *Griffiths vs London Ambulance Service NHS Trust*
Standard of proof	To be found *guilty*, it has to be shown *beyond reasonable doubt* that the *defendant* committed the alleged crime	To be found *liable*, it has to be shown that, *on the balance of probabilities*, it is more likely than not that the *respondent* is responsible for the alleged act
Findings	The defendant can be found guilty or not guilty (or in Scotland a third possibility of 'not proven')	The respondent can be found liable or not liable
Outcomes	A guilty verdict will result in some sort of punishment, such as prison, a fine or community service order being imposed	A liable verdict should result in the situation being 'put right'. This may mean an apology, a change to policy or the awarding of compensation to the claimant

---

Paramedics are subject to the same legislation as any other individual in the UK, and are specifically named in practice notes for particular legislation such as the Mental Capacity Act 2005 (Legislation.gov.uk, 2005).

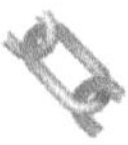 **Chapter 8**, Mental Health: Children, Young People and Adults and **Chapter 14**, Safeguarding Adults, for practical application of the Mental Capacity Act 2005.

In practice, the majority of legislation that impacts on the day-to-day work of the paramedic is dealt with by the paramedic's employing authority. Health and safety, data protection, drugs regulation, medical equipment safety and human rights are all areas that are legislated, and policies and systems are put in place by employers to ensure conformity. Individual paramedics, along with other employees, are required to conform to policies for which they have an individual responsibility, such as data protection and health and safety. This does not mean that all the policies and procedures produced by employers constitute 'the Law' in themselves, rather that legislation has informed the development of such policies. Paramedics are more likely to encounter the civil branch of the law, as opposed to the criminal branch. For example, professional regulation follows the principles of civil law and will be discussed later.

A third branch of the legal system is that of the coroner's inquest. Threats of 'explain it to the coroner' have historically been used to encourage student paramedics to do the right thing when treating patients and when completing records, often portraying the coroner as someone to be feared. This is simply not the case. The role of the coroner in relation to deceased individuals is to establish facts. There are four main facts that the coroner must establish:

- the identity of the deceased;
- the place of death;
- the time of death;
- how the deceased came by their death.

Paramedics may be called upon to provide written witness statements of fact to the coroner and any patient report records that they have completed may also be subjected to scrutiny. In some cases where further clarification is needed, the paramedic may be required to give evidence at a coroner's inquest. Once the paramedic has answered any of the coroner's questions, the coroner may invite any interested parties to question the paramedic. This means that relatives of the deceased, or their representatives, may ask the paramedic questions. This can be a difficult and uncomfortable experience for the paramedic concerned, but it often goes a long way to giving bereaved relatives a greater understanding of what happened to their loved one. In order to make such experiences as pain-free as possible, it is vital that the paramedic thoroughly documents all details of all the calls that they attend.

PROFESSIONAL REGULATION

The paramedic profession is regulated by the Health and Care Professions Council (HCPC). The HCPC's overarching objective is the protection of the public, which it achieves in four main ways:

- The maintenance of a register of health professionals, including paramedics;
- The approval of education programmes leading to eligibility to apply for registration;
- The assessment of continuing professional development (CPD);
- The hearing of Fitness to Practise complaints.

The term 'paramedic' is a protected title, meaning that it can only be used by those whose name appears on the register maintained by the HCPC. Use of the protected title by someone whose name does not appear on the HCPC register is a criminal offence. In order to gain entry to the HCPC register, an individual must demonstrate that they have achieved the threshold requirements of the profession – the *Standards of Proficiency for Paramedics* (HCPC, 2023), generally by completing a programme of study approved by the Education and Training Committee (ETC) of the HCPC. To remain on the register, the paramedic must demonstrate CPD activities and adhere to the *Standards of Conduct, Performance and Ethics* (HCPC, 2024). The implications of failing to do so will be addressed later in this chapter.

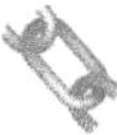 **Chapter 21** for more detail on continuing professional development (CPD).

ACCOUNTABILITY AND CLINICAL NEGLIGENCE

Every paramedic applying to go on the register has to confirm that they have read and agree to adhere to the standards presented in the *Standards of Conduct, Performance and Ethics* (HCPC, 2024). The standards for registrants are outlined in Box 4.2 (adapted from HCPC, 2024). The HCPC also publish *Guidance on Conduct and Ethics for Students* (HCPC, 2016), which outlines to students on pre-registration courses the expectations of the HCPC.

The standards detailed in Box 4.2, along with the *Standards of Proficiency for Paramedics* (HCPC, 2023), form the basis on which registered paramedics will be held accountable, should a complaint be made against them. Any such complaint will be considered by the Health and Care Professions Tribunal Service (HCPTS), the adjudication service for the HCPC. The HCPTS comprises the Health and Care Professions Tribunal – the Panels which hear and determine cases on behalf of the HCPC's three Practice Committees – and the Tribunal Service team, which provides operational support to the Tribunal.

Box 4.2 Summary of the standards expected of registered paramedics

Paramedics must:

- Promote and protect the interests of service users and carers.
- Communicate appropriately and effectively.
- Work within the limits of their knowledge and skills.
- Delegate appropriately.
- Respect confidentiality.
- Manage risk.
- Report concerns about safety.
- Be open when things go wrong.
- Be honest and trustworthy.
- Keep records of their work.

The three Practice Committees are as follows:

1. The *Investigating Committee* looks at every allegation to decide whether there is a case to answer. If a case to answer is apparent, this committee either deals with the case or passes it onto one of the other two committees. It is expected that the investigating committee will always deal with cases of fraudulent or incorrect registration.
2. The *Conduct and Competence Committee* normally deals with cases of misconduct and/or lack of competence. They will also deal with matters arising from police cautions or criminal convictions.
3. The third committee is known as the *Health Committee* and deals with cases of ill health.

Any fitness to practise hearing is based on current impairment to practise at the time of the hearing. The Council, after dealing with each case, has the power to take action against a health professional if a case is established and current impairment is found. Such action may involve removing the paramedic from the HCPC register. Other action may include suspension from the register, restricting the individual's work or publicly cautioning them.

Those prospective paramedics who are trying to join the register will not incur any penalties from the HCPC during education, but will be unable to register if they do not meet the requirements of the HCPC relating to the *Standards of Conduct, Performance and Ethics* in order to apply to be registered with the HCPC. The standards will form part of their educational programme and may be assessed in theory and in the practice environment, depending on the structure and content of the programme approved by the HCPC.

Clinical negligence

Clinical negligence is an area that is often associated with fitness to practise. All paramedics are required by the HCPC to have appropriate professional indemnity insurance, with employees of NHS organisations being covered by their employers' insurance. Those paramedics who undertake private work, or who are self-employed, are required to demonstrate that they have professional indemnity insurance when registering with the HCPC.

Employers are vicariously liable for the actions of their employees, including paramedics. An employer can also be held vicariously liable for an employee's breach of a statutory duty. If the statute imposes a duty on the employee personally, as in the case of the Mental Capacity Act (MCA), and makes no reference to the employer, vicarious liability still applies (*Majrowski v Guy's and St Thomas' NHS Trust* [2006] UKHL 34). If vicarious liability is imposed on an employer, both the employer and employee are held jointly liable, technically enabling the employer to claim a contribution from the employee in respect of any financial loss incurred (Civil Liability (Contribution) Act 1978 (Legislation.gov.uk, 1978)); however, in practice, this does not happen. The NHS Litigation Authority generally deals with claims of negligence relating to NHS staff or organisations.

For a claim in clinical negligence to be successful, three key elements need to be established by the claimant:

- The existence of a duty of care;
- A breach of that duty of care;
- Negative consequences as a direct result of the breach (causation).

The Ambulance Service itself has a duty of care from the point that it has established the location and identity of a patient, a duty which begins before the paramedic has even reached the scene (*Kent v Griffiths* [2000] 2 All ER 474). A paramedic's duty of care is often straightforward to establish and would begin when the paramedic enters into a patient–carer relationship with the patient by engaging in direct contact with them.

A breach of this duty is when a paramedic has failed to carry out their duties to an expected level of care. In negligence claims, this is an area where expert witnesses may be employed to determine if the paramedic had breached their duty by assessing their actions. It is not expected that paramedics provide best-practice care, rather their actions should be those expected of a 'reasonable' paramedic faced with the same circumstances.

The final element, that of causation, is generally the most difficult to establish and it is on the basis of this that a case may or may not proceed to court. Establishing causation relies on proving a link between the breach and the resultant harm using the '*but for*' test (*Barnett v Chelsea and Kensington Hospital Management Committee* [1968] 1 All ER 1068); *but for* the breach, the harm would not have occurred (*Wilshire v Essex AHA* [1988] 1 All ER 871, [1988] AC 1074 (HL)). It is not unusual in clinical negligence cases for duty of care to be established, a clear breach of that duty to be found, but causation not found. An example may be a paramedic who attends a patient and gives the wrong drug during the management of a cardiac arrest, administering a dose of atropine instead of adrenaline. There is a clear duty of care, and the standard of care fell below that reasonably expected in that the paramedic gave the wrong drug. As for causation, in this example, the patient was already in cardiac arrest. Their chances of survival are unlikely to be found to have been reduced as a direct result of the drug error. As such, it is likely that a claim in this case would fail.

The lesson to be learnt from case study 4.1 is that professionals need to demonstrate that they have reflected on their mishaps and developed themselves appropriately. Engagement in such an approach will very likely lessen the chances of an allegation of incompetence going forward to a final hearing. From the litigation aspect, it is worth noting that you may not be aware of a claim made against your employer based on a mistake that you made. Thorough and accurate documentation is essential in the event that such claims are made as the paperwork may be all the evidence that is available.

Case study 4.1

What happened?

A member of the public complains to the HCPC about the treatment of their relative who died following an acute asthma attack. The attending paramedic failed to identify that the patient was asthmatic, treating instead for a drugs overdose. No bronchodilators were administered, and the patient suffered a cardiac arrest. The paramedic failed to maintain the patient's airway and did not attempt intubation.

The employer's perspective

An employer's investigation found that the paramedic had failed to correctly diagnose the patient's condition: a competency issue. This was established through an internal investigation which reviewed the incident, interviewed those present and reviewed all patient report documents. The paramedic reflected on the incident and fully engaged in a period of update training and supervision in practice provided by his employer. He continued to work as a paramedic and self-referred to the HCPC, submitting a full reflective account of the incident and his subsequent update training.

The HCPC perspective

When the case was presented to the HCPTS Investigating Committee Panel, it was considered that there was a reasonable prospect of finding that there had been a lack of competence at the time of the call. When considering the issue of current impairment, however, it was found that the level of insight, remorse and reflection, along with engagement in the remedial plan put in place by the employer, meant that the paramedic's current fitness to practise was unlikely to be found to be impaired. No further action was taken, and the case did not proceed to a full hearing.

The civil litigation perspective

The patient's relative brought a clinical negligence claim against the Ambulance Service. Duty of care and breach of duty were clearly established in that the paramedic should reasonably have been able to differentiate between an asthma attack and a drugs overdose. On the basis of expert evidence, causation was also established because, had the paramedic treated the patient with bronchodilators, it is likely that, on the balance of probabilities, the patient would have recovered and survived. The case was settled out of court with damages being paid to the patient's relatives. The paramedic involved in the initial treatment was not involved in the litigation process at any point.

CAPACITY AND CONSENT

All individuals have fundamental legal and ethical rights in determining what happens to their own bodies – the principle of autonomy. To respect a patient's autonomy, the paramedic has to obtain valid consent in the majority of healthcare encounters. Failure to do so may result in an accusation of assault or battery. A paramedic who does not respect this principle may be liable both to legal action by the patient and to action by their regulatory/ professional body (DH, 2009).

Capacity

The comprehension required for informed consent is based on the patient's capacity to understand the procedure being explained to him or her. Capacity should not be confused with a paramedic's assessment of the reasonableness of the person's decision (DH, 2009). The paramedic must have an understanding of the MCA; indeed, paramedics are among the professional groups named in the Act's Code of Practice (DCA, 2007) who are required to have regard to the Act when carrying out their duties. The Act confirms in legislation that it should be assumed that adults (legally classified as aged 16 or over) have full legal capacity to make decisions for themselves (*the right to autonomy*) unless it can be shown that they lack capacity to make a decision for themselves at the time it needs to be made (see Box 4.3). *Under the MCA, a person is not to be treated as unable to make a decision merely because they make what might be considered an unwise decision.*

Box 4.3 Persons who lack capacity

2   People who lack capacity

(1) For the purposes of this Act, a person lacks capacity in relation to a matter if at the material time he is unable to make a decision for himself in relation to the matter because of an impairment of, or a disturbance in the functioning of, the mind or brain.

(2) It does not matter whether the impairment or disturbance is permanent or temporary.

3   Inability to make decisions

(1) For the purposes of section 2, a person is unable to make a decision for himself if he is unable –

> (a) to understand the information relevant to the deci-
> sion,
> (b) to retain that information,
> (c) to use or weigh that information as part of the pro-
> cess of making the decision, or
> (d) to communicate his decision (whether by talking,
> using sign language or any other means).
>
> (Mental Capacity Act 2005, Part 1, PERSONS WHO LACK CAPACITY;
> contains public sector information licensed under the Open Government
> Licence v3.0)

In the circumstances described above, the Mental Capacity Act 2005 provides a legal framework for how to act and make decisions on behalf of people who lack capacity to make specific decisions for themselves. In order to assess whether the patient understands the information given, the paramedic should explore the individual's ability to decipher what information is relevant in relation to the nature of the decision, to understand why the information is needed, and the likely effects of deciding one way or another or making no decision at all. The Act's Code of Practice advises the practitioner to take time to enable the person to take in the information given to them. It also states that the practitioner must give an appropriate amount of information to the patient and must provide information relating to the risks of any treatment or non-treatment. With respect to taking time with the patient, the Code of Practice provides the following guidance on emergency medical situations:

> *In emergency medical situations, urgent decisions will have to be made and immediate action taken in the person's best interests. In these situations, it may not be practical or appropriate to delay the treatment while trying to help the person make their own decisions. However, even in emergency situations, health-care staff should try to communicate with the person and keep them informed of what is happening. (DCA, 2007: 104)*

The paramedic, in the course of a lifetime career, is likely to come across many difficult and complex situations. Therefore, it is essential that the paramedic has an understanding of the above powers and bodies. It is strongly recommended that any student paramedic or registered paramedic in difficult circumstances and who is having problems with the issue of capacity should ask for advice from their employer through the normal emergency channels within their organisation.

In a time-critical situation, the paramedic should always take the best interests approach to patient care. As long as the paramedic can justify that their actions were, in their professional opinion, in the best interests of the patient, there can be little comeback.

Adult consent

For consent to be valid, a patient has to have the appropriate information and must be able to comprehend the procedure, treatment, intervention and so forth being proposed by the paramedic. This means that the patient must be able to understand not only the procedure or treatment to be carried out, but also the consequences of such actions. This will allow the individual to consider the pros and cons of such situations and provide what is termed 'informed consent'. The depth to which the paramedic will go when discussing these details will be determined by several factors. One may be the severity of the presenting condition and the timescale in which the proposed intervention must take place. The vast majority of invasive interventions are undertaken in circumstances where they are necessary to prevent rapid deterioration of a patient's condition. In such circumstances, it would not be realistic, or expected, for the paramedic to discuss all possible issues surrounding a procedure.

The Department of Health (DH, 2009) advises that consent must be given voluntarily without duress or undue influence from health professionals, relatives or friends. For a patient to give consent, it does not have to be written down, as this does not exclusively prove the consent is valid. Written evidence is used to record the patient's decision and the events which may have taken place. Consent can only be valid if the patient has capacity. Consent can only be valid if the patient has capacity, see case study 4.2 for a more detailed example of the potential complexities.

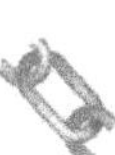

Chapter **8** to explore the issues of mental ill health in more detail; Chapter **14** to read about the complexities of safeguarding adults; Chapter **15** for the variables and complexity associated with establishing consent and capacity when caring for people with dementia; and Chapter **16** for the ethical and legal issues that may arise when caring for people at the end of their lives.

Case study 4.2

What happened?

A paramedic solo responder attends an elderly female patient who is resident at a nursing home. The patient is presenting with mild abdominal pain that she has been experiencing for a number of weeks. The paramedic finds that the patient's observations are normal and suggests that an appointment be made for her own GP to attend. The carers at the nursing home insist that the patient is taken to hospital and say that they have spoken to the patient's son who also wants his mother taken to hospital. The patient is able to understand and retain the information given to her and appears content to await a GP visit, but is anxious not to upset the staff at the home.

The ethical perspective

The patient has demonstrated capacity and therefore is able to give or refuse consent to treatment. Undue influence from the nursing staff and her son may impact on the decision, so it is not entirely autonomous. Similarly, it is not the paramedic's job to convince the patient either way. The paramedic should ensure that sufficient information is given to the patient to allow her to come to her own decision-enabling autonomy. The principle of justice may be considered by the paramedic: would calling an ambulance to convey this patient remove the resource from others who might benefit more, or would leaving an unwell patient at the nursing home divert the attention of the nursing staff away from their other patients? Non-maleficence may also be considered: would conveying this patient to hospital expose them to potential risks from infection or bed sores which would not develop if she were to remain at the nursing home? What course of action would be the most beneficial for the patient? A consideration of beneficence may mean that that the paramedic considers contacting an out-of-hours service rather than waiting for the patient's own GP.

The legal perspective

As the patient has demonstrated capacity, the paramedic cannot remove her to hospital against her will, regardless of the wishes of the patient's family or the nursing staff; to do so would constitute an assault.

Child consent

The *Reference Guide to Consent for Examination or Treatment* (DH, 2009) explains that before examining, treating or caring for a child, the paramedic must seek consent, and the NHS provides a summary of the key points regarding children and young people's consent to treatment (NHS, 2022). Young people aged 16 and 17 are presumed to have the competence to give consent for themselves. Younger children who understand fully what is involved in the proposed procedure can also give consent, although it is better if their parents are involved in the decision at the time it is being made. In other cases, someone with parental responsibility must give consent on the child's behalf, unless they cannot be reached in an emergency. If a 'competent child' consents to treatment, a parent cannot override that consent. Legally, a parent can consent if a child who is deemed competent refuses, but this is rare.

Generally, the complexities surrounding child consent tend to be reserved for debate in a hospital or primary care environment around issues such as immunisation or organ transplantation. It is highly unlikely that paramedics will ever have to deal with a child, or their parent, who refuses a proposed life-saving intervention. If in doubt, adopt the best interests approach.

Patient refusal

In practice, refusal to consent presents a greater challenge for the paramedic. Competent adult patients may refuse treatment (DH, 2009); however, any refusal of treatment must be an informed refusal. The only exception to this rule is where treatment is for a mental disorder/illness and the patient is detained under the Mental Health Acts (Legislation.gov. uk, 1983, 2007). If a patient is not competent, then a paramedic may treat the patient if it is in their best interests. This may include the wishes of the patient when they were competent. People close to the patient may be able to give more information and help the paramedic make a balanced, well-informed decision in such circumstances. Patients may make decisions relating to their future care either verbally or in writing. In cases relating to life-sustaining treatment, any decisions must be in writing and independently witnessed. The MCA introduced 'Advance Decisions', taking the place of advanced directives or living wills. Advance decisions can only refuse consent to certain treatments or interventions in given circumstances; they cannot be used to demand interventions. Case study 4.3 highlights one aspect of patient refusal.

Case study 4.3

What happened?

A paramedic ambulance crew are called to a 45-year-old male patient in cardiac arrest. On arrival, the patient's wife presents the crew with a Lasting Power of Attorney (LPA) document that identifies her as the holder of the LPA. The crew initiate basic life support while the document is checked. It is confirmed that the LPA gives the patient's wife decision-making capacity in aspects of health care and specifically gives decision-making rights in end-of-life situations.

The patient's wife indicates to the crew that she wants them to stop CPR as her husband was terminally ill and would not want to be revived.

The ethical perspective

By appointing an LPA, the patient has delegated their autonomy to their representative. Although the crew may believe that, considering the principle of beneficence, the best course of action for the patient would be to commence resuscitation, the patient has expressed to his representative that this is not what he would want. Even if the crew do not agree with the decision of the patient, expressed through their attorney, they must still respect it as an autonomous decision. Not carrying out resuscitation may be an uncomfortable decision, but it would be ethically justified.

The legal perspective

If the crew reasonably believe the information given to them is true, then they would be legally obliged to respect the wishes of the patient's representative. If there was any doubt regarding the identity of the attorney or the validity of the documentation, then the crew could commence resuscitation and convey the patient while a definitive answer was sought from the Court of Protection. There can be no legal claim for 'wrongful life', meaning that if the crew did successfully revive the patient and it was later discovered that this was against his wishes, the patient would not be able to sue the crew for taking life-saving action.

CONFIDENTIALITY AND DATA PROTECTION

The NHS Code of Practice on confidentiality (DH, 2003: 7) clearly defines a duty of confidence as:

A duty of confidence arises when one person discloses information to another (e.g. patient to clinician) in circumstances where it is reasonable to expect that the information will be held in confidence. It –

a Is a legal obligation that is derived from case law.
b Is a requirement established within professional codes of conduct. and
c Must be included within NHS employment contracts as a specific requirement linked to disciplinary procedures.

The relationship between healthcare professionals and their patients has always been considered especially significant with regard to disclosure of information. Much of the information given to the paramedic is often of a sensitive nature and there is an expectation that this information will not be passed on to others without the consent of the individual concerned. The confidentiality model (see Figure 4.1) advocated by the Department of Health (DH, 2003: 10) may assist paramedics in their main responsibilities regarding patient confidentiality. This model will naturally involve paramedics in other aspects of quality monitoring, such as clinical audit, in order to establish ways to improve their own and others' professional practice.

It is rare that paramedics are the only healthcare professionals involved in the patient's care; an inter-professional approach is the usual practice. It is necessary to disclose information to health and social care professionals when paramedic practitioners, for example, convey patients to the emergency department (ED) to maintain the uninterrupted 'patient care pathway'. In such situations, a copy of the patient record will be left with the relevant ED staff. Patients' consent in such situations should be sought, to enable disclosure of their information wherever possible. When patients are conveyed to hospital, their consent will have been obtained routinely in the vast majority of cases. It is accepted that by agreeing to be taken to

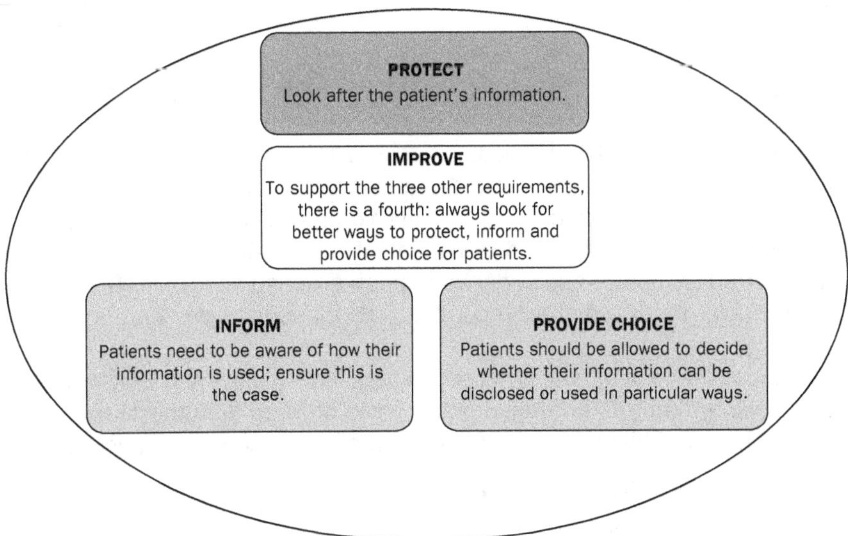

Figure 4.1 The confidentiality model

Source: Adapted from DH (2003: 10).

hospital, disclosure of information relating to the patient will be shared by the paramedic with those entitled to receive it.

There will be situations where the need for confidentiality has to be balanced against what is termed the 'public interest'. Under common law, practitioners are permitted to disclose personal information in order to support detection, investigation and punishment of serious crime and/or to prevent abuse or serious harm to others where they judge, on a case-by-case basis, that disclosure outweighs the obligation of confidentiality. Practitioners should consider each case on its own merits. On occasions, due to the nature of the incident, it may be difficult to make a decision. In such situations, it may be necessary to seek legal or specialist advice from professional, regulatory or employing authorities' legal departments, who will seek further legal advice as required.

The NHS policy relating to confidentiality is based on guidance from Department of Health documents, including *Confidentiality: NHS Code of Practice* (DH, 2003) and *Guidance for Access to Health Records Requests* (DH, 2010), as well as the Information Commissioner's *Use and Disclosure of Health Data: Guidance on the Application of the Data Protection Act 1998* (Information Commissioner's Office, 2002).

Case study 4.4

What happened?

You are in the ambulance station mess room with six colleagues when a paramedic returns from a call. He proceeds to tell those in the room about the call that he has just attended. He says that they went to Kipling Rise where he treated a 14-year-old girl called Mary for severe abdominal pain. He diagnosed an ectopic pregnancy and took the girl straight to the emergency department of the hospital where she was transferred to theatre and underwent an emergency operation. The paramedic is very pleased that he correctly diagnosed the presentation.

You notice that one of your other colleagues is very quiet and looks angry. It transpires that this colleague is the uncle of Mary, and this is the first he has heard of his niece either being unwell or being sexually active.

Has confidentiality been breached?

Patient confidentiality has definitely been breached in this case. From the information disclosed – name, age and address – the patient could easily be identified.

How could this have been avoided?

Mess room discussions and debriefs are an important element of personal and professional development and should be encouraged, as long as confidentiality is respected. There is no breach if there is no disclosure of identifiable data. This case could just as easily have been discussed as a purely clinical presentation with no reference to the patient's name or address. Identifiable data does not only include names and addresses; if the identity of a patient can be determined by the information disclosed, perhaps due to the unique nature of the presentation within a hospital, then confidentiality can be considered to have been breached.

 **Reflection: points to consider**

Have you observed colleagues try to maintain patient confidentiality in public places during an emergency? Think about the strategies you can use to try and maintain confidentiality in emergency situations. Also think about the possible consequences of ignoring the importance of trying to maintain confidentiality.

Case study 4.4 provides one example of a confidentiality breach and how this could have been avoided, please take the time to reflect on your own examples.

Data protection

The Data Protection Acts (Legislation.gov.uk, 1998, 2018) describe the processes for obtaining, recording, holding, using and sharing information. [The later Act is the UK's implementation of the General Data Protection Regulation (GDPR).] The issue of confidentiality and data protection requires careful management by paramedics. When dealing with the public, healthcare professionals, other professions, emergency services or agencies, there is the potential for information to be leaked about patients and their treatment. It is easy at the scene of an emergency call to declare information about a patient that may be overheard by members of the public. Patient records present another risk to patient confidentiality. Patient records completed by paramedics with respect to patient treatment and details must be recorded as accurately as possible and be protected from the view of those not entitled to see them. Safe storage and disposal of these are also a requirement of the Data Protection Acts 1998 and 2018, and healthcare professionals must ensure that they are employing their organisations' policies and procedures.

CONCLUSION

It is accepted that the role of a paramedic brings with it a number of important legal areas within their scope of practice. Paramedics need to be aware of the consequences of their actions and be able to maintain a professional, legal and ethical approach at all times. Understanding the law is particularly important as paramedic practice continues to develop and broaden in scope. The HCPC seeks to provide a framework within which paramedics are able to practise to the highest standards and simultaneously maintain their accountability to patients, clients and other professionals. This chapter presents an overview of some of the most common legal and ethical issues facing the paramedic in the twenty-first century. Many of the areas require further investigation and wider reading in order to obtain a more comprehensive understanding of the issues covered in this chapter, and the list of suggested reading at the end of this chapter will be useful for this.

Chapter key points:

- Ethical dilemmas are part of everyday practice in the NHS.
- Ethical considerations must underpin the clinical approaches undertaken by the paramedic.
- Paramedic ethical dilemmas occur across the lifespan, due to the nature of the role.
- As registered healthcare professionals, paramedics are accountable for their actions.
- Paramedics thus require a good understanding of the law in relation to their role.

REFERENCES AND SUGGESTED READING

Beauchamp, T.L. and Childress, J.F. (2019) *Principles of Biomedical Ethics*, 8th edition. New York: Oxford University Press.

Department for Constitutional Affairs (DCA) (2007) *Mental Capacity Act 2005: Code of Practice*. London: TSO. Available at: https://www.gov.uk/government/publications/mental-capacity-act-code-of-practice.

Department of Health (DH) (2003) *Confidentiality: NHS Code of Practice*. Available at: https://assets.publishing.service.gov.uk/media/5a7c13f0ed915d210ade16fb/Confidentiality_-_NHS_Code_of_Practice.pdf.

Department of Health (DH) (2009) *Reference guide to consent for examination or treatment*, 2nd edition. Available at: https://assets.publishing.service.gov.uk/media/5a7abdcee5274a34770e6cdb/dh_103653__1_.pdf.

Department of Health (DH) (2010) *Guidance for Access to Health Records Requests*. Available at: https://www.careforumwales.co.uk/uploads/Access%20to%20Health-care%20Records%20-%20Dept%20of%20Health%20guidelines%202010.pdf.

Health and Care Professions Council (HCPC) (2016) *Guidance on Conduct and Ethics for Students*. Available at: https://www.hcpc-uk.org/resources/guidance/guidance-on-conduct-and-ethics-for-students/.

Health and Care Professions Council (HCPC) (2023) *Standards of Proficiency for Paramedics*. Available at: https://www.hcpc-uk.org/standards/standards-of-proficiency/paramedics/.

Health and Care Professions Council (HCPC) (2024) *Standards of Conduct, Performance and Ethics*. Available at: https://www.hcpc-uk.org/standards/standards-of-conduct-performance-and-ethics/.

Information Commissioner's Office (2002) *Use and Disclosure of Health Data: Guidance on the Application of the Data Protection Act 1998*. London: HMSO.

Legislation.gov.uk (1978) *Civil Liability (Contribution) Act 1978*. Available at: https://www.legislation.gov.uk/ukpga/1978/47/contents.

Legislation.gov.uk (1983) *Mental Health Act 1983*. Available at: https://www.legislation.gov.uk/ukpga/1983/20/contents.

Legislation.gov.uk (1998) *Data Protection Act 1998*. Available at: https://www.legislation.gov.uk/ukpga/1998/29/contents.

Legislation.gov.uk (2005) *Mental Capacity Act 2005*. Available at: https://www.legislation.gov.uk/ukpga/2005/9/contents.

Legislation.gov.uk (2007) *Mental Health Act 2007*. Available at: https://www.legislation.gov.uk/ukpga/2007/12/contents.

Legislation.gov.uk (2018) *Data Protection Act 2018*. Available at: https://www.legislation.gov.uk/ukpga/2018/12/contents.

NHS (2022) *Children and young people: Consent to treatment*. Available at: https://www.nhs.uk/conditions/consent-to-treatment/children/.

5

Research and evidence-based practice

Julia Williams, Rachael T. Fothergill and Joanna Shaw

In this chapter:

- Introduction
- Why is this relevant?
- The role of the paramedic in research
- What is evidence-based practice?
- What is research?
- Involving service users in research
- Using existing evidence
- Types of research
- The importance of the research question
- An overview of quantitative research
- An overview of qualitative research
- What do we mean by mixed methods research?
- The importance of research ethics and research governance
- Barriers to implementing evidence-based practice
- Conclusion
- Chapter key points
- References and suggested reading
- Useful websites

INTRODUCTION

Research and evidence-based practice are more important in health care today than they have ever been in the history of the National Health Service (NHS) in the UK. Research is no longer an 'optional extra' but is part of the core business for healthcare organisations such as NHS Trusts.

Clinical research is exciting, with the potential to ensure that we are providing our patients with the best available treatments and optimal patient management grounded in the latest scientific evidence. Research can be viewed as the 'disruptive technology' which catalyses necessary changes in clinical practice. Clinical research can progress the development of the paramedic profession, improve patient outcomes and have a positive impact on both patient and healthcare provider experiences. With a renewed emphasis on the value and importance of research in health care, there are increasing opportunities for paramedics to be involved in research studies, and such direct involvement enables paramedics to actively influence the direction of future clinical practices.

This chapter provides an introduction to research and evidence-based practice, with a brief overview of some of the key components of these concepts. Further reading will be required in order to fully appreciate and understand the complexities of the processes described.

WHY IS THIS RELEVANT?

Research and evidence-based practice are central to the role of any healthcare professional and have a direct effect on paramedic practice, regardless of which sector paramedics are employed in. Research impacts clinical guidelines and protocols, healthcare systems and policies, and the treatment options and clinical management of patients.

As part of professional registration with the Health and Care Professions Council (HCPC) in the UK, all paramedics are expected to meet specific standards of proficiency (HCPC, 2023) in relation to professional practice. Several of these standards are related to the knowledge of research and evidence-based practice:

- 'use research, reasoning and problem-solving skills when determining appropriate actions' (2023: 4.7);
- 'demonstrate awareness of the principles and applications of scientific enquiry, including the evaluation of treatment efficacy and the research process' (2023: 12.2);
- 'principles of evaluation and research methodologies which enable the integration of theoretical perspectives and research evidence into the design and implementation of effective paramedic practice' (2023: 12.10);
- 'recognise a range of research methodologies relevant to their role' (2023: 13.8);
- 'recognise the value of research to the critical evaluation of practice' (2023: 13.9).

HCPC-registered paramedics must ensure that they have an understanding of the evidence that underpins their professional practice.

THE ROLE OF THE PARAMEDIC IN RESEARCH

As an absolute minimum, paramedics need to be research-aware and use current evidence in their professional practice. Some will take their interest in research further, contributing in a number of ways, such as assisting with research project design, providing clinical expertise, collecting data or providing recommendations for change. Others will want to follow a full-time clinical research career pathway as outlined in the College of Paramedics' *Career Framework* (CoP, 2024; Figure 5.1).

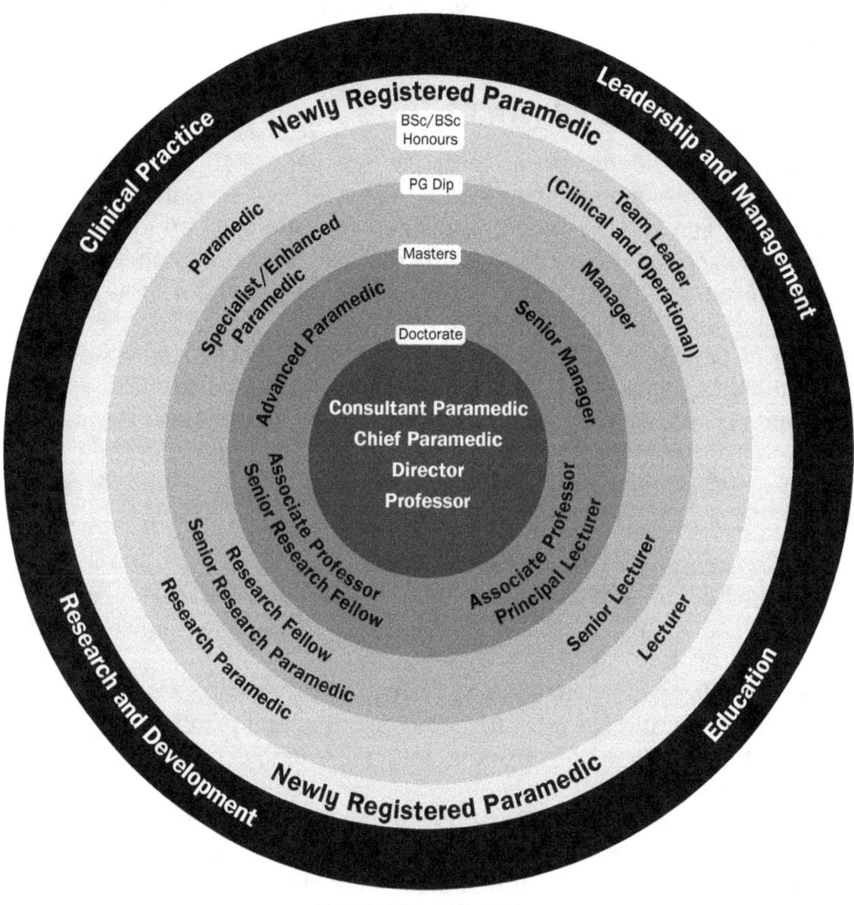

Figure 5.1 College of Paramedics, *Career Framework* (Revised 2024)

WHAT IS EVIDENCE-BASED PRACTICE?

Evidence-based practice started its journey as 'evidence-based medicine' and is defined by Sackett et al. (1996: 71) as

> *the conscientious, explicit, and judicious use of current best evidence in making decisions about the care of individual patients. The practice of evidence-based medicine means integrating individual clinical expertise with the best available external clinical evidence from systematic research.*

Over time, evidence-based medicine, originally aimed at doctors, expanded to include other healthcare professionals, moving away from the term 'medicine' towards 'evidence-based practice', 'evidence-informed practice' or 'evidence-based health care'. Evidence-based practice has become synonymous with high-quality patient care.

WHAT IS RESEARCH?

Research aims to generate new knowledge and is vital in health and social care to provide the evidence needed to transform services and improve patient care. In order to demonstrate that new interventions and developments offer the most effective care and the best possible outcomes for patients, they must be based on research evidence. However, the pace of development of many out-of-hospital unplanned, urgent and emergency care treatments and practices has been so rapid that it has surpassed the supporting evidence base. While the evidence base is growing rapidly, there are still gaps and many questions to be answered. As a result, the research of other professions often needs to be used while the paramedic profession continues to build its own evidence.

INVOLVING SERVICE USERS IN RESEARCH

In recent years, there has been an increase in the involvement of service users and the general public in healthcare research. Many healthcare organisations have their own Patient and Public Involvement (PPI) groups that assist research teams with developing research questions, and designing and undertaking the research itself, as well as promoting findings and helping to ensure the study's relevance to patient care (Hirst et al., 2016; Irving et al., 2018). For the first time, the 2023 edition of the *Standards of Proficiency for Paramedics* included the need to 'engage service users in research as appropriate' (HCPC, 2023: 13.11). The National Institute for Health Research (NIHR) Centre for Engagement and Dissemination builds on the work of the INVOLVE programme and provides a range of resources to facilitate both researchers and the public to participate in these activities effectively (NIHR, 2020).

 **Reflection: points to consider**

Identify a research study that you know about which is relevant to paramedics. How were service users involved in this study? Can you think of other ways that this could be done?

USING EXISTING EVIDENCE

The paramedics' regulatory body, the Health and Care Professions Council, expects paramedics to 'critically evaluate research and other evidence to inform their own practice' (2023: 13.10). To start to meet these requirements, it is therefore essential that paramedics possess the skills to find and evaluate relevant published research evidence.

Sourcing research evidence

There are multiple electronic databases available to search for published research evidence. PubMed, CINAHL (Cumulative Index to Nursing and Allied Health Literature) Plus and Science Direct are just a few that might be relevant to the paramedic profession. In addition, to facilitate research and evidence-based practice, all NHS employees have the opportunity to set up an Athens account for easy access to many journals.

To enhance a search, it is possible to look for multiple relevant search terms, or specify terms you do not wish to be included. Box 5.1 outlines the most common BOOLEAN operators which help to narrow or broaden your search.

Once articles are found, it is beneficial to search through the reference lists to find further relevant sources. It is also possible to search by author if you know the names of specialists in your area of interest, and hand-search the contents pages of relevant journals. Some electronic databases also allow you to set up citation alerts to send a message if an article you are interested in is cited elsewhere. Grey literature, such as government reports and guidelines, also provide sources of evidence that may be of interest and can be found on databases such as OpenGrey.

> ## Box 5.I Common BOOLEAN operators
>
> - **AND:** Narrows your search to return only articles that include all of your search terms.
> - **OR:** Broadens your search to return articles that include any of your search terms (can be used when there are several terms for a certain aspect).
> - **NOT:** Limits your search to articles that include relevant terms.

Critical appraisal

Not all published articles present well-designed and robust research, which means it is important for a paramedic to be able to critically appraise the evidence to determine its relevance and validity. By studying the research methods used, any potential limitations can be understood and a judgement made as to the quality of the research and whether the research is relevant and applicable to paramedic practice.

Various tools are available to appraise research articles, some specific to certain research methods while others are more generic checklists. When reading research evidence, it is helpful to consider the general points in Box 5.2.

> ## Box 5.2 Points to consider when reading research evidence
>
> - Was the purpose of the research clearly explained?
> - Do you agree with how the research was done? For example, the intervention the patients received? Was the research design appropriate?
> - Do the results/findings sound reasonable, or is there something about them that is not explained?
> - Are the conclusions justified? Have the authors provided adequate evidence to support the conclusions?
> - What do you think are the positive points about the study in general?
> - Are there any negative aspects or limitations? For example, is the research specific to the country or healthcare system where it has been undertaken?

- Is it a worthwhile piece of work or has it got the 'so what?' factor? Does it provide valuable evidence that contributes to existing literature?
- Would you recommend changing what you do based on this research?
- Do you trust the findings?
- Does the research identify any 'gaps' for future research?
- If you were asked to do the same project, is there anything you would change?

TYPES OF RESEARCH

Research can be broadly categorised as quantitative or qualitative. However, mixed methods research is increasingly being used within health care to examine phenomena from a variety of perspectives. Research is often confused with other types of projects such as clinical audit, service evaluation and quality improvement, as outlined in Box 5.3.

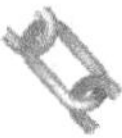

Clinical audit is discussed in **Chapter 3** where you will find more detail about what it is, its importance and the clinical audit process.

Box 5.3 Definitions of research, clinical audit, service evaluation and quality improvement

- *Research*: Research generates new knowledge by answering a clearly defined question. It typically requires extra data compared to that which is routinely collected and may involve interventions not used in standard practice.
- *Clinical audit*: Clinical audit measures the current standard of clinical care against a benchmark standard. It is used to inform the delivery of best care.
- *Service evaluation*: Service evaluation examines a service or interventions already in practice. It generally uses existing data, without reference to a standard.
- *Quality improvement*: Quality improvement specifically focuses on making continual small changes to improve a service that is already in use.

THE IMPORTANCE OF THE RESEARCH QUESTION

Never underestimate the importance of a good research question, or the length of time it might take to refine that question. It is essential that the research question, and any associated aims and objectives, are as clear as possible as these will inform the subsequent decisions about choice of research design and methods. As with many areas of research, there is no single way of writing questions, and it is beyond the scope of this chapter to identify all the conventions used because many textbooks on research will cover these areas. However, it is worth drawing attention to the FINER framework (see Box 5.4).

Box 5.4 Characteristics of a good research question

- *Feasible*: Can the study actually be completed? Can it be done in a reasonable time? Do you have the necessary funding? Do you have access to appropriate expertise? Do you have access to an adequate sample size? Is it manageable in scope?
- *Interesting*: Do you and your colleagues think it is interesting? What are the views of patients, funding bodies and other interested parties?
- *Novel*: Will this add to existing knowledge? Does it fill a 'gap' in existing literature?
- *Ethical*: Have you considered all ethical aspects of your study? Would it be approved by a research ethics committee?
- *Relevant*: Has your study got the 'so what?' factor?

Adapted from: Hulley et al. (2013).

You must ask yourself: does my research add to existing knowledge? Is it relevant? Is it needed? Will it influence clinical practice? Will it improve patient experience or outcomes? If you answered 'no' to any of these questions, then you should think again before investing further energy and resources in the research.

AN OVERVIEW OF QUANTITATIVE RESEARCH

Quantitative research is generally defined as the collection of numerical data or data that can be enumerated. It is often associated with inductive reasoning where the researcher aims to prove or disprove existing theories. Quantitative research includes both experimental studies such as randomised controlled trials and experiments, and non-experimental studies such as surveys, observational studies, correlational studies and case studies (Cutter, 2012). The gold standard of quantitative research is usually deemed to be the randomised controlled trial.

An illustration of the general stages involved in quantitative research is provided in Figure 5.2.

Some examples of frequently used approaches to data collection in quantitative research are presented in Box 5.5. There are many data collection

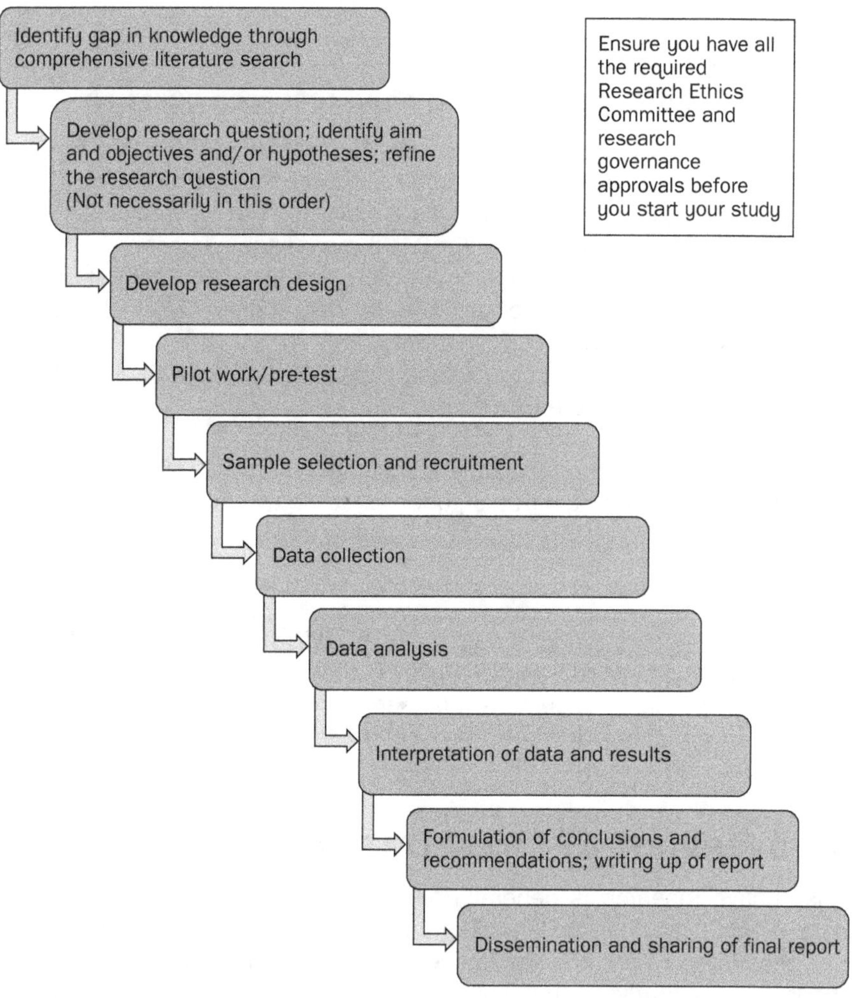

Figure 5.2 Linear process of activities commonly observed in quantitative research

Reflection: points to consider

Find a recently published quantitative research article related to the paramedic profession that you find interesting. As you read it, map the key stages identified in this section to your chosen paper and identify the similarities and/or differences between this framework and what the researcher(s) used in your chosen paper.

strategies and most research texts will give you additional information relating to the strengths and limitations of each of these.

Box 5.5 Examples of frequently used approaches to data collection in quantitative research

- Questionnaires/surveys that use 'closed-ended' questions – there is increasing use of online platforms such as SurveyMonkey, Qualtrics and Online surveys
- Various measurement tools, including scales to measure knowledge, skills, attitudes, etc.
- Likert scales
- Structured observational measurement
- Physiological measurement tools
- Trial/experiment proformas for recording research data, such as additional information boxes added to existing patient report forms for the duration of the trial
- Highly structured interviews

AN OVERVIEW OF QUALITATIVE RESEARCH

Qualitative research focuses on attributing meaning to human behaviours and experiences, and exploring motivations for people's actions. It is associated with inductive reasoning, which 'means that theory or interpretation emerges from the data rather than the researcher trying to *test* some external theory or prior interpretation from the outset' (Williams, 2012: 74). Qualitative research designs include various approaches, such as grounded theory, action research, interpretive description, phenomenology, ethnography, case studies and generic qualitative research, to name a few.

An illustration of the general stages involved in qualitative research is provided in Figure 5.3.

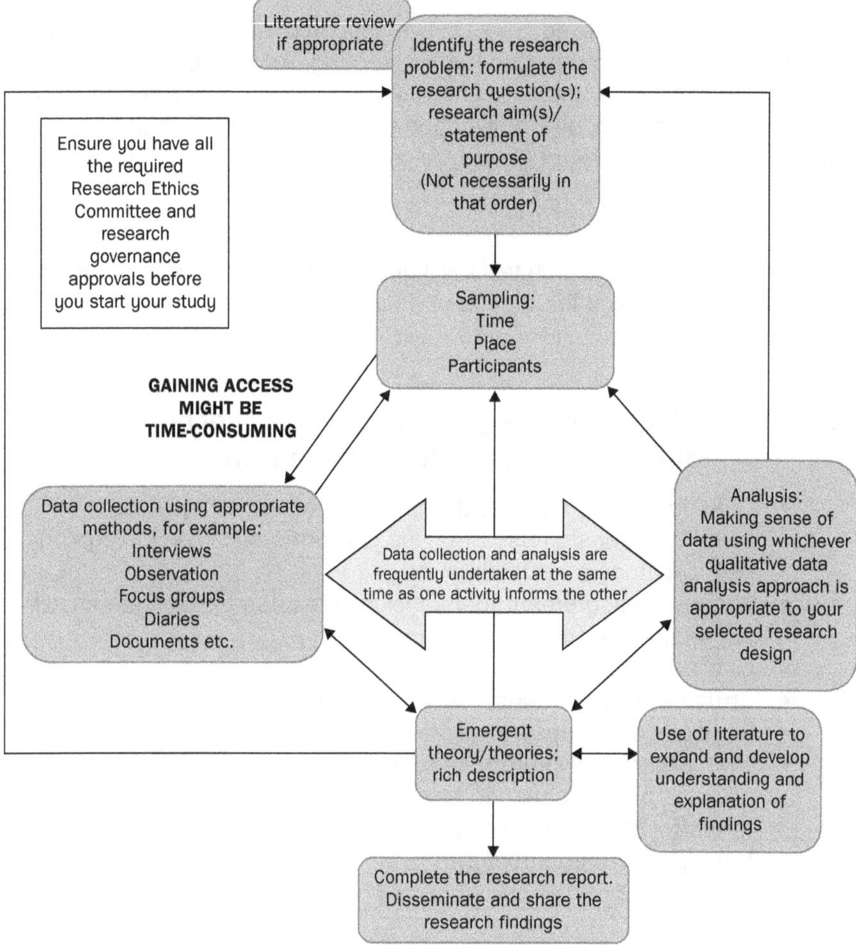

Figure 5.3 Cyclical process of activities commonly observed in qualitative research

Source: Adapted from Williams (2012: 77).

Qualitative research contains similar activities to those found in quantitative research (Figure 5.2) but their sequencing may not be the same. Due to its flexible nature, and because data collection and analysis are often undertaken simultaneously, the emerging findings from qualitative analysis may lead the researcher to revisit parts of the research cycle to gather additional data, or include a different sample group, or add in another type of data collection to investigate new themes as they emerge during the study.

This potential flexibility is not a licence for researchers to explore areas in an unsystematic manner. An unstructured approach is not the same as being unsystematic. In qualitative research, it is essential that the researchers document, in the form of a research diary (sometimes called a research log), all the factors that influence the emergent research design as this forms part of the research audit trail, essential to enhancing the rigour of the research study.

 **Reflection: points to consider**

Find a recently published qualitative research article related to the paramedic profession that you find interesting. As you read it, map the key stages identified in this section to your chosen paper and identify the similarities and/or differences between this framework and what the researcher(s) used in your chosen paper. Do not forget that when writing up qualitative research, given the word limitations for publishing in journals, it is possible that the cyclical nature may not be completely obvious within the article.

Box 5.6 Examples of frequently used approaches to data collection in qualitative research

- Interviews – usually semi-structured or unstructured – either online, on the phone or face-to-face
- Focus groups – usually face-to-face, otherwise online
- Questionnaires using 'open-ended' questions – often using online platforms (see Box 5.5)
- Online discussion forums
- Social media, including Facebook, X (previously Twitter), Instagram, texts, etc.
- Observation: participant and/or non-participant
- Diaries
- Photographs
- Videos/films
- Biographies

Table 5.1 Summary of common characteristics and differences of qualitative and quantitative research

Qualitative	Quantitative
Inductive reasoning	Deductive reasoning
Focuses on unknown issues	Focuses on known issues
Purpose is to explore, describe and/or understand	Purpose is to measure, test or predict
The study design is cyclical, flexible and emergent	The study design is fully developed before data collection, usually a linear process
Gathers non-numerical data	Gathers numerical data or data that can be assigned a numerical value
Methods are frequently semi-structured or unstructured, flexible	Methods are predetermined, highly structured, standardised, inflexible
Researcher frequently interacts with the people being studied, therefore seen as more subjective	Researcher is distanced from subjects, therefore seen as more objective
Criteria used to evaluate methodological rigour usually include credibility, dependability, confirmability and transferability	Criteria used to evaluate methodological rigour usually include reliability and validity
Findings may be transferable to other settings	Results may be generalisable to other populations
The research process is systematic	The research process is systematic

There are many data collection strategies that are appropriate for qualitative research (examples of which are given in Box 5.6). The common characteristics and differences between qualitative and quantitative research are presented in Table 5.1.

WHAT DO WE MEAN BY MIXED METHODS RESEARCH?

Mixed methods research design is gaining popularity in healthcare research. However, there is some discussion as to how this all fits together philosophically in relation to mixing research methodologies, and different authors interpret the term 'mixed methods' differently. Recently, Whitley et al.

(2020) explained the benefits of using mixed methods to gain insight into complex clinical issues within emergency medical service settings, arguing that the flexibility within mixed methods approaches is a good match for the unpredictability of this environment. 'Mixed methods' is most often taken to mean adopting both qualitative and quantitative approaches in the same study. Other terms, however, are also used to describe the adoption of both qualitative and quantitative methods in the same study, including 'multi-method' or 'mixed methodology' (Creswell and Creswell, 2018).

THE IMPORTANCE OF RESEARCH ETHICS AND RESEARCH GOVERNANCE

During the course of history, there have been some horrific practices under-taken in the name of research, including medical experiments on prisoners in Nazi concentration camps, without the subjects' consent (United States Holocaust Memorial Museum, 2016). Such ethical atrocities coming to light began a movement which saw the development and implementation of governance frameworks that included the Nuremberg Code (BMJ, 1996), the Declaration of Helsinki (WMA, 2013), Good Clinical Practice Guidance (ICH, 2016) and the *UK Policy Framework for Health and Social Care Research* (NHS HRA, 2017). Each framework aims to ensure the safety of research participants through the key ethical principles of autonomy, beneficence, non-maleficence and justice. It is a requirement of all NHS Trusts to adhere to ethical and research governance requirements, and for all relevant research to be reviewed by an independent research ethics committee (REC) to protect the rights, interests and safety of participants.

Before your project can commence, you will need to establish which approvals apply to your research and ensure that all relevant approvals are obtained (such as NHS Research Ethics approval, Confidentiality Advisory Group approval, the local research approvals process and Information Governance approval). You need to be crystal clear which governance and ethics permissions and approvals are needed for your study. If you have any doubts, you should approach the research units within your Trust or organisation where you intend to undertake your research. They have staff who will be able to advise you and who are familiar with the frameworks and systems. Additionally, a useful resource is the Health Research Authority's decision tool, called 'Is my study research?', which helps you decide whether your research will need NHS REC approval (www.hra-decisiontools. org.uk/research/index.html). It is important to note that even if the HRA decision tool does not consider your project to fall within their definition of research (for NHS REC purposes), your project will still, most likely, be defined as research by your NHS organisation and will need to go through their local research approvals process.

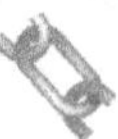 **Chapter 4** for more detail on ethical principles.

BARRIERS TO IMPLEMENTING EVIDENCE-BASED PRACTICE

The process of implementing evidence-based practice requires careful consideration, and the decision to use research to change any healthcare practices and/or systems must not be undertaken lightly and would rarely be the sole responsibility of any one individual clinician.

While paramedics have been shown to be receptive to evidence-based practice as a concept (Simpson et al., 2012), as with other healthcare professions, there are many barriers to its implementation (Williams et al., 2015). One of the common challenges is a conflict between guidelines and evidence, which is thought to arise from delays in producing new evidence, finite resources for guideline development and a lack of quality criteria for guidelines (Clark et al., 2006).

Rosser (2012) also identifies time as being a potential barrier and discusses this in relation to clinicians not having or being afforded adequate time to access and review current literature. Furthermore, she suggests that not having relevant skills and knowledge to effectively critically appraise published literature is an obvious barrier to the implementation of research findings into practice.

Despite these challenges, it is encouraging to see evidence-based practice being successfully implemented in the rapidly developing field of paramedic science with results and findings from research studies being used to make changes in many areas. Some examples are given in Box 5.7.

Box 5.7 Examples of areas being influenced by research related to paramedic practice

- Healthcare service provision
- Policy development
- Clinical skills
- Clinical management and treatments

- Clinical pathways and ambulance response options
- Medical devices and pharmacology
- Inter-professional working
- The health and wellbeing of paramedics and other emergency medicine staff
- Educational development and provision
- Expanding roles and scope of practice
- Service users' experiences
- The experiences of paramedics and other emergency medicine staff

Reflection: points to consider

How can you become involved in supporting the development and implementation of evidence-based practice in your NHS Trust? Are there any clinical trials happening that you could sign up to in order to enrol patients? Are there any working groups or committees for research projects that you might be able to join? Does your Trust employ research paramedics and is this something you could aim for?

CONCLUSION

This chapter has highlighted some of the complexities of research and evidence-based practice. It is an exciting area which has direct relevance to paramedic practice and the paramedic profession. Research as a career choice for paramedics is gaining traction and employing research paramedics is becoming far more frequent within healthcare organisations.

Research in paramedic practice continues to develop and we are still learning about research philosophies, methods and approaches within critical inquiry. In part, that is what makes it such a challenging and exciting discipline.

Chapter key points:

- Research and evidence-based practice are concepts which have direct relevance to the paramedic profession.
- Research is essential to achieve evidence-based patient care and management of the highest quality.

- HCPC paramedics must have an awareness of research methodologies and be able to evaluate existing research and other evidence.
- Research is core business for NHS Trusts and is not an optional activity.
- There are increasing opportunities for paramedics to engage in research activities at a variety of different levels, from having an awareness of research findings, to following a full-time clinical research career pathway.
- It is important to be aware of the characteristics of quantitative and qualitative research and what makes a good research question.
- There is continual growth and development in research methodologies. Decisions about the most appropriate research design/approach must be driven by the research question itself; choosing the 'best' way to answer the research question(s), meeting the study's aim(s) and achieving the objectives and/or test hypotheses.
- Service users should be involved in the development of healthcare research to increase its clinical relevance.

REFERENCES AND SUGGESTED READING

BMJ (1996) Nuremberg Doctor's Trial, *British Medical Journal*, 313 (7070): 1445–74.

Clark, E., Donovan, E.F. and Schoettker, P. (2006) From outdated to updated, keeping clinical guidelines valid, *International Journal of Qualitative Health Care*, 18 (3): 165–66.

College of Paramedics (CoP) (2024) *Paramedic Career Framework 2022*, 5th edition, revised. Bridgwater: College of Paramedics. Available at: https://collegeofparamedics.co.uk/COP/ProfessionalDevelopment/post_reg_career_framework.aspx (accessed 7 April 2024).

Creswell, J.W. and Creswell, J.D. (2018) *Research Design: Qualitative, Quantitative and Mixed Methods Approaches*, 5th edition. Los Angeles, CA: Sage.

Cutter, J. (2012) Quantitative research in paramedic practice: an overview, in P. Griffiths and G.P. Mooney (eds.) *The Paramedic's Guide to Research: An Introduction*. Maidenhead: Open University Press.

Greenhalgh, T. (2014) *How to Read a Paper: The Basics of Evidence-Based Medicine*, 5th edition. Chichester: Wiley.

Health and Care Professions Council (HCPC) (2023) *Standards of Proficiency for Paramedics*. Available at: https://www.hcpc-uk.org/standards/standards-of-proficiency/paramedics/.

Hirst, E., Irving, A. and Goodacre, S. (2016) Patient and public involvement in emergency care research, *Emergency Medicine Journal*, 33 (9): 665–70.

Hulley, S.B., Cummings, S.R., Browner, W.S., Grady, D.G. and Newman, T.S. (2013) *Designing Clinical Research*, 5th edition. Philadelphia, PA: Lippincott, Williams & Wilkins.

International Council for Harmonisation of Technical Requirements for Pharmaceuticals for Human Use (ICH) (2016) *ICH Harmonised Tripartite Guideline Integrated Addendum to ICH E6(R1): Guideline for Good Clinical Practice E6(R2)*. Available at: https://database.ich.org/sites/default/files/E6_R2_Addendum.pdf (accessed 7 April 2024).

Irving, A., Turner, J., Marsh, M., Broadway-Parkinson, A. et al. (2018) A coproduced patient and public event: an approach to developing and prioritizing ambulance performance measures, *Health Expectations*, 21 (1): 230–38.

National Institute for Health and Care Research (NIHR) (2020) *NIHR launches new Centre for Engagement and Dissemination*. Available at: https://www.nihr. ac.uk/news/nihr-launches-new-centre-for-engagement-and-dissemination/24576 (accessed 7 April 2024).

NHS Health Research Authority (HRA) (2017) *UK Policy Framework for Health and Social Care Research, v3.2*. London: NHS Health Research Authority.

Olaussen, A., Bowles, K. A., Lord, B. and Williams, B. (2023) *Introducing, Designing and Conducting Research for Paramedics*. Chatswood, NSW: Elsevier Health Sciences.

Rosser, M. (2012) Evidence-based practice in paramedic practice, in P. Griffiths and G.P. Mooney (eds.) *The Paramedic's Guide to Research: An Introduction*. Maidenhead: Open University Press.

Sackett, D.L., Rosenburg, W.M.C., Muir Gray, J.A., Haynes, R.B. et al. (1996) Evidence-based medicine: what is it and what it isn't, *British Medical Journal*, 312: 71. Available at: https://doi.org/10.1136/bmj.312.7023.71.

Simpson, P.M., Bendall, J.C., Patterson, J. and Middleton, P.M. (2012) Beliefs and expectations of paramedics towards evidence-based practice and research, *International Journal of Evidence-Based Healthcare*, 10 (3): 197–203.

Siriwardena, A.N. and Whitley, G.A. (2022) *Prehospital Research Methods and Practice*. Bridgwater: Class Professional Publishing.

United States Holocaust Memorial Museum (2016) *Nazi medical experiments*. Available at: https://encyclopedia.ushmm.org/content/en/article/nazi-medical-experiments (accessed 9 April 2024).

Whitley, G.A., Munro, S., Hemingway, P., Law, G.R. et al. (2020) Mixed methods in pre-hospital research: understanding complex clinical problems, *British Paramedic Journal*, 5 (3): 44–51.

Williams, B., Perillo, S. and Brown, T. (2015) What are the factors of organisational culture in healthcare settings that act as barriers to the implementation of evidence-based practice? A scoping review, *Nurse Education Today*, 35 (2): e34–41.

Williams, J. (2012) Qualitative research in paramedic practice: an overview, in P. Griffiths and G.P. Mooney (eds.) *The Paramedic's Guide to Research: An Introduction*. Maidenhead: Open University Press.

World Medical Association (WMA) (2013) World Medical Association Declaration of Helsinki: ethical principles for medical research involving human subjects, *Journal of the American Medical Association*, 310 (20): 2191–94.

USEFUL WEBSITES

Open Athens: www.openathens.net/ (accessed 9 April 2024).

CINAHL (Cumulative Index to Nursing and Allied Health Literature) Plus: https://www.ebsco.com/products/research-databases/cinahl-database (accessed 9 April 2024).

Council for Allied Health Professions Research (CAHPR) – hub: http://cahpr.csp.org.uk/ (accessed 9 April 2024).

Critical Appraisal Skills Programme (CASP) – Making sense of evidence: www.casp-uk.net/ (accessed 9 April 2024).

EQUATOR Enhancing the Quality and Transparency of Health Research: www.equator-network.org/ (accessed 9 April 2024).

Is my study research?: www.hra-decisiontools.org.uk/research/index.html (accessed 9 April 2024).

Library & Knowledge Service for NHS Ambulance Services in England (LKS ASE): https://ambulance.libguides.com/home1 (accessed 9 April 2024)

NIHR Evidence: https://evidence.nihr.ac.uk/ (accessed 12 April 2024).

OpenGrey: www.opengrey.eu/ (accessed 9 April 2024).

PubMed: www.ncbi.nlm.nih.gov/pubmed/ (accessed 12 April 2024).

Science Direct: www.sciencedirect.com/ (accessed 12 April 2024).

Human Factors in paramedic practice

Christopher Matthews (for Isabella and Emilia)

In this chapter:

INTRODUCTION

This chapter provides an overview of Human Factors (HF) and non-technical skills (NTS). It includes some of the important components that fall under the umbrella term 'HF/NTS'. Although these specific skills are still to be embedded within all paramedic education and Ambulance Trust organisations, thankfully their importance is being more widely understood and considered.

WHY IS THIS RELEVANT?

HF and NTS encompass the cognitive and social skills that enable clinicians to deliver safe and effective care, and directly enhances or hinders clinical interactions and patient safety (Poranen et al., 2022). Health Education

England (HEE) (2023) suggests that HF principles aim to understand the connection and relationship between a clinician, and their environment and equipment, including situational awareness, communication, leadership, decision-making and teamwork. The importance of these factors is increasingly being understood, especially within high acuity incidents such as a resuscitation (Resuscitation Council UK, 2021).

Many incidents of patient harm across the NHS are attributable to the failure of NTS, rather than technical skills (with 1 in 20 hospital admissions having some form of preventable error). Human error is a normal part of everyday life, but recognising one is fallible is the first step to improving patient safety (Brennan and Oeppen, 2022).

The College of Paramedics (CoP) is aware that HF/NTS are fundamental to ensuring effective team performance and reducing human errors and improving patient outcomes (CoP, 2019).

HF is already an established discipline within many other safety critical industries, such as aviation, which understands the importance of HF/NTS in the management of emergencies (Jenkins, 2015). Although the NHS is better at harnessing HF, it appreciates that there is further learning that must be adopted and adapted to optimise human performance in health care, thereby minimising the risk to patients (HEE, 2019); this is especially important considering studies have demonstrated improved patient care can be achieved when clinicians undergo HF training (Casali et al., 2019).

COMMUNICATION

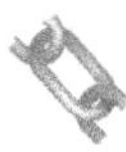 **Chapter 1** for more on interpersonal communication.

Communication is an important aspect of paramedic practice. To comprehend an incident scene or assist with a differential diagnosis, one must be able to effectively communicate with patients, relatives, bystanders and colleagues. History taking is an important part of a paramedic's role, and understanding types of communication will be of benefit in obtaining and passing on information.

A paramedic must be aware of the different forms of communication. Although verbal communication skills are immensely important in paramedicine, one must also be mindful of such factors as non-verbal/body language, listening and written communication skills.

It is important that a paramedic completes a legible and accurate patient report form. The patient report form is often the document that hospital doctors will consult for an accurate, honest and non-biased account of what happened prior to arrival at hospital. Paramedics ought to be aware of this when completing it.

Case study 6.1

George has been working all night and receives a 999 call at 03:30 to attend an elderly gentleman suffering from chest pain. Henry is 87 and George has previously attended him on several occasions for minor, non-cardiac chest pain. George is a professional paramedic who tries to do his utmost for his patients, but he is now tired, hungry and cold.

On entering the property, George and his colleague find Henry sitting on his bed, holding his chest. He tries to tell the ambulance crew that this pain is different and is crushing and radiating, and woke him up. George stands over Henry looking down at him. He has both hands in his pockets and his facial expression reflects that he is tired, on autopilot and would rather not be there.

Although George greets Henry using the correct words and terminology that are associated with professional politeness, Henry is innately aware of the many non-verbal clues/actions that have betrayed George's true feelings.

This, in turn, leads Henry to feel uncomfortable and may prevent him from expanding on his history/presenting condition. It might also impact his decision to call an ambulance in the future when suffering from cardiac pain, possibly leading to further complications in his failing health.

Non-verbal communication plays a significant role in establishing a good rapport between a paramedic and their patient (McGlashan and Crawford, 2022). It may be argued that non-verbal communication is as important as verbal communication; regardless of what words a clinician articulates, their body language can betray their true thoughts and feelings, as seen in case study 6.1.

COMMUNICATION STYLES

Communication can be broken down into several different 'styles'. This section focuses on the main four styles: passive/submissive, aggressive, passive-aggressive and assertive. It is important that a paramedic is aware of the differences and recognises which style they most often adopt. Paramedics must be able to alter their communication style dependent on the situation. This section highlights some important differences between these styles and offers examples for you to consider (see case study 6.2).

Case study 6.2

Bella is a newly qualified paramedic who has previously worked as a phlebotomist and is an expert at cannulating children. She is a member of the second crew dispatched by control to the scene of a 14-year-old having a seizure. On entering the first ambulance, she notices the first paramedic crew are readying an intra-osseous (IO) drill and needle for the patient, who is now no longer seizing. The crew inform Bella that they have had a quick look, but are unable to find a vein to cannulate, so will be 'using the drill'.

Passive/submissive communication

Passive/submissive communicators seek to please others, avoid conflict and have an 'easy life'. They are apologetic in their communication and may speak softly, avoiding eye contact. They develop a pattern of avoiding expressing their opinions/feelings to make things less stressful for themselves. If they are unable to step outside of their communication style, they will fail to assert themselves and may become anxious, depressed and resentful.

Case study 6.2.1

After the crew inform Bella that they are about to IO the patient, she looks at the floor, hunches her shoulders and quietly responds by saying, 'Okay, I suppose so'.

Whilst it is usually not a problem being a passive communicator on a day-to-day basis, in certain situations, it can lead to poor patient outcomes, as can be seen in case study 6.2.1. It can also lead to the communicator feeling negative and wishing they could have communicated more effectively.

You can see from case study 6.2.1 how this form of communication has led to this patient receiving suboptimal treatment, with Bella not stopping or challenging the first crew's decision to insert an IO.

Aggressive communication

Aggressive communicators express their feelings and opinions in a way that projects that any other view is not worth considering or is incorrect. They stand up for themselves and directly express their thoughts in an unhelpful manner, becoming angry or aggressive in their body language if they do not get their way. They may use fixed eye contact, raise their voice and have an overbearing or intimidating posture. Aggressive communicators may use humiliation to control others or seek to force colleagues to agree with them.

Case study 6.2.2

Once the crew have stated they are going to insert an IO needle, Bella glares at them and adopts a 'square-on' intimidating posture. She snaps at them and, in a raised and aggressive tone, says: 'It's ridiculous you can't cannulate them, they are 14. I can easily see an obvious vein from here and it will be easy for me. Move out the way and I will fix the problem'.

Not only will this form of communication be detrimental to building a good rapport with colleagues and other healthcare professionals, but it will also appear unprofessional in front of the patient and family members. It is not the most appropriate way of ensuring the best outcome for the patient or for building colleague relationships.

Passive-aggressive communication

Passive-aggressive communicators appear passive on the surface but are displaying anger in a subtle/indirect way. They tend to mutter to themselves rather than confront an individual or problem directly. Their facial expressions may not match their feelings, as they may smile when angry. Often using sarcasm, they feel powerless, resentful and incapable of dealing directly with the object of their resentment.

Case study 6.2.3

Bella turns to the crew with a smile on her face and states in an overtly friendly, but sarcastic tone, 'Okay, then, don't worry that I could cannulate this patient and that they don't even need an IO right now. Do whatever you want, as you won't listen to my ideas and it obviously doesn't matter that the patient isn't even fitting'. After the incident, Bella criticises the crew in front of other clinicians.

This form of communication is not conducive to effective teamwork or patient care. It will also lead to further conflicts when the crew hear about the negative conversations Bella has had with others about them.

Assertive communication

Assertive communicators clearly, respectfully and appropriately convey their thoughts and feelings, advocating for their rights without showing aggression towards others. These individuals usually have high self-esteem and listen to the views of others without interrupting. They feel in control of themselves and make good eye contact. They display confidence in their communication, not allowing others to abuse or manipulate them, and show respect for others and their points of view, as can be seen in Case study 6.2.4.

Case study 6.2.4

When the crew state they will insert an IO needle, Bella turns to face them, displaying confident body language and eye contact. She addresses them in the ideal middle ground between aggressive and passive communication: 'Whilst I understand your thought process, I am a trained phlebotomist as well, and have good cannulation rates in children. As the patient is not currently seizing, if you don't mind, I can have a look at their veins to see if I can insert a cannula to save the requirement for an IO, which would be the best course of action for the patient'.

Assertive communication is thought to be the most effective style of communication. Ensuring we have 'stood up' for ourselves and our patients allows us to take care of our own mental wellbeing, as well as ensuring good relationships with colleagues and patients (UCL, 2012; Bennett et al., 2020).

There will be times when the paramedic needs to adapt their communication style so as to be commensurate with the circumstances. It is essential that paramedics are aware of their usual style of communication and have the flexibility to alter this when necessary.

Consider your own approach to communication, and which style you adopt most of the time. If you fall within one of the styles other than assertive, do not be disheartened as this is common. What is important is that you can recognise this and learn the required skills and abilities to step into the assertive communication style when required.

Here are some tips to assist with assertive communication (UCL, 2012):

- What do you want to gain?
- What is the problem?
- Consider/describe your thoughts and feelings.
- Explain what it is you need.
- Be persistent but flexible.
- Recognise there won't always be a solution.
- Recognise the difference between what you want and what the other party wants, as they may not always be the same.
- Practise communicating in an assertive manner whenever you can.

SITUATIONAL AWARENESS

Situational awareness is an important skill for a paramedic to learn and develop. Whilst many will have begun their career with some form of this skill, it is important to expand and hone this attribute.

Cognitive capacity, or bandwidth, is an important concept for all paramedics to be aware of. There is a finite amount of information we can absorb at any given time and one's cognitive load is only able to accommodate so much. While long-term memory has unlimited capacity, at any given time, a paramedic's working memory will only be able to process a limited amount of new information (Society for Education and Training, 2023).

A paramedic's bandwidth will only be able to hold and assimilate a certain volume of information. Once capacity is reached, they will start to lose situational awareness, suffering from tunnel vision. In a clinical setting, this bandwidth-overload will be reflected in:

- a loss of hearing;
- a loss of peripheral vision;

- becoming task-focused;
- increased stress and panic.

If any of the above develop, the efficiency of the paramedic as well as the wider team will be impacted. Cognitive overload can occur almost instantaneously on arrival at an incident or develop later. Whilst everyone has a finite bandwidth, it can be expanded through education, experience and exposure to different incidents.

For example, a cardiac arrest incident can be a stressful environment with a high cognitive load due to the number of higher-order cognitive processes that are required. If the paramedic has efficient technical skills, they may then have a reduced individual cognitive load, freeing up cognitive resources for HF and technical skills. It has been shown that individuals with high levels of technical skills may demonstrate better NTS performance and vice versa (Riem et al., 2012).

It is as important to be aware of the phenomenon of cognitive overload (being 'maxed out') to combat and alleviate the problems associated with it. If a paramedic is aware of their own limitations, they can stay alert and be aware of the warning signs that their cognitive limit is approaching.

You may decide to allocate certain technical skills to others or instruct someone else to take a temporary overview of the scene, enabling you to take a step back from the immediate scene to 're-group', re-organise your thoughts and look at the bigger picture. This will help reduce cognitive overload. The sharing of cognitive load can be witnessed in many circumstances, including Helicopter Emergency Medical Services (HEMS) systems. HEMS clinicians use the above knowledge to their advantage. For instance, the doctor might be the individual undertaking a certain advanced technical skill, taking up most of their cognitive capacity, while the paramedic takes an overview of the scene and directs scene management, focusing on NTS, thereby sharing the load and freeing up bandwidth.

TEAMWORK

The ability to work within a cohesive team is invaluable for a paramedic. Teamwork is essential in ensuring high-quality patient care, especially at larger, more complex incidents. It has been shown that the ability of a team to work cohesively is directly correlated with patient safety (RCN, 2017).

It is important to remember that each team member will have their own strengths and weaknesses. There are different roles that team members can fulfill, but in the fast-moving, dynamic pre-hospital environment, there is usually little time to designate those roles: resource investigator, team worker, coordinator, plant, monitor evaluator, specialist, shaper, implementer and completer finisher (Belbin, 1993). Another compounding factor is that pre-hospital teams don't tend to have the same mix of people. Due to the nature of paramedicine, crews will change, with different crews arriving in support of each other, meaning it is even more important that pre-hospital clinicians are flexible, with the ability to adapt and overcome the many challenges of teamwork they will encounter. With this is in mind, followship is an important aspect of HF.

Followship does not mean that a senior clinician will automatically take the leadership role, with less senior colleagues in the followship roles. Followship is an art, requiring a person to be adept at following direction, allowing whoever is in the lead role to lead, ensuring proactive and appropriate support is available.

An example of good followship might be when an advanced paramedic arrives at an incident that is already being competently and appropriately led by another paramedic. If there is no requirement for the advanced paramedic to take the lead, they can easily slot into a followship role and follow the direction of the other paramedic, while offering support and guidance when required.

Undoubtedly, there will be times when the team does not form as cohesive a unit as one might want. This could, for example, be due to individual conflicts, disagreements regarding the plan/management of the patient/ scene, or different clinicians vying to be the leader of the team. If this occurs, it is down to the individuals within the team, as well as the team leader, to ensure that the patient is at the heart of any conflict and that any issues and disagreements are dealt with later.

The team should work towards the same goal, with the same mental model. This can be carried out through skilful communication, ensuring that everyone is aware of the plans and goals. It is important that the team leader shares information with the team, and that the leader asks the other team members for their thoughts and opinions. Team members must be able to work under direction, as well as assisting the team leader in decision planning if required.

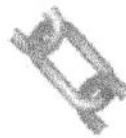

Chapter 17 for more on leadership style and **Chapter 18** for theories of decision-making.

GRADED ASSERTIVENESS

Unfortunately, not all incidents will run smoothly and, regardless of clinical grade or seniority, each and every clinician must challenge inappropriate or dangerous practice and behaviours – a possibly daunting prospect. However, all clinicians must feel empowered to voice their concerns and, if required, escalate these until they are addressed and acted on.

It may be a case that the challenging party does not fully understand the plan or treatment being proposed or undertaken. It may be due to the challenging person not having been party to pertinent information. If this is the case, the individual being challenged should simply, and without hostility, inform the 'challenger' of their plans and reasoning for their actions. However, it is justifiable for an individual to seek clarification if there is uncertainty or concern surrounding patient safety and care.

If there is a genuine concern and an individual's practice needs to be challenged, the challenger may be required to escalate this to the appropriate level to ensure compliance and, ultimately, patient safety.

There are several ways of doing this, with various mnemonics being used to assist with assertive communication, including PACE: **P**robe, **A**lert, **C**hallenge, **E**scalate (Besco, 1999). This system uses escalating levels of graded assertive communication to highlight a concern. It is important that all clinicians are aware of how to escalate assertive communication, as this will ensure that any difficult and potentially dangerous/unsafe situations can be averted in a professional manner, which leaves little room for individual uncertainty or confrontation. An example of how to use the PACE mnemonic (Besco, 1999) is given in case study 6.3.

Millie is 'probing' to see if Sophia is aware of the 'bigger picture' as well as highlighting her concerns in a simple, non-confrontational manner. When Sophia doesn't respond to her comment, continuing to try to ventilate in the same manner, Millie steps up her assertiveness, with a slight increase in volume:

> *I think there is an airway obstruction. Can we have a look with a laryngoscope to check, as it is vital that the patient does not become more hypoxic?*

By now, Sophia is displaying signs of cognitive overload and is fixated on squeezing the bag-valve-mask as hard as possible. As her 'bandwidth' is overloaded, she does not register Millie's 'alert'. Millie realises there is an urgent need to clear a possible foreign body obstruction (FBO) in the airway to enable adequate ventilation of the patient; she moves next to Sophia and 'challenges' her in a louder, more assertive tone. Although Millie has already informed Sophia of the importance of her concerns, she continues this further and informs her of the danger to the patient (whilst holding out the laryngoscope and Magill forceps she has been preparing):

> *Please stop squeezing the bag. You need to undertake laryngoscopy to see if there is an obstruction. You need to do this now, as the patient is becoming increasingly hypoxic and will be at risk of a hypoxic brain injury soon.*

Although Sophia is not purposefully ignoring Millie, this 'challenge' is not acted upon, with Sophia continuing to fixate on squeezing the bag-valve-mask as hard as possible. Millie realises that she needs to escalate her level of assertiveness even further, highlighting the 'emergency' need to clear any obstruction and ventilate the patient. She uses tactile stimulation (if not already undertaken) and places a hand on Sophia's shoulder, addressing her by name (or rank) in a direct, assertive, yet professional tone:

> *Sophia, STOP trying to ventilate the patient, as you are causing serious harm. Move to the side, as I am going to carry out laryngoscopy to look for an obstruction.*

Sophia takes note of this, realising her loss of situational awareness and admitting to herself and Millie that she is struggling with the airway. Sophia moves to the side, allowing Mille to carry out laryngoscopy and the subsequent removal of an FBO, allowing for adequate ventilation of the patient.

LEADERSHIP

Clinical leadership is a key component of paramedic practice, and the hope/increasing expectation is that the application and importance of clinical leadership will become established throughout paramedic education programmes (CoP, 2019). Importantly, this is not simply a paramedic-driven expectation and has arisen from the wider NHS Clinical Leadership Competency Framework (NHS Leadership Academy, 2011; NHS Improvement, 2019).

By the very nature of the role, all paramedics will find themselves in a leadership position. Many will never have experienced this prior to being required to 'step up' during clinical practice. Therefore, it is important that one is aware of many of the NTS that help when undertaking clinical leadership. Although leadership is, itself, a component of HF, there are many NTS which will aid the paramedic in this role. The clinical lead must be able to draw upon many of these NTS-aspects to ensure a competent and expert leadership style is delivered.

Communication plays an important role within leadership. Some incident scenes may be loud and hectic. It is important that any direction or message that you pass on as the leader is understood and acted upon promptly. Miscommunication can occur when the leader thinks the other clinician has heard and understood the command/request, but they have in fact not, which may not be beneficial for the patient.

Closed loop communication is one way to avoid this and does not have to be done with the rigid formality that some always associate with this communication technique. Simply put, the sender verbally sends a message to the receiver. The receiver verbally accepts they have heard and understood the message by repeating it back to the sender. Finally, the sender closes the loop by confirming what the receiver has said is correct (see case study 6.4).

Case study 6.4

Rachel (lead paramedic): *Tim, can you administer 500mL of sodium chloride to this patient. Please let me know when this has been completed.*
Tim (second paramedic): *I will administer 500mL of sodium chloride and inform you when this is complete.*
Rachel: *Thank you.*

As well as differing communication styles, each of us tends to have a preferred leadership style. Although there are as many as 12 different leadership styles, this section will focus on three. These can be interchangeable, and an accomplished leader will be able to alter their leadership style to achieve their goals.

Autocratic leadership

This is an extreme form of transactional leadership. Members of the team will have little to no input in making decisions or even suggestions, even if these are in the best interest of the patient. Although autocratic leadership may alienate the team, leading to feelings of resentment or lack of appreciation, one might choose to use this sometimes-efficient style during a high-acuity, stressful incident, when decisions must be made quickly and without dissent (Barr and Dowding, 2022).

Democratic leadership

Democratic leaders usually adopt a more approachable and inclusive style than autocratic leaders. The democratic leader will be more open to team members offering up ideas and engaging in the decision-making process. However, democratic leaders still make the final decision. Although this style seems to motivate and empower team members during incidents, it may hinder a hectic, time-critical scene where speed/efficiency is essential (Barr and Dowding, 2022).

Laissez-faire leadership

'Leave it be' leaders appear more easy-going, allowing their team to work independently. Although the laissez-faire leader will offer support with resources and advice, they will not otherwise become involved (unless clinically required) and will leave decision-making to team members. There is a place for this leadership within an experienced, skilled team and it has been shown to lead to high job satisfaction and increased productivity. However, it can be counter-productive and possibly dangerous to patients if the team members do not manage their skills, time or themselves appropriately – especially if they do not possess the correct level of knowledge, skills and motivation to do their work effectively (Barr and Dowding, 2022).

As you can see, each of the styles has its own positive and negative aspects and it will be up to the leader to ensure they adopt the optimal style for the moment.

CONCLUSION

It is evident that NTS are an important aspect of paramedicine. To be an effective and safe clinician, it is vital that you develop a good understanding of the different aspects of HF. Self-reflection on your adopted communication and leadership styles is important and you should challenge yourself to use other styles when appropriate.

Consider how you would interact and feel if you were one of the individuals discussed in the case studies provided throughout this chapter.

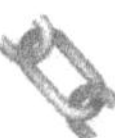 **Chapter 2** for more on reflection and **Chapter 17** for more on leadership styles.

You will not always achieve the desired result or the objective in the most appropriate way. When this occurs, you must have the ability for self-reflection in order to develop your NTS, ensuring you do not repeat the same mistakes during the next situation.

Chapter key points:

- Human Factors (HF) are an essential and important component of paramedicine.
- There are many aspects to HF.
- Failures in HF can be attributed to many patient harm incidents.
- Be aware of the different communication and leadership styles, and become adept at moving between the styles when necessary.
- Be aware of the importance of non-verbal communication.
- Develop your ability as an assertive communicator.
- Be aware of your situational awareness and understand that your 'bandwidth' is finite. However, with experience, expertise and continued education, your bandwith can be expanded and honed.
- Teamwork is essential in ensuring high-quality patient care.
- Be aware of the different roles that form a cohesive team and develop the ability to know which one to adopt in any situation.
- Competent followship can be as essential as strong leadership in ensuring the effectiveness of the team.
- The ability to calmly, professionally and assertively challenge colleagues and escalate concerns is important for patient safety.
- Find an approach to escalating concerns that suits you, then practise and develop it.
- Leadership is a key component of paramedic practice.
- Competent and strong leadership can be developed and honed with practice and experience.

REFERENCES AND SUGGESTED READING

Barr, J. and Dowding, L. (2022) *Leadership in Health Care*, 5th edition. London: Sage.

Belbin, R.M. (1993) *Team Roles at Work*. Oxford: Butterworth-Heinemann.

Bennett, R., Mehmed, N. and Williams, B. (2020) Non-technical skills in paramedicine: a scoping review, *Nursing and Health Sciences*, 23 (1): 40–52.

Besco, R. (1999) PACE: Probe, Alert, Challenge, and Emergency Action, *Business and Commercial Aviation*, 84 (6): 72–74.

Brennan, P. and Oeppen, R. (2022) The role of human factors in improving patient safety, *Trends in Urology & Men's Health*, 13 (3): 30–33.

Casali, G., Cullen, W. and Lock, G. (2019) The rise of human factors: optimising performance of individuals and teams to improve patients' outcomes, *Journal of Thoracic Disease*, 11 (suppl. 7): S998–1008.

College of Paramedics (CoP) (2019) *Paramedic Curriculum Guidance*, 5th edition. Bridgwater: College of Paramedics.

Health Education England (HEE) (2019) *Human Factors and healthcare. Evidencing the impact of Human Factors training to support improvements in patient safety and to contribute to cultural change. A report for Health Education England by the Chartered Institute of Ergonomics & Human Factors.*

Health Education England (HEE) (2023) *Human factors.* Available at: https://www.hee.nhs.uk/our-work/human-factors (accessed 9 April 2024).

Jenkins, B. (2015) Training and assessment of non-technical skills in the operating theatre: Where next?, *Journal of the Association of Anaesthetists of Great Britain and Ireland*, 70 (8): 897–902.

McGlashan, J. and Crawford, C. (2022) Paramedic and patient: lessons from my double life, *Journal of Paramedic Practice*, 14 (9): 386–88.

NHS Improvement (2019) *Clinical leadership: A framework for action.* Available at: https://www.england.nhs.uk/publication/clinical-leadership-a-framework-for-action/ (accessed 9 April 2024).

NHS Leadership Academy (2011) *Clinical Leadership Competency Framework.* Coventry: NHS Institute for Innovation and Improvement. Available at: https://www.leadershipacademy.nhs.uk/ (accessed 7 April 2024).

Poranen, A., Kouvonen, A. and Nordquist, H. (2022) Perceived human factors from the perspective of paramedics – a qualitative interview study, *BMC Emergency Medicine,* 22: 178. Available at: https://doi.org/10.1186/s12873-022-00738-x.

Resuscitation Council UK (2021) *Education guidelines.* Available at: https://www.resus.org.uk/library/2021-resuscitation-guidelines/education-guidelines (accessed 9 April 2024).

Riem, N., Boet, S., Bould, M., Tavares, W. et al. (2012) Do technical skills correlate with nontechnical skills in crisis resource management? A simulation study, *British Journal of Anaesthesia*, 109 (5): 723–28.

Royal College of Nursing (RCN) (2017) *Teamwork.* London: RCN.

Society for Education and Training (2023) *The importance of cognitive load theory (CLT).* Available at: https://set.et-foundation.co.uk/resources/the-importance-of-cognitive-load-theory (accessed 9 April 2024).

University College London (UCL) (2012) *Session 5: Communication Styles.* London: Division of Psychiatry, UCL.

7

Introduction to psychology and child development

Jackie Whitnell and Carol Lloyd

In this chapter:

- Psychology: an introduction
- Why is this relevant?
- Psychology: what is it?
- Different approaches to psychology
- Child development
- Why is this relevant?
- Theories of development
- Psychological approaches linked to practice
- Atypical development
- Conclusion
- Chapter key points
- References and suggested reading

PSYCHOLOGY: AN INTRODUCTION

There are several different approaches that psychologists or psychiatrists adopt in their attempt to better understand human behaviour and consciousness. Some approaches to behaviours appear similar, such as cognitivism and learning theory (or behaviourism) and some approaches are very different and relate to individual or diverse personality development. Psychology is the study of behaviour, personality and mental processes. A person's actions and why they do or say what they do is psychology. This chapter will endeavour to provide the reader with an introduction to the understanding of psychology to enhance the care and compassion offered to individuals.

WHY IS THIS RELEVANT?

Psychology is a core subject for the paramedic, as it serves to underpin their professional knowledge of and responses to health and health behaviours. The majority of 999 calls are psychosocial in origin, with only a small percentage of life-threatening emergencies, thus highlighting the importance of knowledge and understanding of psychosocial health behaviours. In order that paramedics and healthcare professionals can help people who are ill or disabled, it is important that they understand how humans function when they are healthy and understand individual patterns of behaviour and the difficulties associated with behaviour change.

To work successfully in the paramedic profession, you will need a thorough grasp not only of how an individual person functions but also how they interact with other individuals and in groups. It is especially useful to understand those who are potentially vulnerable, such as babies, children, the mentally ill and elderly, plus those who have a disability or learning needs (neurodiverse), among others. As a healthcare professional you will spend many hours caring for those who are socioeconomically disadvantaged and those who find it difficult to cope with life's complexities. You will also be aware that in the West today, people are living longer, and so you will find yourself caring for people with chronic illness and life-limiting conditions. Consequently, a grasp of the breadth of psychology can help you understand human development and reactions to events, in particular the trauma suffered by children in an emergency situation (Marks et al., 2021).

PSYCHOLOGY: WHAT IS IT?

There are many factors that determine our behaviour and personality, including:

- the genes we are born with;
- our physiological system (brain, nervous system, endocrine system);
- our cognitive system (thoughts, perception, memory);
- the social and cultural environments in which we develop over time;
- our life experiences, including those from childhood;
- our personal and individual differences, including our IQ, personality and mental health.

Reflection: points to consider

You are called to a nightclub following the collapse of a man from an altercation outside the establishment. Which of the following do you think might apply?

1. The attacker has inherited his genes from his parents and has anger management issues (genetics and physiology).
2. The attacker experienced violence in his childhood in his family home (learned behaviour).
3. The attacker has a history of personality disorder and is experiencing mental health problems (social/cultural experiences).
4. The attacker was frustrated with the other person and this made him angry and aggressive (cognitivism).
5. The attacker thought the other person was insulting his family, and, in his culture, it is acceptable to defend your family in that way (social/cultural).

Having reflected as above, you are likely to filter your thoughts from your own world view. The study of psychology can be usefully applied in order to be more objective in perceiving different situations and life experiences. For the purposes of this chapter, psychology will be considered in brief to provide the reader with a thirst for further exploration of the subject and an appraisal of difficult emergency and caring situations. Psychology is not a single subject; rather, it is a coalition of different specialisms.

There are many different schools of thought, as the example in the reflection box above shows, and include biological, cognitive, developmental, social, health and clinical psychology, to name but a few. With psychological knowledge, we can gain greater insight and prepare to react in the most helpful way. This chapter will provide an overview of psychology and child development, which will include a discussion on atypical development. Chapter 8 will further discuss atypical psychology, and child and adolescent mental health, as well as adult mental health. These areas have been chosen not because they are essentially more important than others but because paramedics and allied health professionals in their day-to-day working life will benefit from an understanding of the theoretical underpinning of these topics, thus linking theory to practice.

Psychology is an academic discipline and characterised by many different theoretical approaches to behaviour, personality and the mental functioning of individuals. Psychology has evolved from Freud's talk therapy, or psycho-analysis, emerging as a distinct discipline approximately 150 years ago. It has its roots in physiology, physics and philosophy, and relies on abstract and scientific theories of consciousness and developmental patterns to understand how people behave and think, and attempts to make predictions about how processes, such as memory, occur. In order to do this, some psychologists design and undertake carefully planned experiments and observations and use specific scientific methods to collect data, which – after careful analysis – enables them to make such predictions. However, theories are constantly evolving, and depending on their specific theoretical orientation, psychologists may modify them over time when they continue to investigate their chosen approach/approaches (Marks et al., 2021). Theorists investigate from many different viewpoints. Some viewpoints or approaches that are important in current psychology are biological, psycho-dynamic and learning theory as well as cognitivism and humanism.

Psychology is concerned with many aspects of human beings but the nature of 'the human' is subject to much debate. Questions have been asked as to whether a person is a product of pre-wiring (according to laws of innate nature and constructivism) or develops from their nurturing environment (laws of extrinsic behaviour), in that humans are a product of the interaction between creativity, free-will and being responsible for their own actions versus the social influences of others. This question has, over decades, been transposed into what is commonly called the 'nature/nurture' debate. It is a long-standing debate among philosophers, psychologists and educators concerning the importance of heredity and sociocultural learning.

Theoretical perspectives also vary in terms of the timespan that psychologists consider; for example, psychologists, including Freud, consider past experiences to explain present behaviour, including experiences in childhood, and the effects of abuse and family break-up. However, the focus could be on the present, observing behaviour here and now and how that behaviour is shaped by reward and reinforcement (operant conditioning). This chapter continues with a brief introduction to some of the approaches in psychology.

DIFFERENT APPROACHES TO PSYCHOLOGY

Biological theory

This approach seeks to explain human functioning in terms of underlying physical structures and biochemical processes; it seeks to explain behaviour in terms of its physiology, its development, its evolution and its function (Kalat, 2023).

Psychobiologists argue that the causes of behaviour arise from within the nervous system and are pre-wired, affected by hormones and biochemical brain structures. The trigger for action comes from chemical and electrical activity that takes place within and between nerve cells. Biological theory is often considered reductionist, whereby individual components are examined to understand behaviour instead of understanding behaviour as an embodied whole.

Psychodynamic approach

Sigmund Freud (1856–1939) is a name that often springs to mind when people think of psychology. Freud was credited for making the concepts of consciousness and the unconscious worthy of serious inquiry in the development of personality. His talking therapy techniques (used to investigate people who had mental health problems), termed psychoanalysis, involved free association and dream analysis. Freud, in essence, proposed that these techniques led him to an understanding of the patient's perceived problems and by bringing that source out in dialogue, into conscious awareness, the emotional release (or catharsis) would assist in helping the patient towards a solution to the problem and emotional regulation. However, he has been criticised for his theory being one of mythology, drama and legend as opposed to a sound empirical theory. Freud's ideas, methods and evidence have been open to many differing interpretations as therapies and the psychology of personality have evolved, and cannot be tested or verified in the way that modern scientific/empirical psychology claims to be essential. However, it could be argued that Freud's research and semantics were limited to sexual connotations. Freud's views of the human mind, personality and behaviour have highly influenced psychological thinking over time, although they are not central to it and have been adapted and developed by other theorists in this field, including Erikson, Jung and Klein. Other approaches have also evolved over time, including the humanistic and transpersonal.

Learning theory (behaviourism)

Learning theory argues that the process of learning involves a relatively permanent change in behaviour or behaviour potential as a result of experience. From 1912 onwards, Watson, Pavlov and Skinner were influential theorists who dedicated their studies to observable behaviour, working with animals and then with humans. They argued that our capacity for learning depends on both genetic heritage and the nature of our environment. The study of learning has been dominated by the behaviourist approach, as represented in their work. Two main areas of study are those of classical conditioning and operant conditioning.

Social cultural theory

This theory was developed by contemporary social scientists during analysis of the social origins of mental processes. In this view, mental functioning of the individual can be understood only by examining the social and cultural processes (e.g. the family, environment, culture) from which the individual derives. Humans are nurtured in a world full of social and cultural diversity, which must have an impact on their behaviour and adaptation. Development commences with a human being totally unconscious, dependent and supported in learning a new skill ('scaffolding'), then being facilitated and guided (guided participation) to becoming independent in a new skill.

Cognitivism

Cognitivism has its origins in learning theory with an emphasis on controlled observation of behaviour but with different considerations, such as how people think, make decisions and so on, often known as mentalisation. Since the inception of computers, researchers have examined the ways in which people mentally process and store information. The term cognitivism usually refers to a range of processes from mental representation of events, to the interpretation, prediction and evaluation of the environment, as well as beliefs, thoughts and expectations (Marks et al., 2021). The so-called 'cognitive revolution' has emerged over the past few decades as a direct challenge to learning theory, and cognitivism is unconcerned with intrapsychic dynamics as in psychodynamic and humanistic theory.

There has been much critique of this perspective and it is argued by cognitive theorists that a person's life can be programmed like a computer; however, it can also be argued that emotions all too often can ruin one's life plan! For instance, people are not usually emotionally moved by things they see or experience literally, but more by the view, or interpretation, they make of what they see or experience.

Humanism

Known as the 'third force' in psychology and developed in the US in the 1950s, the humanistic approach is an alternative to psychodynamic and learning theory. Humanistic psychologists hold neither the Freudian view that people are driven by forces, nor the behaviourists' view that they are manipulated by the environment. Humanism argues that people learn from internal individual experiences, their personal view of events and from the life histories of other people, and concludes that this leads to a better understanding of the meaning of life experience. Humanistic psychologists argue that people are active creatures, essentially good and capable of choice.

The two main contributors to humanism were Carl Rogers and Abraham Maslow; both argued that human health, growth and positive self-concept come from individual natural tendencies. Maslow developed a humanistic psychology of motivation; he argued that the individual has a need for self-actualisation, is personally responsible and free-willed, and will strive towards personal growth and fulfillment. In Maslow's hierarchy, basic needs must first be granted, then the individual can move on, through the other needs, to reach their peak in performance and personality (see Figure 7.1).

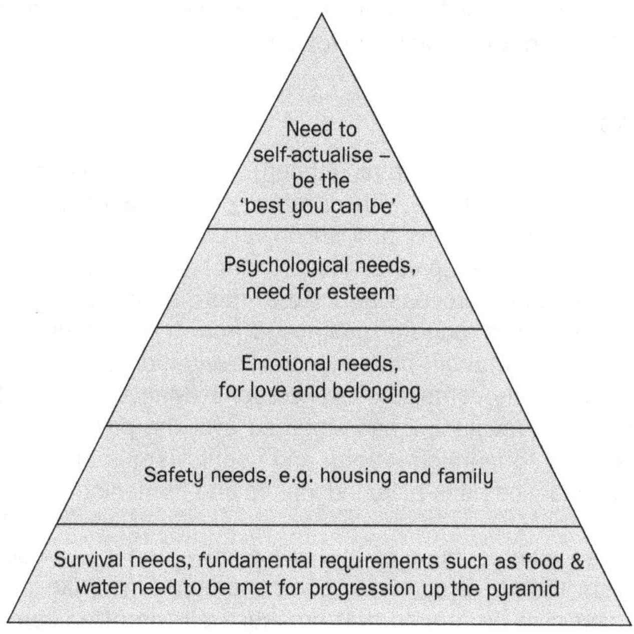

Figure 7.1   Hierarchy of needs

Source: Based on Maslow (1970).

Social constructionism

Social constructionism is a non-scientific approach to psychology along with humanism. This approach assumes that our knowledge of ourselves and of others is socially constructed. In other words, social construction is about understanding the behaviour of human beings based on what the current thinking is; so what we call facts are simply versions of events that are acceptable in modern-day society. Social constructionism argues that human beings are always a product of their cultural and personal histories and of their immediate social contexts. This approach directs study away from individual behaviour, towards a study of relationships, examining human practices and discourses (experiences and language). Social constructionism informs us of how to behave in a given group.

Summary

The approaches discussed briefly above are not exhaustive; they have been chosen to provide readers with an awareness of the topic of psychology, and hopefully encourage them to undertake further reading. Theories often contradict, but sometimes complement, each other. However, they all pursue the accumulation of knowledge. In psychology, there are many theories based on several schools of thought or approaches. In order to relate the perspectives discussed above to the practice of the paramedic, this chapter will now focus on a case study that will analyse a situation using some of the discussed perspectives. Hopefully, this will aid the reader in terms of the application of psychology to practice.

Case study 7.1

David is a 21-year-old first-year student at university. He is doing well in his studies and is enjoying his programme so far. However, he finds it extremely difficult to participate in seminars and workshops, and experiences extreme stress prior to these sessions and suffers physiological symptoms of nausea, sweating, stammering, dry mouth and cough. At these times, David feels faint and gets angry with himself, as he has no control over these bodily experiences.

While reading Case study 7.1, you may well conclude that David suffers from anxiety; you would be correct.

Reflection: points to consider

What would the differing approaches to psychology above make of David's experience?

Psychodynamic approach

From a psychoanalytic view, David's anxiety may well be a symptom of problems dating back to his childhood. He may have had difficulty in speaking out in the family home; it may be that one of his parents was very dominant and David found it easier to remain silent. It could be that David experienced conflict at the stage of development during which he was attempting to find his own identity when trying to establish sexual, political and career identities or was confused about what roles to play. Identity crises can create storm and stress. A psychotherapist could help David to come to terms with his anxiety or repressed issue, and help him to alter his responses to the situational factors that make him anxious, bringing about new consciousness and resilience (Turner-Cobb, 2014).

Learning theory (behaviourist approach)

In his early life, David could have experienced a situation in which he felt extreme anxiety in a classroom: that could be enough to generate anxiety in similar future situations. This is known as a conditioned emotional response or learned behaviour, and arises, according to learning theory, from classical conditioning. Classical conditioning (in essence) occurs when a stimulus (event or situation) triggers anxiety because it has previously been associated with another threatening stimulus and negative response.

Behaviourists would be most concerned with the circumstance in which the anxiety occurs – the antecedent (A), the behaviour itself (B) and the consequence (C), and not David's thoughts and feelings. This is termed as a functional analysis of behaviour. It may also be that David has previously experienced, for argument's sake, a situation in which he gave a presentation and forgot his note cards and felt very embarrassed, which produced anxiety. This experience would have negative consequences for further presentations. This behaviour is brought about by operant conditioning based on the law of effect (Mukherji and Dryden, 2014).

Cognitivist approach

The cognitivist would consider David's situation in terms of his previous experience, like the behaviourist, but would want to know how David interprets the problem and how he has processed the information that causes the anxiety, and why he gets angry with himself. A cognitivist would consider the interpretation as the basis for changing the way David thinks about the problem that causes the anxiety. If the anxiety was such that it became debilitating, David might be offered cognitive behaviour therapy (CBT).

Humanist approach

The humanist would be interested in David's self-esteem (Banyard et al., 2019). How does he perceive his abilities? Does David have a perception of himself as a failure when having to 'speak out' in public? The humanist may consider that David would benefit from client-centred therapy and may refer him to the student counselling service. This would provide David with the opportunity to talk through his fears and to gain insight into what worries him and why. The intended outcome would be that David gains confidence and feels better about himself, and in the future, he would experience far less anxiety when participating in seminars or workshops and speaking out in class.

Psychology and the approaches to therapeutic help vary depending on the theory and can be considered a difficult subject to understand in one chapter. However, the study of human behaviour can be divided in two perspectives: one that deals in absolute scientific reality, learned through experimentation, and the other that appears to be common sense – logical and easily understood – which is socially constructed and can change over time and in different situations and circumstances. The study of human behaviour has, over many years, enabled psychologists to understand how certain psychological problems may arise and how they can be managed. In terms of providing wider health care, the understanding of how people think and why they behave as they do can support paramedics in their care practice and be a valuable resource.

Hopefully, this introductory section of the chapter has given you a taste of the exciting subject of psychology and a thirst for more. Psychology is a core subject for the paramedic, along with sociology, mental health and physiology. However, it can be a difficult subject to follow in terms of its relevance to health care. Psychologists like to debate differing ideas; if you have an interest in psychology, you will join this interesting debate (Banyard et al., 2019).

 **Reflection: points to consider**

Consider the differing approaches. Which do you think makes most sense? Which do you think aligns with your practice best? Challenge the basic assumptions and ask your own questions.

CHILD DEVELOPMENT

The lifespan approach is commonly used in developmental psychology – from conception onwards. This introductory section will consider child development from birth to young adulthood; however, we would advise you to take time to read about the important development that occurs at conception and throughout pregnancy. Development through pregnancy will also have an effect on an infant's postnatal development.

Research can be conducted over different time spans, from a few seconds or minutes of observation to months, years or even an entire lifetime, as with longitudinal research. This is seen in developmental psychology and is vital in terms of understanding what can occur at periods in a child's development. This section of the chapter will first look at the importance of the paramedic understanding child development (developmental psychology). Having previously taught this subject to student paramedics, I (J.W.) am often greeted in the first instance with a query as to why they need this knowledge, therefore I am taking this opportunity to provide an answer, with the intention that this part of the chapter will not be skipped! This chapter will also consider, albeit briefly, atypical development, also referred to as learning disabilities or neurodiversity, to provide the reader with an overview of the diversity of children's development.

WHY IS THIS RELEVANT?

Having considered some of the approaches of psychology earlier in the chapter, you could ask, 'How will the theory link to my practice?' The answer is that you may, for a short, yet extremely valuable period of time, be caring for children and their family members. In that time, your knowledge of human behavioural theories and approaches to intervention as to how a child develops and what constitutes atypical development will likely be essential.

Reflection: points to consider

Before reading further, note down why you think it is important for you to have an understanding of child development?

Below, we outline why knowledge of child development is of paramount importance. If you have an awareness of normative child development, you will be in a better position to do the following:

- Understand why children and families behave the way that they do.
- Have an awareness of what to expect in terms of the child's language, in an appropriate manner, in accordance with a range of expected development, which will aid communication in order to obtain accurate information regarding the child's health needs.
- Make a more accurate assessment regarding learning needs, special needs, disability, pain and so on. Only the child can tell you how they feel (if able to express it, aiding accuracy of assessment).

- Help the carer describe what they have seen or heard.
- Observe the child's behaviour and social interaction with their carer. This can be extremely valuable information, especially if non-accidental injury is a concern.
- Identify inappropriate extreme or adverse behaviour for the expected range of development of the child and be able to inform the professional of your worries when handing over the child's care (Mukherji and Dryden, 2014).
- Use evidence-based knowledge from differing perspectives of child development, including psychosocial influences when caring for the child.
- Be aware of children's rights (Jones and Welch, 2018).
- Inform emergency department staff and other healthcare professionals of concerns, in order that the child can be followed up appropriately, safeguarding the child at all times.
- Be able to complete appropriately, and with child development knowledge, the patient report form and, if necessary, the safeguarding children report form.

Reflection: points to consider

Review your last call out to a child of any age.

- Were you confident communicating with the child?
- Was your knowledge of the stage and range of development expected for their age clear to you?
- How well did you do with assessment?
- Could it have been improved? If so, how?

THEORIES OF DEVELOPMENT

Attachment theory

Most infants' early learning is in social development. There are two main aspects of this early learning that are very important: sociability and attachment. As a paramedic, you will observe relationships between child and carer and you may well try to administer care to the infant/child. You may experience a crying child, clinging to its carer and trying to get away from you; this could be due to what is termed 'stranger awareness'. The child may instinctually cling to the secure person when in fear. This usually occurs around the age of 4–6 months when the child develops object permanence (Gale, 2015c; Bradford, 2021).

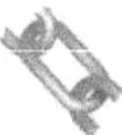

Piaget's sensori-motor stage of development is discussed later in this chapter.

At this stage, the child knows the difference between a familiar face and that of a stranger; this highlights that the child's cognitive development and social development is taking place. At approximately 6–10 months, most children will try to cling on to their carer if a secure attachment has developed. When you try to remove them for a short while, they will cry out, but will stop crying and smile almost as soon as you pass them back to their familiar carer. There has been much research on attachment theory and you might like to read Mary Ainsworth on infant–mother attachment, where she discusses what she termed 'strange situations' and differing attachment behaviours (Gale, 2015c).

John Bowlby (1907–1990) was a child psychiatrist and Freudian-trained psychoanalyst, and one of the first theorists to describe the importance of attachment in human development. His interest in the study of animal behaviour led to his theory that human children, like young animals, have a need for a figure that provides a source of safety, comfort and protection (Gale, 2015c).

Bowlby (1979) identified the 'critical period' and argued that although the main attachment of an infant is usually to its mother, strong bonds occur with significant others with whom the infant has regular contact. If as a paramedic, it is essential you administer treatment to a child, it would always be better (if possible) for you to have the person to whom the child is attached to help you; this may make the administering of care a lot easier. Look up the work of Bowlby to improve your knowledge of attachment theory, in particular attachment styles and behaviours (Krumwiede, 2014).

Reflection: points to consider

Consider the relationships between parent and child that you have cared for. Have they always been warm and caring? As a paramedic, you are in a prime position to notice the interaction between the child and carer and it is important that you report anything that is untoward or inappropriate when you hand over the care of the child. You will note that not all attachment is positive.

According to Bowlby, in the first three years of life, bonding must occur. In contrast, Ainsworth (1979) found that the relationship between mother and baby develops over time, rather than being fixed shortly after birth. In reality, not all infants and children are parented sensitively or responsively. As a paramedic, you will observe many different/diverse parenting skills. Deprivation can lead to long-term difficulties when it occurs due to problems with social relationships, more than from ill health. Bowlby (1979) argued that the adverse effects of maternal deprivation are usually irreversible. Cultural differences in parenting practices reflect differences in terms of adults' cultural expectations and values. Parental acceptance and rejection can vary in different cultures but, in the main, rejection is generally associated with poor outcomes in children, including low self-esteem, delinquency and limited educational attainment. However, it is incumbent upon me to say that most infants in most cultures have a secure attachment, and as a paramedic, you will most often see positive attachment between child and carer throughout your daily practice. Case study 7.2 encourages you to relate your learning to a practical example.

Case study 7.2

You are tasked to attend a 999 call for a 2-year-old who has been hot and unwell for three days and has a rash. On first assessment, the child is alert, appears to be breathing normally, is well perfused and has a widespread blotchy rash on the visible areas of her arms and legs. However, the child is very clingy to her mother and makes it quite clear she does not want to be examined. Consider the following:

- What are the necessary assessments and investigations you must undertake?
- How can you balance distressing the child against your professional duty of care?
- How does the child's developmental stage influence your plan of care?
- To what extent is observing the behaviour and interactions between the carer and child important for your assessment and why?

Psychoanalytical and learning theory

Grand theories are comprehensive theories that have inspired and directed thinking about development over decades, but are no longer considered as influential as they once were.

During the first half of the twentieth century, two opposing grand theories dominated the child development 'scene':

1. Psychoanalytic theory in two strands: psycho-sexual = Freud, and psychosocial = Erikson.
2. Learning theory (behaviourism) = Thorndike/Watson/Skinner/Pavlov/Harlow.

These began as psychological theories and later were applied to human developmental psychology theories more broadly. A fundamental assumption of psychoanalytic theory is that development over the lifespan is determined during early childhood.

Psycho-sexual theory

Freud was interested in the role of unconscious mental processes and inner forces (id, ego and superego) that he considered influenced people's behaviour. Freud argued that urges are gratified by three parts of personality, through stages of development which reflect erogenous zones (see Table 7.1). These underlying forces (id, ego and superego) and urges influence people's thinking and behaviour, from the smallest decisions to crucial life changes. (Storr, 2001).

Drives and motive provide foundations for universal stages of development in human experience. A critique of this theory of development is that it is one-sided, with an emphasis on sexuality as the dynamic factor in development. Theorists from other approaches acknowledge Freud's thinking even though it is considered empirically weak, as mentioned earlier in the chapter. An important example of radical reformulation of psycho-sexual development theory is Erikson's psychosocial theory.

Psychosocial theory

Erik Erikson (1902–1994) was a Jewish German developmental psychologist who coined the phrase 'identity crisis'. He was one of Freud's followers

---

Table 7.1 Freud's stages of psycho-sexual development

Stage	Average age	Development
Oral	0–18 months	Eating and sucking provides satisfaction
Anal	18–36 months	Anal area is interesting and satisfying
Phallic	3–5 years	Satisfaction from the genitals
Latency	6 years to puberty	Boys and girls spend little time together
Genital	Onset of puberty	Main pleasure from genitals

who accepted some of Freud's theory and expanded it to consider people's lifestyle and culture.

Erikson acknowledged the importance of the unconscious; he agreed that unresolved childhood conflicts at certain stages affect adulthood, but expanded and modified Freud's ideas. Erikson proposed eight developmental stages, each characterised by a particular challenge or developmental crisis, which is central to that stage of life. He placed the emphasis on a person's relationship to their family and culture, not just sexual urges.

Erikson's stages are as follows:

1. Trust vs. mistrust (birth to 1 year): babies learn either to trust that others will care for their basic needs, including nourishment, warmth, cleanliness and physical contact, or will lack confidence in the care given by others.
2. Autonomy vs. shame and doubt (1 year to 3 years): children learn either to be self-sufficient in many activities, including toileting, feeding, walking, exploring and talking, or they may doubt their own abilities.
3. Initiative vs. guilt (3 years to 6 years): children want to undertake many adult-like activities, sometimes overstepping the limits set by parents; this can lead to the child feeling guilty, thus resulting in poor self-esteem.

 **Reflection: points to consider**

As a paramedic, you will identify stages 2 and 3 in terms of children who have attempted something that may well have been out of their stage or range of development, which results in an accident.

4. Industry vs. inferiority (6 years to 11 years): children either learn to be competent and productive in mastering new skills, or instead feel inferior and unable to do anything well, thus leading to the potential for child and adolescent mental health issues (e.g. depression).
5. Identity vs. role confusion (adolescence): adolescents try to figure out who they are. They establish sexual, political and career identities or may be confused about what roles to play. Identity crises can create storm and stress for the young person. Sociological theory suggests that changes within social roles cause conflicts,

   e.g. girlfriend and daughter, schoolgirl and work experience. In addition, the mass media and peers can create conflicting values at this age. It can be a very difficult time for the young person going through this stage of development.

6. Intimacy vs. isolation (early adulthood): at this age, people are working on establishing intimate ties with others; however, if they have experienced earlier attachment problems, some young adults cannot form close relationships and remain isolated.

7. Generativity vs. stagnation (middle adulthood): this stage involves giving to and guiding the next generation through childrearing, caring for others and reproduction. If a person cannot achieve this, they may experience an absence of meaningful accomplishment.

8. Ego integrity vs. despair (late adulthood): this is the final stage where people reflect on the kind of person they have been and have become. Integrity comes from feeling that life is worth living. However, older people who are not happy with their life fear death (Berger, 2021).

Learning theory (behaviourism)

Learning theory holds the view that all development involves a change in an individual. It avoids reference to the unconscious which cannot be observed. Behaviourism and the law of learning theory are based on the premise that learning can be explained by the forming of associations. Learning involves a *stimulus* (action which elicits a response) and *response* (instinct or learned action in response to the stimulus) through *conditioning*. There are two types of conditioning associated with behaviourism: classical conditioning and operant conditioning.

- **Classical conditioning:** John Watson (1876–1958) was opposed to Freud and Erikson's ideas on development and offered a new type of psychology. He argued that psychologists should study only what they could see and measure, not the unconscious. According to Watson, anything could be learned; in the right environment, he could train anyone to be anything regardless of talents, tendencies, abilities, vocations and cultures. He argued that the study of actual behaviour is objective and far less difficult than the study of unconscious motives and drives. Watson extended Pavlov's research with dogs and showed that classical conditioning also occurred in humans (Whitnell and Preston, 2019).

- **Operant conditioning:** This conditioning occurs when behaviour produces a consequence. The principle is that the consequence (effect) of behaviour will determine how likely it is to re-occur; for example, if the consequence of a behaviour is useful/pleasure/relieving (a positive reinforcement, such as medication), a child will take the medication again, when instructed, to achieve that same consequence (effect). Conditioning is used quite widely in the behaviour management of children and in managing people who suffer with phobias.

Reflection: points to consider

If a child experiences an asthmatic attack and is given a nebuliser, which makes the child feel much better and less scared, the child will be happy to use it again. Reinforcement and reward are very useful when managing a child who is scared; learning theory used in practice can be very useful. The child using the nebuliser has learned that the response to her difficult breathing comes from the positive reward = operant conditioning.

Social learning theory

Conditioning does not adequately explain where new behaviour comes from; social learning theory may help to explain this. This approach argues that not all learning has occurred from the child's experience of direct classical or operant conditioning (behaviourism). Children learn to behave in ways that are rewarding and avoid ways that are punished by others. Social learning theory, a more recent approach, accepts that children learn from reinforcement and punishment but also suggests that they learn by observing, imitating and modelling others. Modelling occurs when the observer is uncertain or inexperienced and models themselves on a more senior, admired or powerful role model (Bandura, 1977).

Reflection: points to consider

If a child needs medication or a plaster, for example, you could consider this theory to aid administration. You could use modelling in terms of pretending to give the medication to the child's doll or teddy or put the plaster/bandage on the doll or teddy. Upon seeing this and with the intention of modelling the behaviour, the child may have more confidence in your care.

Cognitive theory

Jean Piaget (1896–1980) was a biologist and zoologist from Switzerland. Piaget's basic idea was that it is more useful to understand how a child stores and uses information than how much knowledge and intellect a child has.

His work covered three main areas:

- how the senses take in information about things around us;
- how the brain processes and stores information;
- how the subsequent behaviour changes as a result of stored information = cognitive theory of development.

Piaget was a very influential and extraordinary intellectual leader/researcher who fashioned the framework of cognitive theory. Piaget argued that development does not occur through what has been forgotten (Freud and Erikson's ideas) or what has been learned (Pavlov and Skinner's ideas), but from what and how children think and understand at different ages and stages.

Piaget argued that children develop in stages. There are four age-related stages of development in which changes take place: (1) sensorimotor, (2) pre-operational, (3) concrete operational and (4) formal operational. The first – the sensorimotor stage – is the most dynamic in a child's life. Let us now look at these stages in turn.

Sensorimotor stage, 0–2 years

Most changes take place during this stage, from simple physical reflexes to beginning to symbolise. Initially, an infant's interactions are basic and reflexive, they are unconscious but forming neural connections of understanding. After a very short time, however, the baby will learn to use some muscles and limbs for movement and will begin to understand some information received through the senses (Sharma and Cockerill, 2014).

Reflection: points to consider

What are the senses? Jot them down and consider why they are important.

The first ideas babies develop are around how to deal with their world; these are called 'action schemas' (constructing representations of events, people and relationships from the real physical world). Babies are totally egocentric; they are unable to take anyone else's needs or interests into account. They start to develop fine and gross motor skills, become social beings and develop language (for detail on the development of these skills over the first weeks, months and early years, see Sharma and Cockerill, 2014). Infants learn about objects and what they can be made to do. Some intellectual behaviour occurs; for example, they will hold a rattle and shake it, then throw it and watch what happens to it. Objects start to have meaning and babies/infants begin to do more with them. This is the time when object permanence occurs.

Pre-operational stage, 2–7 years

Operations at this stage will require combining schemas in an orderly, sensible and logical way, although at this stage, they will be somewhat limited. The child's vocabulary and imagination are expanding at 2 years, seen in the use of words in play such as 'house', 'mummy', 'car', 'bird', 'dog', 'cat' and so on, although they may not be heard clearly. At the beginning of this stage, the child understands much of what is being said to them but can find it difficult to express themselves, which results in frustration. Vast differences in development can be seen from 2 years to 7 years. See case study 7.3 for a practical example of cognitive development, where you can assess your own understanding

During this stage, the child begins to use:

- **Symbolism:** children's thought processes are developing; they are starting to make sense of their world and make use of symbolisation – for instance, a thumbs-up symbol for agreement/happiness.
- **Egocentrism:** children generally see things from their own point of view.

 **Reflection: points to consider**

You could use a doll or teddy to aid you when caring for a child at age 2–7 years. Not all children at this stage are egotistical; if the task is simple, the child may be able to see it from others' perspectives depending on where the child is in this stage of development.

- **Animism:** the child holds the belief that everything that exists has some kind of consciousness, relative to their own feelings and world view. For example, if the car won't start, the car is tired; if the child is hurt in a collision with a chair, they will blame the 'naughty chair'.

- **Moral realism:** towards the later stage, the child thinks that their way of thinking about what is right and wrong will be shared by everyone else. They will have respect for rules. The use of moral realism may well help you to administer treatment, if you explain that the treatment is essential.

Case study 7.3

You are called to a 5-year-old boy who has developed paraphimosis (a painful and retractile foreskin which constitutes a medical emergency). Considering different theories and stages of the boy's development, what conclusions might you reach on the nature of this condition being idiopathic, self-inflicted or symptomatic of abuse? What would be your plan of care?

Concrete operational stage, 7–11 years

At this stage, you will experience a child with more rational and adult-like thinking. There is more logical reasoning and grasp of the idea that illness and death have biological causes. At this stage, the child recognises their own mortality. This is an easier stage in the child's life, where you can explain what has happened and what you are going to do about it.

Children can think logically, if they can manipulate the actual object that they are thinking about. At this stage, the child learns that objects are not always what they appear, for example, conservation, number, volume, length and mass.

Formal operational stage, 11–16 years

At this stage, children can manipulate their own thoughts, and do not need the real object at hand. Around puberty, the ways in which children think change again. They work things out in their heads, without seeing the object; they think more abstractly, consider a range of societal issues and can take others' reasons for behaviour into account. However, not all young people, or indeed some adults, can do this, as they may not have developed to this stage cognitively.

Contemporary thinking on child development tends to lean towards ranges of development as opposed to stages (Berger, 2021). Children develop different skills at differing times. Each child is unique!

Table 7.2 highlights the areas of development according to the main domains: biosocial, cognitive and psychosocial.

Table 7.2 Domains of development

Biological	Cognitive	Psychosocial
Genes	Perception	Temperament
Hormones	Memory	Family
Information processing	Imagination	Culture
Motor skills	Learning	Values
Fine motor skills	Thinking	Beliefs
	Decision-making	School
	Hearing and speech	Socialisation and play
		Significant others

 **Reflection: points to consider**

Jot down from memory what is expected in terms of physical gross and fine motor skills according to the ages and stages of child development, from birth to 5 years. It would be valuable for paramedics and other health professionals who encounter children to understand the range of 'normal' development milestones to aid assessment of children. See the useful text entitled *Child Development: A Practical Introduction* (Crowley, 2017), which breaks down the stages and ranges of development in detail.

Piaget was criticised by social constructivists for his underestimation of the role of social and cultural factors in knowledge development, hence the emergence of the sociocultural theory of development (Vygotsky, 1962).

Sociocultural theory

Lev Vygotsky (1896–1934) was one of the most important Russian psychologists of the twentieth century. He is famous for research into the development and structure of human consciousness, and the theory of signs, which explains the way children internalise language in the course of their social and cultural development.

The sociocultural theory is relatively new when compared with the grand theories of development. Vygotsky argued that development results in a dynamic interaction between child/learner and people, surroundings and culture (normally parents, teachers, peers) that provides instruction and support to the

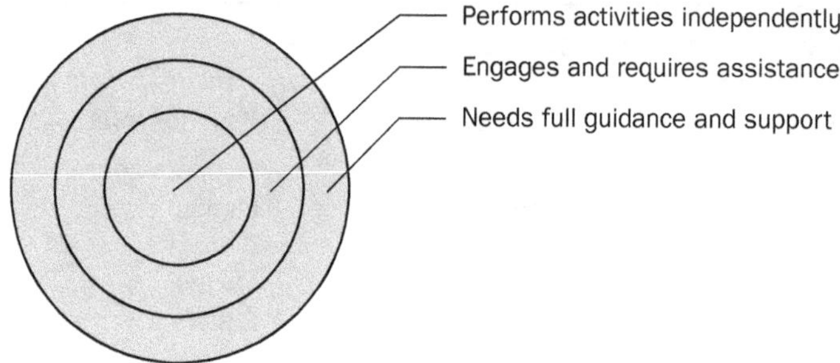

Figure 7.2   Process of proximal development

Source: Based on Vygotsky's Zone of Proximal Development.

child in order that they can acquire knowledge and capabilities. This theory considers the importance of social factors; children are apprentices in thinking. The concepts of 'scaffolding' and 'guided participation' in acts of everyday life are important for children to draw on. This is acquired through the child learning from experienced members of a social group. Vygotsky developed the concept of the Zone of Proximal Development (ZPD), shown in Figure 7.2.

Figure 7.2 highlights the process a child goes through, in terms of learning. The child moves through the learning process from the outer zone (being totally dependent and supported) through the middle zone (being facilitated) to the inner zone where the child becomes fully independent.

Vygotsky (1962) also emphasised the importance of language as a learning tool for children and language being valuable in terms of communicating feelings. He argued that inner speech is a form of language spoken to oneself; for instance, in an examination, a student could use inner speech to talk through the answer to a question before beginning writing.

This chapter has provided the reader with an understanding of children's development. It will be apparent that there are not only different theoretical approaches to child development but also different stages/ranges at which the child develops. Below are examples of two situations that can be related to children of different ages, in terms of practical care.

PSYCHOLOGICAL APPROACHES LINKED TO PRACTICE

When caring for children at different ages and stages of development, there will be differing ways to approach the child in order that you can care appropriately. The age and stage examples below provide a guide to the range of development, bearing in mind that each child is unique.

Below, we highlight the different ways in which you may care for a child with breathing difficulties who is in need of an oxygen mask, and make the link between a developmental theory and the management:

- At 6–9 months of age, you may show the child what the mask looks like on a teddy or doll before attempting to use it on the child so that they allow you to care for them. A child will copy/mimic behaviour if it appears to be 'okay'. This aligns to modelling behaviour within social learning theory.
- At 5 years of age, the child grasps and understands that illness has a biological cause and that they need help, but may be assertive and refuse. It is necessary to explain to a child of this age the importance of the mask and the reasoning behind its use in quite simple terms. The child may want to take control of the mask. This situation in terms of development aligns with cognitive theory; this child is likely to be at the pre-operational stage of development. This child's efforts to act independently can lead to pride or failure. At this age, the child is at the initiative vs. guilt stage within psychosocial theory.
- At 12 years of age, this child would be within the formal operational stage of cognitive development. Their thinking is more refined and they can comprehend more immediate risks, and will accept help and try to understand why they require the oxygen via a mask to make their breathing easier.

Below, we highlight the different ways in which you may care for a child who is experiencing pain at different ages while considering the theories of development:

- At 2 years of age, the child may cry out 'it hurts' or 'sore' and possibly hold the painful area while crying. At this age, the child is unlikely to communicate clearly verbally. You will need this child's comforter to help settle them if possible. This child will be 'stranger aware' and cling to the carer; you may need to administer the treatment to the child in the carer's arms. This child is at the end of the sensorimotor stage according to Piaget, and has become attached to the carer.
- At 5 years of age, the child will show you where the pain is on their body by pointing to the area that hurts. The child will be able to point at a pain chart of images/faces to gauge the amount of pain they are experiencing; they may also be able to show you on the teddy or doll where the pain is. According to the cognitive

pre-operational stage of development, this child may have a cognitive understanding of moral realism.

- At 11 years, the child will be able to rate on a scale of 1–10 how bad it is. Pain experience can be mediated by sociocultural factors (e.g. verbal/non-verbal cues given by the carer). However, it is imperative that as a paramedic, you always believe what the child says until the child is investigated. If the child has been rewarded for their behaviour previously, they may have learned to behave in this way. The theory behind this idea comes from positive reinforcement/operant conditioning. This child may have experienced pain in the past and had a positive outcome after being medicated, in which case the child may be happy to accept pain relief; this situation links with the theory on classical conditioning.

ATYPICAL DEVELOPMENT

As a paramedic, you are likely to care for and transport children with special needs or neurodiversity. As this is an introductory text, this chapter includes limited discussion of emotional, behavioural and social problems, and learning disabilities that children can experience. Therefore, the section will include an example of disorders that lead to atypical development such as attention deficit hyperactive disorder (ADHD) and autistic spectrum disorder, and an example of Down's syndrome. It is important that you understand the diversity of children's development in order that you care for them appropriately. In the first instance, it is important to highlight that children with learning disabilities should be considered as children in the first instance, with needs and rights similar to those of any other child. Their disability and care needs are secondary. They will have other special needs but the understanding and management of those needs (albeit in some instances challenging) will affect the outcome. There are many difficulties that all children can face, and it is important that paramedics are aware of the potential additional risk of harm to children with learning disabilities and the need to protect them and consider their rights as with other children (Jones and Welch, 2018). We hope that this section will offer 'food for thought' and that you will be interested enough to search for further information on children with atypical development by way of self-directed learning.

The study of developmental psychopathology is thought of as a relationship between psychology and the study of childhood disorders. A range of functions will be considered when assessing a child's development, including biological, genetic, sociocultural and cognitive. Psychologists generally assume a continuum of behaviour, with the child's behaviour somewhere along it (Comer and Comer, 2021). There are a number of factors that may contribute to, or result in, learning disabilities. The preconceptual, prenatal, perinatal and postnatal periods are distinct periods, before and during pregnancy and after birth, when learning disabilities can occur, as these are the times when possible causative factors are in operation. These factors are either hereditary or environmental:

- **Heredity:** the gene is a discrete segment of the chromosome and the basic unit for the transition of heredity instructions, e.g. hair and eye colour traits. The chromosome is the carrier of genes. An example of chromosomal abnormality is Down's syndrome; see the section on Down's syndrome in this chapter for further details.
- **Environment:** during and after pregnancy – toxic agents, birth trauma, oxygen starvation, nutrition.

How do professionals diagnose children with atypical development? How do they know when normal behaviour ends and developmental psychopathology begins? Children differ considerably in their rate of development, and it makes sense to continue to think in terms of the stages of development that most children go through at around the same ages. However, these stages are less relevant to those children who, for a number of reasons, are not developing as per the 'normal' age and stage/range.

There are many ways of determining whether someone has a learning disability; however, no one criterion will provide a definitive answer. Over time, psychiatrists and researchers have highlighted the confusion of diagnosis and the use of different tools. Defining learning disability is difficult as it means different things to different people. Generally, it is agreed that learning disability comprises sub-average intellectual functioning that co-exists with below-average social functioning that manifests before the age of 18 years (Atherton and Crickmore, 2022).

Children with learning disability fall into three main areas and can be assessed using differing diagnostic tools:

1. Intellectual ability (Intelligent Quotient = IQ) (APA, 2022); Child Behaviour Checklist (Achenbach, 2013); DSM-5 (APA, 2022) and ICD-11 (WHO, 2022);
2. Legislative definitions: Mental Health Acts (Legislation.gov.uk, 1983, 2007);
3. Social competence criterion.

Children who have a learning disability will have an IQ that is below the average IQ of 100. IQ is useful only up to the age of 18 years. IQ within the population is evenly distributed, therefore it is possible to measure how far an individual is from what is considered 'normal'. Using this system, a child who has an IQ of less than 70 is said to have a learning disability (scores more than two standard deviations (SD) from the average of 100; score of 15 = 1 SD).

- 70–84 = borderline of intellectual functioning;
- 50–69 = mild learning disability (25–30 people in UK per 1000 population);
- 35–49 = moderate learning disability;
- 20–34 = severe mental retardation (3–4 people in UK per 1000 population);
- <20 = profound mental retardation (people with complex additional disabilities, e.g. sensory, physical or behavioural).

(adapted from NICE, 2015)

In legislative terms, children who have physical and sensory impairment – for example, who are blind or deaf or suffer from cerebral palsy – are considered to have a learning disability (Legislation.gov.uk, 2007).

Children with emotional and behavioural problems, such as autistic spectrum disorders (including Asperger's disorder) and attention deficit hyperactivity disorder (ADHD), are likely to have impaired social functioning and may be assessed using the social competence criterion (Wilmshurst, 2022).

Diagnostic tools

An example of a diagnostic tool is given in Box 7.1.

Box 7.1 Diagnostic Statistical Manual of Mental Disorders (DSM-5-TR)

DSM-5-TR uses categories to classify behaviour, signs and symptoms logged to enable diagnosis. DSM-5 is not concerned with classification, more with the behaviour expressed; suggesting this helps to remove the negative stigma of labelling which only leads to derogation and uninformed understanding.

Critique: DSM-5-TR considers developmental issues but does not consider changes in children over time. Disorders can occur as a function of age and change at different ages, e.g. ADHD = in young child; more hyperactivity than in older child (APA, 2022).

Another useful diagnostic tool is shown in Box 7.2.

Box 7.2 Child Behaviour Checklist (CBCL)

The Child Behaviour Checklist (CBCL) is a component of the Achenbach System of Empirically Based Assessment (ASEBA). The CBCL is dimensional and provides information about the way and how much the individual shows disturbance. Deviation is viewed as continuous from normal (continuum). It allows for changing behaviour. The CBCL looks at internal and external scales. Internal disorders include anxiety and depression; external disorders involve 'acting out' a form of distress, including aggression and delinquency. Children can show both, e.g. be sulky and aggressive at the same time.

Critique: CBCL does not include some major disorders, e.g. autism and eating disorders, which DSM-5-TR includes (Achenbach, 2013).

It can often be difficult to confirm a diagnosis of behaviour because co-morbidity (where two different conditions are present in one child) may be present. For some children with learning disabilities, a precise diagnosis is not possible and a more comprehensive, multi-agency assessment of the child's needs is required. This is obtained using the Early help assessment tool (NSPCC, 2023). This assessment includes parents' need for support with caring for the child.

CHILDHOOD DISORDERS

This section will consider a small sample of childhood disorders that children experience that will bring into being learning disabilities of one form or another; during your working practice, it is very likely you will care for children with developmental disorders or who may have experienced some form of trauma in their life.

Attention deficit hyperactivity disorder (ADHD)

The signs and symptoms of ADHD include:

- unable to sit still for any length of time (pattern of restlessness/overactivity);
- loses things;
- cannot concentrate on tasks, even fun tasks;
- easily distracted;

- doesn't appear to listen (inattentive);
- much energy, fidgets, runs, climbs, talks incessantly;
- shows anti-social behaviour (impulsive, always late, angry);
- interrupts conversation.

(adapted from APA, 2022)

ADHD is an externalising form of maladjustment. The name of this disorder highlights the issues that arise. It involves the ongoing presence of inattention and hyperactivity with impulsiveness, all of which are beyond the norm and are more frequent and severe. In true ADHD, symptoms are evident in children younger than seven years of age and the behaviour occurs at school and at home.

Case study 7.4

You are called to a 14-year-old child who has punched a brick wall and has suspected fractures to the fingers and hand. The child is both aggressive and uncooperative and finds it difficult to articulate how they feel. A carer introduces herself and explains that the child has ADHD. Consider how you would assess and treat this young child.

It is difficult to diagnose ADHD in toddlers, as at this age, you would expect inattention, but it can be detected if extreme, frequent and chronic. It is easier to detect in middle childhood, as one would expect a child to have more control in their activities, be socially competent and be able to concentrate for a period of time. These children can show antisocial behaviour in adolescence and young adulthood; consequently, this disorder may go hand in hand with conduct disorder (co-morbidity). Case study 7.4 highlights an example of such behaviour. Conduct disorder is defined as 'a repetitive and persistent pattern of behaviour in which the basic rights of others or major age-appropriate societal norms or rules are violated' (APA, 2022). Indeed, co-occurrence of conduct disorder and ADHD and their symptoms is so strong that researchers have questioned whether they are separate disorders.

Autism

Autism lies at the extreme end of the autistic spectrum and is characterised by a triad of social communication difficulties. Vygotsky (1962) stated that language, thoughts and social interaction are inextricably linked by around 2 years of age. Consequently, this disorder may not be detected in infancy. These children have impaired communication and socialisation, and restricted and repetitive interests, movements and activities. The factors suggested for this disorder are prenatal (genetics/uterine environment, brain structure and function), perinatal (birth trauma) and postnatal (vaccination = MMR, food intolerance) (Boucher, 2022).

The signs and symptoms of ADHD include:

- deficits in sociability and empathy;
- deficits in communicative language;
- deficits in cognitive flexibility;
- delayed speech development;
- restricted, repetitive and stereotyped patterns of behaviour, interests and activities;
- detectable before the age of 3 years;
- 70 per cent of children have an IQ < 70.

Asperger's syndrome

The signs and symptoms of Asperger's syndrome include:

- poor social skills, lack of insight;
- behavioural inflexibility, narrow range of interests;
- IQ > 70: it is important to note that these children have an IQ that is higher than the criteria for learning disability and indeed can have strengths in verbal areas (Wilmshurst, 2022);
- no delay with speech; often well-developed vocabulary basis but deficit in communication at a social level;
- visual motor clumsiness with typical stiff gait and posture.

The word 'autism' was first used by the Boston physician Leo Kanner in 1943. The characteristics that form the triad of social communication of this disorder are:

1. Social interaction – poor eye contact and use of gestures and facial expressions. These children have no interest in others or joining in. They cannot understand the effect of their behaviour on others and have no insight into their own or others' behaviour.
2. Communication – there is delay in speech. These children misinterpret sarcasm, jokes and non-verbal cues. They also take things literally.
3. These children have restrictive, repetitive patterns of behaviour, interests and activities. They are excessive in rituals and routines and have unusual interests. These children can be prone to self-injury, e.g. head banging or biting.

There is another form called pervasive developmental disorder (PDD) that is not otherwise specified. PDD applies to less severely affected children who do not meet the criteria for either autism or Asperger's syndrome (APA, 2022).

Autism can be co-morbid with:

- a learning disability;
- epilepsy;
- speech and language difficulties;
- ADHD;
- dyspraxia (motor coordination problems);
- tics and Tourette's syndrome;
- feeding and eating difficulties (refusal, hoarding, overeating) (www.nas.org.uk).

Parents are usually the first to note that their child's development is unusual and are relieved to know there is a reason/diagnosis. However, it should not be underestimated that raising a child with autistic spectrum disorder (like other disorders) can cause considerable stress. Three things are particularly stressful to parents and child alike: (1) a societal lack of understanding (stigma and challenging behaviour); (2) poor service provision (pre-school and school provision); and (3) the permanency of the condition (relationships and work). However, an emerging political movement of autistic people is gaining media attention in the hope that society will alter its attitudes towards autistic spectrum disorder (Atherton and Crickmore, 2022).

Prior to the inclusion of Asperger's disorder in the DSM, there was considerable controversy regarding differential diagnoses among disorders and syndromes that share common features, such as autism, Asperger's syndrome and semantic pragmatic disorder. Even though these disorders now sit within a spectrum of pervasive developmental disorders, it remains difficult to distinguish between Asperger's and 'high-functioning autism' (Wilmshurst, 2022).

Down's syndrome

British physician John Langdon Down (1828–1896) first described the abnormality of chromosome 21 in 1866, hence the name Down's syndrome. It is the most common chromosomal disorder leading to a learning disability (Atherton and Crickmore, 2022). Definitive diagnosis is available by obtaining a small sample of cells from the tissue of the placenta from the pregnant woman, called chorionic villous sampling by amniocentesis.

There are three types of chromosomal abnormality resulting in Down's syndrome:

- **Trisomy 21:** accounts for 94 per cent of people with Down's syndrome. The individual has three instead of two copies of chromosome 21.
- **Translocation:** the individual has two normal copies of chromosome 21 and a third fused with another chromosome (either chromosome 15 or 13).
- **Mosaicism:** this condition is extremely rare and involves the individual having cells with two copies of chromosome 21 *as well as* cells with three copies of chromosome 21.

The signs and symptoms of Down's syndrome include (Comer and Comer, 2021; Atherton and Crickmore, 2022):

- IQ between 35 and 49 (level of intellectual impairment differs in individuals);
- may have difficulty with pronunciation due to protruding tongue and intellectual disability;
- may develop slower than expected range of development;
- the child will age quickly so may look older than his or her biological age;
- may develop dementia in older age (40–50) due to genes of dementia being located close to each other on chromosome 21 (ongoing research);
- facial features = small head, flattened facial appearance, high cheekbones, hair is dry and sparse;
- congenital heart disease affects around 40 per cent of individuals;
- thyroid disease occurs in about 20 per cent of individuals.

A useful website is: www.downs-syndrome.org.uk. Many different characteristics are associated with Down's syndrome, but it should be noted that not all children and adults with this condition will exhibit them all.

 **Reflection: points to consider**

As a paramedic, you are in a prime position to notice differences and atypical behaviour in terms of a child's development. Some things to think about include:

- A child may not be developing according to the age and expected range of development; this is where your knowledge

> of the well child and stages/ranges of development will be very useful.
> - You need to pick up cues from the carer and from the responses that you get from the child when communicating with them. (For ideas on communication, see Chapter 1.)
> - Make sure you collect whatever enables the child to maximise their ability to understand, if possible, and most certainly allow the child to take their comfort, e.g. toy, doll, blanket. Remember that this child may have an 'unusual' interest in an object – for example, the batteries in a toy rather than the toy itself.
> - May become over stimulated in an emergency situation

How to relate to a child/adult with learning disability

Children and adults with learning disability, like the rest of the population, display a range of behaviours. As a paramedic, you will need to use your acute assessment and communication skills in order to establish a rapport and maximise communication with the child/adult/family/carer as soon as possible. This is so that you get the best from them and they trust your professional care. As a paramedic, you will use the clues around you, in terms of the domestic situation and how the carer communicates with the child/adult, to determine how you should communicate with them, in either a child-like or adult-like manner. Children can show challenging behaviour towards you; indeed, this can be a characteristic of a child with learning disability, such as ADHD or autism. You would be wise to seek the assistance of the carer who will know how best to manage the child. In contrast, children with Down's syndrome, for example, are very often known to have a loving nature and publicly demonstrate that love (Whitnell and Preston, 2019).

> ## Reflection: points to consider
>
> While children with Down's syndrome are generally happy and loving and are often keen to express their love (even to strangers), this can be a disadvantage as it can make them vulnerable.

You may be called to a person with a learning disability who lives alone, in a supported community, with carers or with family as back-up support.

Observation of the environment in which the person lives may provide you with clues about how independent they are. If a person with a learning disability lives in a supported community, it is likely that they may have been encouraged with and taught some social and practical skills to enable them to live relatively independently. If, however, a person with a learning disability lives with their family, it may be that they are unable to live independently or have not been given the opportunity to do so.

People with learning disabilities who have been socialised to be more independent may have been taught to curb their affections with strangers. However, in general terms, if a person, especially a child, with a learning disability takes a liking to your personable nature, they will generally cooperate with you in your assessment and possibly even treatment. In contrast, if a child or adult with a learning disability does not want to cooperate, they can be extremely stubborn and possibly obstructive.

CONCLUSION

We hope that we have provided a taste of what psychology and child development cover. In order for the paramedic to assess and treat patients accurately and effectively, it is important to have knowledge and understanding of why children and families behave in the way that they do.

In addition to providing you with information on the many approaches to psychology and child development theory, this chapter also considered atypical development to provide you with an overview of the diversity of children and young adults and their needs. There are many positive changes that have occurred in the care of children and adults with learning disabilities. However, change needs to continue if this group is to be included, valued and afforded an equal status in society.

Chapter key points:

- Paramedics require an understanding of psychology and child development theory in order to care holistically for patients/clients and their families.
- An understanding of the work of the key child development theorists will help you understand more about the development and behaviour of clients requiring your care and treatment.
- In addition to 'normal' development, paramedics also require an understanding of atypical development and neurodiversity, in order to provide holistic care to the patient.

REFERENCES AND SUGGESTED READING

Achenbach, T.M. (2013) *Assess Adaptive and Maladaptive Functioning: Achenbach System of Empirically Based Assessment (ASEBA)*. London: Harcourt Press.

Ainsworth, M.D.S. (1979) Infant-mother attachment, *American Psychologist*, 34 (10): 932–37.

American Psychiatric Association (APA) (2022) *Diagnostic and Statistical Manual of Mental Disorders*, DSM-5-TR, 5th edition, text revision. Philadelphia, PA: APA. Available at: www.dsm.psychiatryonline.org/doi/book/10.1176/appi.books.9780890425596 (accessed 9 April 2024).

Atherton, H. and Crickmore, D. (2022) *Intellectual Disabilities: Toward Inclusion*, 7th edition. London: Elsevier.

Bandura, A. (1977) *Social Learning Theory*. London: Prentice-Hall.

Banyard, P., Davies, M.N.O., Norman, C. and Winder, B. (2019) *Essential Psychology: A Concise Introduction*, 3rd edition. London: Sage.

Berger, K.S. (2021) *The Developing Person through Childhood and Adolescence*, 12th edition. New York: Worth Publishers.

Boucher, J. (2022) *Autism Spectrum Disorders: Characteristics, Causes and Practical Issues*, 3rd edition. London: Sage.

Bowlby, J. (1979) *Attachment and Loss*, vol. 1. Harmondsworth: Penguin.

Bradford, H. (2021) *The Wellbeing of Children Under Three*. London: Routledge.

Comer, R.J. and Comer, J.S. (2021) *Abnormal Psychology*, 11th edition. New York: Worth Publishers.

Crowley, K. (2017) *Child Development: A Practical Introduction*. London: Sage.

Department for Education (DfE) (2023) *Working together to safeguard children: A guide to multi-agency working to help, protect and promote the welfare of children.* London: TSO. Available at: https://assets.publishing.service.gov.uk/media/65cb4349a7ded0000c79e4e1/Working_together_to_safeguard_children_2023_-_statutory_guidance.pdf.

Dogra, N., Parkin, A., Gale, F. and Frake, C. (2009) *A Multidisciplinary Handbook of Child and Adolescent Mental Health for Front-Line Professionals*, 2nd edition. London: Jessica Kingsley.

Frost, N., Abbott, S. and Race, T. (2015) *Family Support: Prevention, Early Intervention and Early Help*. Cambridge: Polity Press.

Gale (2015a) *A study guide for psychologists and their theories for students: Albert Bandura*. Farmington Hills, MI: Gale Cengage Learning.

Gale (2015b) *A study guide for psychologists and their theories for students: Jean Piaget*. Farmington Hills, MI: Gale Cengage Learning.

Gale (2015c) *A study guide for psychologists and their theories for students: Mary Salter Ainsworth*. Farmington Hills, MI: Gale Cengage Learning.

Gates, B. (2011) *Learning Disabilities: Towards Inclusion*, 6th edition. London: Churchill Livingstone.

Gerrig., R.J., Zimbardo, P.G., Svartdal, F., Brennen, T. et al. (2013) *Psychology and Life*. Harlow: Pearson Education.

Hayes, C. (2023) *The Early Years Handbook for Students and Practitioners: An Essential Guide*, 2nd edition. London: Routledge.

Jones, P. and Welch, S. (2018) *Rethinking Children's Rights: Attitudes in Contemporary Society*, 2nd edition. London: Continuum.

Kalat, J.H. (2023) *Biological Psychology*, 14th edition. Belmont, CA: Wadsworth.

Krumwiede, A. (2014) *Attachment Theory According to John Bowlby and Mary Ainsworth*. Munich: GRIN Verlag.

Legislation.gov.uk (1983) *Mental Health Act 1983*. Available at: https://www.legislation.gov.uk/ukpga/1983/20/contents.

Legislation.gov.uk (2007) *Mental Health Act 2007*. Available at: https://www.legislation.gov.uk/ukpga/2007/12/contents.

Levine, P.A. and Kline, M. (2018) *Trauma through a Child's Eyes: Awakening the Ordinary Miracle of Healing*. Berkeley, CA: North Atlantic Books.

Marks, D.F., Murray, M. and Estacio, E.V. (2021) *Health Psychology: Theory, Research and Practice*, 6th edition. London: Sage.

Maslow, A.H. (1970) *Toward a Psychology of Being*, 3rd edition. New York: Van Nostrand.

Mukherji, P. and Dryden, L. (2014) *Foundations of Early Childhood: Principles and Practice*. London: Sage.

National Institute for Health and Care Excellence (NICE) (2015) *Challenging behaviour and learning disabilities: Prevention and interventions for people with learning disabilities whose behaviour challenges*, NICE Guideline (NG11). Available at: https://www.nice.org.uk/guidance/ng11?unlid=1062136304201610142380.

National Institute for Health and Care Excellence (NICE) (2018) *Learning disabilities and behaviour that challenges: Service design and delivery*, NICE Guideline (NG93). Available at: https://www.nice.org.uk/guidance/ng93.

The National Society for the Prevention of Cruelty to Children (NSPCC) (2023) *Early help and early intervention*. Available at: https://learning.nspcc.org.uk/safeguarding-child-protection/early-help-and-early-intervention.

Sharma, A. and Cockerill, H. (2014) *Mary Sheridan's From Birth to Five Years: Children's Developmental Progress*. London: Routledge.

Storr, A. (2001) *Freud: A Very Short Introduction*. Oxford: Oxford University Press.

Turner-Cobb, J. (2014) *Child Health Psychology: A Biopsychosocial Perspective*. London: Sage.

Vygotsky, L. (1962) *Thought and Language*. Boston, MA: MIT Press.

Whitnell, J. and Preston, C. (2019) Introduction to psychology and child development, in A.Y. Blaber (ed.) *Blaber's Foundations for Paramedic Practice: A Theoretical Perspective*, 3rd edition. London: Open University Press.

Wilmshurst, L. (2017) *Child and Adolescent Psychopathology: A Case Book*, 4th edition. London: Sage.

Wilmshurst, L. (2022) *Abnormal Child and Adolescent Psychology: A Developmental Perspective*, 2nd edition. London: Routledge.

World Health Organization (WHO) (2022) *ICD-11 International Classification of Diseases, 11th Revision. The global standard for diagnostic health information*. Geneva: WHO. Available at: www.who-int/standards/classifications/classification-of-diseases (accessed 9 April 2024).

Mental health
Children, young people and adults
Jackie Whitnell and Carol Lloyd

8

INTRODUCTION

The field of mental health and atypical psychology is the area of psychological investigation directly concerned with understanding mental health and the nature of individual pathologies of mind, mood and behaviour. Atypical psychology focuses on the causes and treatment of psychological disorders and adjustment problems, including mood, personality and dissociative disorders, colloquially referred to as 'mental health problems/ disorders' or 'mental ill health'. Defining mental health and illness is difficult. In western society, the word 'mental' has negative connotations and, over time, has been used as a term of abuse. Estimates of the prevalence of mental ill health in Britain vary. The Mental Health Foundation (MHF, 2018) and mental health statistics from Baker and Kirk-Wade (2023) put the figure at one in six adults at any one time. The one-in-six figure represents those people defined as having 'significant' mental health problems. Following the COVID-19 pandemic, Suleman et al. (2021) presented evidence regarding the effects the pandemic had on children and young people's mental health, as well as other groups (i.e. disabled people, ethnic minority communities, care home residents, homeless people and prisoners) who have been more affected by mental health problems than others. Mental health problems are common at all ages, affecting one in four people at some point in their life. Just over one in three children and young people with a diagnosable mental health condition get access to NHS care and treatment. There is untold stress and burden on the young person's significant others, but also on the NHS itself. Around 18 per cent of children aged 7–16 had a probable mental health condition in 2022, up from 12 per cent in 2017. In addition, in 2021–22, 3.25 million people accessed NHS mental health, learning disability and autism services. However, the waiting times for NHS talking therapies vary from 4 days to 229 days depending on where you live in England (Baker and Kirk-Wade, 2023).

Box 8.1 Guidance for assessment of atypical behaviour

1. *Distress or disability*: an individual experiences disabled functioning or personal distress which puts them at increased risk of psychological deterioration.
2. *Maladaptiveness*: an individual acts in ways that hinders lifestyle and thus hinders the personal wellbeing of self or others.
3. *Irrationality*: an individual talks or acts in ways that are incomprehensible or irrational to others.
4. *Unpredictability*: an individual behaves erratically or unpredictably, experiencing loss of control.
5. *Unconventionality and statistical rarity*: an individual behaves In a way that is rare, that violates social norms.
6. *Observer discomfort*: an individual creates discomfort in others, making them feel distressed or threatened.
7. *Violation of moral and ideal standards*: an individual violates expectations for how they ought to behave in the normal social world.

Adapted from: Gerrig et al. (2013) and DSM-5-TR (APA, 2022).

How do health professionals decide what is atypical behaviour? The distinction between normal and atypical is not a difference between types of behaviour; it is more a matter of the extent to which a person's actions resemble a set of agreed criteria of atypicality (APA, 2022). Mental disorder is best thought of as a continuum, as normal and atypical are relative and not absolute. One end of the continuum defines optimum mental health;

at the other end are behaviours that define minimal mental health and in between are gradations of maladaptive behaviours (Gerrig et al., 2013). For guidance on assessment of atypical behaviour, see Box 8.1.

Professionals are more confident in labelling behaviour as 'atypical' when more than one criterion is present and valid (Gerrig et al., 2013). The frequency of mental health problems is well documented statistically. However, these figures need to be considered with some caution. Often widely differing figures will be given for the same mental health problem, making it difficult to determine exactly how common the problem is. This is partly because these figures are not always measuring the same thing. There have been controversial challenges to the DSM-5 (Field and Cartwright-Hatton, 2015). For example, in order to reflect the fact that mental health is not fixed but likely to change over time, a variety of different figures are used. The most common are:

- **Prevalence:** this measures the number of people with a particular diagnosis at a given time.
- **Lifetime prevalence:** this measures the number of people who have experienced a particular mental health problem at any time in their lives.
- **Incidence:** this measures the number of new cases of a particular mental health problem that appear over a given period of time (Comer and Comer, 2021).

Often these figures are compared to provide further information about a mental health problem. For example, comparing the number of new cases (the incidence) with the number who are ill at any one time (the prevalence) can give us a rough idea of the average amount of time a mental health problem is likely to last. Another important factor is the kind of sample used to arrive at a particular figure. Sometimes, the number of people treated by health professionals is used to determine how common a mental health problem is. However, this excludes those people who have not come into contact with services. Furthermore, psychiatric diagnosis is often far from straightforward – a person's diagnosis may be changed several times during their treatment.

Mental health problems may be associated with, provoked by and maintained by alcohol or other substances, or traumatic experiences, possibly making the care of these individuals difficult. Indeed, while some patients will volunteer to accept your help, others will not and may need to be compelled to receive an assessment and treatment, possibly against their will, using the powers of legislation (Legislation.gov.uk, 2005, 2007). You may notice that this legislation is somewhat old. In 2022, the government published a draft Mental Health Bill to make changes to the current Act. The Bill was considered by a committee in parliament (GOV.UK, 2022a). The committee listened to organisations like MIND and gave recommendations for how to improve the Bill. Government is yet to respond to the recommendations. (See the MIND website for information on the recommendations and for what MIND considers is wrong with the Bill.)

Due to the introductory nature of this text, this chapter will provide the reader with only a brief overview of mental ill health. The chapter will start with an overview of child and adolescent mental health before discussing the various mental health disorders that people can suffer.

Children can experience most of the disorders that adults experience. This chapter cannot cover them all, so instead will consider the mental health issues around deliberate self-harm, depression, eating disorders and anxiety. It is important that when assessing and caring for children, the age and stage of development is taken into account (Wilmshurst, 2017; Laver-Bradbury et al., 2021) (see Chapter 7).

WHY IS THIS RELEVANT?

It is extremely important that paramedics have at least an understanding of some of the most common mental illnesses which children, young people and adults may have, and knowledge of some of the signs and symptoms that the client/patient may exhibit in order to make an evidence-based assessment (Laver-Bradbury et al., 2021). Paramedics will be in the position of caring for clients with mental ill health and will make assessments during their working practice. It is the aim that this overview will at least provide some information and excite an interest and thirst for further exploration of this area of ill health.

CHILD AND ADOLESCENT MENTAL HEALTH (CAMH)

It is now recognised that many mental health problems can manifest in childhood. Young people's mental health and wellbeing has never been so important. One in three mental health conditions relates directly to adverse childhood experiences (Kessler et al., 2010; APA, 2022). There are a wide range of mental health problems that can affect children and adolescents. One in six children aged 5–16 were identified as having a probable mental health condition in July 2021, a marked increase from the one in nine in 2017. That equates to five children in every classroom (ONS, 2023a). Some 2 per cent of children suffer from more than one type of disorder (co-morbidity); this poses a greater challenge in terms of diagnosis and in the care the child should receive. Children who experience three or more stressful life events, such as serious illness, family bereavement or divorce, are significantly more likely to develop emotional and behavioural disorders. Many studies have been conducted to identify the number of individuals experiencing specific problems. These studies generally use one of two classifications and sets of diagnostic criteria – DSM-5 (APA, 2022) or ICD-11 (WHO, 2022). Studies will give different results depending on the measures used and the cultural context in which they are used. Results will also differ depending on other variables, such as different populations and environments. Consequently, there are widely varying rates of recorded prevalence of mental health problems in young people today.

An NHS survey of children and young people's mental health in England was undertaken in 2017 and followed up in 2020, 2021 and 2022. It was found that 18 per cent of children aged 7–16 had a probable mental disorder in 2022, up from 12.1 per cent in 2017. The biggest rise was among those aged 17–19 years: 10.1 per cent had a probable mental disorder in 2017, rising to 17.7 per cent in 2020; a similar rate was then recorded in 2021, before increasing again to 25.7 per cent in 2022 (ONS, 2023a). These statistics could be linked to the isolation necessitated as a result of the COVID-19 pandemic (Baker and Kirk-Wade, 2023). Indeed, a survey conducted by King's College London identified a concerning number of longitudinal studies and systematic reviews which have highlighted the overwhelmingly negative impact of the pandemic. NHS England (2018) found that nearly half of the 11–12-year-olds in the cohort (44 per cent) reported an increase in symptoms of depression, and a quarter (26 per cent) reported an increase in post-traumatic stress disorder (PTSD) symptoms since the start of the pandemic (NHS England, 2020).

Further evidence suggests that some children and young people's mental health and wellbeing was massively impacted during the pandemic. For example, 83 per cent of young people with mental health needs believed that the pandemic had made their mental health worse (Young Minds, 2021). Between March and June 2020, a period when schools were closed to most pupils, symptoms of depression and PTSD were found to have significantly increased in children and young people aged between 7 and 12 years old compared to immediately before the pandemic. However, some pupils reported sleeping and feeling better and primary aged children were more likely to report that they felt happier and less lonely during the lockdown than secondary aged pupils. During these months, some parents and carers reported an overall increase in mental health problems in their children. By September 2020, relative to the March to June 2020 lockdown, reported behavioural, attention and emotional difficulties in children had returned to, and stabilised at, previous levels (GOV.UK, 2022b).

Read the section on atypical development for more information on child-related conditions in **Chapter 7**.

Deliberate self-harm

Although children as young as 7 have been found to self-harm, the average age at which children start self-harming is 13 years. Deliberate self-harm (DSH) is common in the 10–14-year age group. One other important factor is that DSH is four times more common among girls; however, until the age of 12 years, boys are more likely than girls to self-harm. Whilst it is sometimes assumed that suicide is a leading cause of death in the younger age groups, this is in fact not the case. In 2022, the highest registered suicide rates were among people aged 50–54 years, both males and females (ONS, 2023b). In fact, people 10–24 years have the lowest suicide rate of all age groups. But that should not detract from the seriousness of deliberate self-harm and the impact it has on families and friends.

Deliberate self-harm is considered an intentional act of self-injury with a non-fatal outcome in which an individual acts in one of the following ways:

- ingests a substance in excess of the prescribed dose or generally recognised therapeutic dose;
- initiates behaviour (e.g. self-cutting, jumping from a height) that they intend will cause self-harm;
- ingests a recreational drug or illicit substance that the person regards as self-harm;
- ingests a non-ingestible substance or object.

Reflection: points to consider

Before continuing, jot down some of the risk factors for mental health problems in children and young people.

There are a number of environmental, family and individual factors that can lead to a higher level of risk of mental health problems in children and young people. These include living in families where there is unemployment, having a parent with a mental illness and having some form of intellectual disability. Other possible causes are genetic predisposition, stress at home or school, over-protective parents and an over-controlling environment (Field and Cartwright-Hatton, 2015)

It is estimated that 80 per cent of children and adolescents with mental health problems are also likely to experience family life and relationship difficulties. Thankfully, suicide is rare in childhood and early adolescence, but it becomes more frequent with increasing age. Suicide is the most common cause of death among boys aged 5–19 and the second most common among girls of the same age. The relationship between psychiatric disorders and adolescent suicide is now well established. Previous suicide attempts, mood disorders and substance misuse are strongly related (Dogra et al., 2017; ONS, 2023a).

Depression in childhood

The criteria for depressive disorders are the same or similar for children and adults (depression in adults will be discussed later in this chapter). However, there are differences in how this disorder shows itself across the age range. Depression is thought to occur in 1 per cent of children and young people, with children as young as 5 suffering signs and symptoms of depression (Achenbach, 2013a, 2013b; RCP, 2022) (see Box 8.2).

Box 8.2 Depression in childhood – signs and symptoms at different stages

- *Infant/toddler* – loss of developmentally appropriate behaviour (e.g. toilet training and intellectual function).
- *Pre-school* – sad appearance or irritable, regression to earlier behaviours (e.g. separation anxiety and sleep problems).
- *School age* – exhibiting eating and sleep disturbances, being self-critical and having low motivation. Showing less or no interest in self-care. They may act out their distress.

In terms of gender and depression in childhood, prior to age 12, males report greater rates of depression, following which girls begin to be diagnosed more often than boys (Dogra et al., 2017). In puberty, more girls than boys suffer with depression and the same is true into adulthood. By mid-adolescence, approximately 2–3 per cent of children will be diagnosed with a depressive disorder. Girls internalise their feelings and depression tends to be reflected in mood state, whereas boys externalise their feelings and act out (Dogra et al., 2017) (Box 8.3). Consequently, one could argue that as girls express this disorder more outwardly in their mood, it is more noticeable and easier to detect. One approach used to explain the occurrence of depression in childhood derives from attachment theory. Since the effects of trauma on young children are more physiological in their immediacy, because the child's ability to process cognitively is less developed than that of an adult, regulation and treatment are very different. Interventions are unique and specific (Levine and Kline, 2018). This suggests that insecure attachment can lead to depression in infants, children and adolescents. Feeling insecure leads to unworthiness and a feeling of being unloved can predispose children to being vulnerable, fearing disapproval and abandonment. A further consideration from the social cultural theory suggests the cause could derive from problems in the home, at school or with peers (Whitnell, 2012; Berger, 2021; Young Minds, 2021).

Box 8.3 Depression in childhood

The signs and symptoms of depression in childhood include:

- sadness or irritability, withdrawing from friends;
- tiredness;
- self-pity, hopelessness;
- loss of appetite;
- disturbed sleep pattern;
- thoughts of death.

Source: Whitnell (2019).

Other specified feeding or eating disorders

In 2023, 12.5 per cent of 17–19-year-olds were considered to have an eating disorder, with a rate four times higher in young women (20.8 per cent) than young men (5.1 per cent). In addition, 2.6 per cent of 11–16-year-olds had an eating disorder, with girls (4.3 per cent) four times more likely to be affected than boys (1.0 per cent). Finally, 5.9 per cent of 20–25-year-olds were considered to have an eating disorder, with similar rates evident in women and men.

Anorexia nervosa is rare: over a 12 month period, the prevalence in females was reported to be 0.4 per cent (APA, 2013). However, this figure is likely to be an underestimation, as many cases of eating disorder go unreported or undiagnosed. For anorexia, there is evidence to suggest that in the younger age group (7–14 years), up to 25 per cent of cases are boys (MHF, 2018).

The impact of starvation has physical implications that can have serious consequences. Studies on the mortality rate of young people with anorexia suggest that it is between 5 and 10 per cent, particularly if there is rapid weight loss with 0.1 per cent of cases culminating in suicide (Culbert et al., 2015; Field and Cartwright-Hatton, 2015). Bulimia nervosa is a more common condition, with around 1–1.5 per cent of females presenting, again with the same ratio of boys to girls as anorexia nervosa. Binge eating disorder is assessed at 1.6 per cent of females and 0.8 per cent of males. There are overall better outcomes for binge eating than for bulimia and anorexia nervosa. The causes of eating disorders include: heredity, prenatal stress and birth trauma, adverse childhood experiences and social/cultural factors, including the idealism of the thin model (Field and Cartwright-Hatton, 2015). For guidelines on reporting eating disorders, visit the BEAT Eating disorders website.

Anxiety in childhood

Anxiety is an illness that becomes problematic enough to interfere with a child's or adult's ability to function effectively or enjoy everyday life. Anxiety produces an intense, often unrealistic, and excessive state of apprehension and fear. This may or may not occur during, or in anticipation of, a specific event, and may be accompanied by a rise in blood pressure, increased heart rate, rapid breathing, nausea and other signs of agitation or discomfort.

The different types of anxiety include:

- specific phobias;
- obsessive-compulsive disorder (boys > girls);
- separation anxiety disorder;
- emotional disorders;
- social phobia;
- panic disorder (girls > boys).

Anxiety in adults will be discussed in more detail later in the chapter.

 **Reflection: points to consider**

You may attend to and transport a child/adult who suffers from anxiety. What would your approach be? How would you try to calm them so as to care for them and transport them safely?

When children and young people present with mental health problems, the solution to their difficulties is rarely straightforward as children often present with more than one problem. The most frequent number of problems experienced is four or five, while half of the children referred to CAMH services have at least two severe problems (co-morbidity) (Field and Cartwright-Hatton, 2015; ONS, 2023a). As a paramedic, you will attend and possibly transport children and adolescents with mental health problems. It is important that you have a good understanding of the types of issues and difficulties facing these children, and report your findings of interactions you observe between the child/young person and significant others, noting anything that you find unusual, inappropriate or unsafe (AACE/JRCALC, 2022).

AN OVERVIEW OF ATYPICAL PSYCHOLOGY

Self-harm and suicide

The incidence of self-harm, which has always been high, does not seem to be abating. Attempted suicide and self-harm are considered the same entity: called 'suicide-related behaviour'. The term 'suicide-related behaviour' is used to describe all behaviours where the person intended to kill or harm themselves. Deliberate self-harm is frequently encountered by paramedics and healthcare professions alike; it is a hidden health problem worldwide (Rees et al., 2015). Self-harm is one of the five leading causes of acute medical admission for women and men. The myth around self-harm is that it is a cry for attention; this is not totally accurate. While deliberate self-harm can communicate to others the person's suffering, it can also express that the individual needs help and is in crisis. Self-harm is commonly completed in private. It is true to say that family, friends and therapists may be unaware of the episodes of self-harm a person is inflicting (Whitnell, 2012; MHF, 2018).

There is no doubt that there is no greater problem facing mental health practitioners than suicide-related behaviour. Since the mid-1970s, the data gathered has consistently indicated that suicide is a leading cause of death in young people. Contributing factors might include:

- decriminalisation of the Suicide Act in 1961;
- drug-prescribing increase since the 1960s;
- the rise in unemployment at the end of the 1970s and early 1990s;
- the influence of social media;
- after-effects of the COVID-19 pandemic.

There is one death from suicide every 90 minutes across the UK and Ireland (ONS, 2017). Almost three-quarters of these suicides are among men. Suicide rates for men are higher than for women in all age groups, and currently, men are almost three times more likely than women to commit suicide. Altogether, 5,642 suicides were registered in England and Wales in 2022. Suicide rates are measured as an age-standardised mortality rate (ASMR): 5,642 suicide deaths equates to 10.7 deaths per 100,000 people. This rate remained the same in 2021 (ONS, 2023b).

The likelihood of a person committing suicide depends on many factors: social problems – especially those related to family stress, separation, divorce, social isolation, death of a loved one and unemployment (an unemployed man is two to three times more at risk of suicide than the general population); mental and physical illness; and access to the means of suicide. Certain occupational groups, such as public sector workers and IT workers, appear to be at a higher risk of suicide, but it is a complex, multi-factorial issue (for more detail, see ONS, 2024). Alcohol and drug use are also factors which can influence suicide risk. Men are known to have far higher drug and alcohol consumption rates than women, and the figures are particularly high for younger men (ONS, 2023b). Suicide by self-poisoning is a leading cause of death worldwide. A substantial proportion of those with a fatal outcome may come into contact with a paramedic and/or emergency department before they die. Box 8.4 highlights some risk factors for suicide.

A variety of tools are available for use by specialist paramedics and approved mental health professionals (AMHP), and the paramedic has a professional responsibility and should be encouraged to expand and update their knowledge of mental health assessment to improve their competence and confidence. Such knowledge may aid their skill of appropriate referral and subsequently the care of patients. An example assessment tool used by paramedics in practice can be found in AACE/JRCALC (2022).

Box 8.4 Suicide – a serious mental health and public health problem

Facts about suicide

- Suicide rates vary by culture.
- Among males, in 2022, the age-specific rate of suicide was highest in those aged 90 years or over (32.1 deaths per 100,000), followed by those aged 45–49 years (23.0 deaths per 100,000) (ONS, 2023b).
- In all cultures, men are more likely than women to complete suicide.
- Among females in 2022, the age-specific rate of suicide was highest in those aged 50–54 years (7.8 deaths per 100,000);

in 2021, the highest rate was for those aged 45–49 years (7.7 deaths per 100,000) (ONS, 2023b).
- People with mental disorders, especially depression, schizophrenia and borderline personality disorder, are at high risk for suicide.

Risk factors

- Past history of attempted suicide, including inter-generational/ family history of suicide
- Talking about committing suicide
- A clear plan to commit suicide
- Available means (e.g. access to a gun, drugs)
- Depression
- Substance abuse
- Hopelessness
- Impulsivity
- Stressful life events
- Lack of social support
- Saying goodbye to people
- Giving away personal items

Adapted from: Whitnell (2012: 38–44).

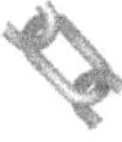

Chapter 21 for your continuing professional development responsibilities.

Anxiety disorders

MIND (2024b) estimates that 6 per cent of adults experience generalised anxiety disorders (GAD) (not including depression) at any one time. It is an anxiety disorder in which the individual feels anxious or worried most of the time for at least 6 months when no threat is apparent (Field and Cartwright-Hatton, 2015). A further 8 per cent of the population has mixed anxiety and depression (MIND, 2024b). Mood, stress-related and anxiety disorders are the most common groups of problems and often represent the extremes of normal emotion. They are recognised by a set of symptoms (adapted from APA, 2022):

- depressed mood (to be discussed further later in the chapter);
- emotional – fear, worry;

- physical – shortness of breath, sweating, upset stomach, heart pounding;
- cognitive – fear of dying, losing control, 'going crazy'.

Anxiety is a usual part of our everyday lives. However, how do we differentiate between 'normal' or manageable fear from anxiety and impairment due to unmanageable anxiety? A disorder can be classified when there is fear and anxiety in response to something that is not inherently frightening or dangerous (see Box 8.5). This may be termed the 'target of fear'.

Box 8.5 Anxiety disorder

Anxiety disorders have four things in common:

- Each is defined by a specific target of fear – this is the situation/item the person is afraid of.
- Encountering the target of fear may induce anxiety or panic attacks.
- The sufferer avoids the target of fear.
- Anxiety disorders tend to be persistent, so are chronic in nature, rather than being episodic.

Adapted from: Whitnell (2012: 38–44).

The different types of anxiety disorder are:

Specific phobias: fear and avoidance of a particular object or situation (e.g. dogs, heights, flying). People can live a 'normal' life by avoiding their phobia, unless they are asked to confront their fear. Phobias are experienced by 18 per cent of adults and 1 per cent of children, and more by females than males. It is estimated that 10 million people in the UK have phobias (Field and Cartwright-Hatton, 2015; ONS, 2023a).

Social phobia: tends to be more impairing as it involves significant social isolation. People with this type of phobia are afraid of rejection and negative evaluation, so they avoid it at all costs. Such phobia can be mild (fearful of public speaking – see case study 7.1 of David in Chapter 7) or severe (fearing all social interaction).

Panic disorder: can be debilitating, especially when accompanied by agoraphobia. Panic disorders are related to anxiety: an anxiety disorder in which sufferers experience unexpected, severe panic attacks that begin with a feeling of intense apprehension, fear or terror. The anxiety begins with panic attacks that occur 'out of the blue'. The disorder gets worse when people worry about having another panic attack and begin to avoid places and situations associated with the panic attack. Panic disorder is experienced by 2–3 per cent of the population with an onset in childhood or adolescence; it is often co-morbid with another disorder (RCP, 2022).

Obsessive-compulsive disorder (OCD): can be quite specific but can also cause obsessive domination and impairment of someone's life. Symptoms include unwanted, persistent, intrusive, repetitive thoughts, also typical ritualistic repetitive behaviours that a person feels compelled to engage in, including hand washing, checking, counting and hoarding. It is traditionally regarded as a neurotic disorder, like phobias and anxiety states (Comer and Comer, 2021).

Post-traumatic stress disorder: see separate subsection below.

Generalised anxiety disorder: is characterised by a period of over six months of chronic, uncontrollable worry about numerous things. Sufferers are always worried and tense, easily irritated and have trouble sleeping and concentrating.

Post-traumatic stress disorder (PTSD)

Post-traumatic stress disorder (PTSD) is characterised by the persistent re-experience of traumatic events through recollections, dreams, hallucinations or flashbacks. It is one of the anxiety disorders but is worthy of specific attention due to the nature of the role of a paramedic.

 **Reflection: points to consider**

Consider the local and global situations that people have found themselves in over recent years that may predispose them to suffering from PTSD.

Box 8.6 Post-traumatic stress disorder

The signs and symptoms/presentation of PTSD include:

- Fear of the trauma itself creates anxiety, so the person will avoid anything associated with the trauma (avoidance).
- The person may lose their memory of the event, or be plagued with intrusive and unwanted thoughts, such as flashbacks and nightmares (re-experience).

- People tend to be psychologically numb, emotionally 'shut down', find no pleasure in things and cannot look to the future (emotional numbing).
- Conversely, the person may have symptoms of 'hyper-arousal' – startle easily, cannot sleep or concentrate, and be irritable and easily angered.

Specifically in relation to children and young people:

- Do not rely wholly on an adult's assessment; if possible, ask the child or young person to explain how they feel and what they are experiencing.
- Ask the adult/child about patterns of sleep and any significant changes that have occurred.

Sources: NICE (2018) and RCP (2022).

PTSD was first noted among war veterans. It is also seen in victims of trauma and in others who either witnessed or were involved in the event. Stress is the cause of PTSD (Box 8.6). Up to 80 per cent of adults experience a traumatic event in their life which may develop into PTSD. Sufferers have a high suicide rate (Dogra et al., 2017). It can present in children following a traumatic event such as the divorce of their parents, seeking asylum, child abuse and/or living with domestic abuse. Emotionally, the responses to PTSD can occur in an acute form immediately after the trauma and may not subside for several months. Globally people are migrating and seeking asylum, hence refugees are a vulnerable group (Levine and Kline, 2018).

Anxiety and COVID-19

A survey by Young Minds (2021) of 2,438 young people aged 13–25 to examine the impact of the pandemic, carried out between 26 January and 12 February 2021, showed:

- 75 per cent of respondents agreed that they found the current lockdown harder to cope with than the previous ones, including 44 per cent who said it was much harder (14 per cent said it was easier, 11 per cent said it was the same).
- 67 per cent believed that the pandemic will have a long-term negative effect on their mental health. This included young people who had been bereaved or undergone traumatic experiences during the pandemic, who were concerned about whether friendships would

recover, or who were worried about the loss of education or their prospects of finding work (19 per cent neither agreed nor disagreed, 14 per cent disagreed).
- 79 per cent of respondents agreed that their mental health would start to improve when most restrictions were lifted, but some expressed caution about restrictions being lifted too quickly and the prospect of future lockdowns.

As stated earlier in the chapter, between March and June 2020, a period when schools were closed to most pupils, symptoms of depression and PTSD were found to have increased significantly in children aged between 7½ and 12 years compared to immediately before the pandemic. However, some pupils reported sleeping and feeling better and primary aged children were more likely to report that they felt happier and less lonely during the lockdown than secondary aged pupils. During these months, some parents and carers reported an overall increase in mental health problems in their children By September 2020, relative to the March to June 2020 lockdown, reported behavioural, attention and emotional difficulties in children had returned to, and stabilised at, a lower level (King's College London, 2022).

Depression in adults

Depression is considered to be the 'common cold' of psychopathology, and aligns to learned helplessness. In psychology, learned helplessness is a state that occurs after a person has experienced a stressful situation repeatedly. They believe that they are unable to control or change the situation. It occurs frequently and almost everyone has elements of this disorder at some time in their life. Depression with anxiety is experienced by one in six adults living in the UK. All neurotic disorders are more common in women than men, except panic disorder, which is diagnosed equally in both. Women have a higher prevalence of mood disorders; however, studies suggest depression occurs as often in men. Although women are twice as likely to be diagnosed and treated for depression, men are four times as likely to die from suicide, suggesting that many men have undiagnosed mental health issues. It is argued that men tend to express their symptoms differently, for example, through the use of alcohol and drugs, and are unwilling to admit to the symptoms of depression. Stigmatisation may be particularly strong among men with male-typical depressive symptoms since they are most likely to adhere to socially constructed gender norms. Other indicators of undiagnosed mental health issues in men can manifest in aggressions, irritability, violence or somatic complaints, none of which are included in the DSM-5. It is interesting to note that the figures for men are rising faster than the figures for women. This may indicate that men now are more likely to admit to feeling depressed (WHO, 2022).

Mood disorders may have some common symptoms, but they have very different causes and prevalence to other disorders. Unipolar depression or major depressive disorder is one of the most common (see Box 8.7). Less prevalent are the bipolar disorders (otherwise known as manic depression). Depression is a disorder that affects people of all age groups, including children (Dogra et al., 2017; Wilmshurst, 2017). The age of onset of major depressive disorder is reducing; early onset predicts a worse course of depression over time. Depression follows a recurrent course. Most people have multiple episodes that become worse with time, while some may have isolated episodes. Mild depression with a few symptoms may indicate the person will suffer with more serious depression later. The feelings of major depressive disorder should not be negated. Some 15 per cent of depressed people commit suicide, due to the feelings of hopelessness and long-term suffering (MHF, 2018).

Box 8.7 Unipolar depression/major depressive disorder

The primary symptom is sad or depressed mood, but it is much more than this. Other symptoms include:

- lack of interest or pleasure in things that are usually enjoyed;
- changes in appetite;
- changes in sleep habits;
- low energy levels, poor concentration and extreme fatigue;
- feeling bad about themselves, low self-esteem, negative self-concept; self-reproach and blaming themselves for what has 'gone wrong' in their life, 'paralysis of will' (Gerrig et al., 2013);
- hopelessness about the future;
- preoccupation with ailments and death – suicidal ideation.

Adapted from: Whitnell (2012: 38–44).

Bipolar affective disorder commonly known as manic depression

Bipolar disorder is a mood disorder characterised by alternating periods of depression and mania (MIND, 2024a). Most studies give a lifetime prevalence of 2 in 100 people for bipolar disorder and equal prevalence rates for men and women. Bipolar is a common health problem affecting between 1 and 2 per cent of the population and it affects people of all ages (see Box 8.8). However, hospital admission rates are much higher owing to the recurrent nature of the illness. It is a serious mental illness, but if it is well managed with help from family, friends, support groups and health professionals, a person with bipolar can lead a productive and satisfying life. Manic depression has no known cure; a person may require psychiatric treatment for the rest of their life, although people who have a first episode of manic depression may not get another (MIND, 2024a). It is considered that sufferers of bipolar depression have a predisposition genetically, but the manic state can be triggered by the stresses and strains of everyday life, or a traumatic event. Sufferers experience a sudden onset that can last one or two days or weeks or even months.

Box 8.8 Bipolar affective disorder

The signs and symptoms/presentation of bipolar affective disorder include:

- Highs and lows are increasingly disconnected from everyday events and out of control.
- People feel excessively self-important, expansive and over-confident with inflated self-esteem or grandiose ideas.
- There is an increase in goal-directed activity.
- The person may become sexually promiscuous, excessively religious, financially irresponsible, intolerant, verbally aggressive, irritable, over-communicative and incapable of listening to or empathising with other people.
- They may suffer from hallucinations, delusions and paranoia in extreme depression.
- The person may suffer from sleeplessness and over-active behaviour.

Adapted from: Whitnell (2012: 38–44).

The symptoms of this disorder may only be spotted with the onset of a severe crisis in a person's life and may require compulsory treatment under the Mental Health Act (Legislation.gov.uk, 2007). It may only be then that the person is referred to a psychiatric unit and diagnosed for treatment.

Postnatal disturbance or depression

Another form of depression that is seen less frequently is that of postnatal depression. The most common form of postnatal disturbance is the 'baby blues', which is said to be experienced by at least half of all Western mothers. This usually lasts between 12 and 24 hours, generally occurring between the third and sixth day after the birth. This is perfectly normal and the mother and family may just need reassurance. An incidence of 10 per cent of all new mothers is most often quoted, with other studies showing a figure between 3 and 22 per cent. It is likely that around 50 per cent of these cases will never come to medical attention. However, puerperal or postpartum psychosis is a severe and relatively rare form of postnatal depression that can affect someone soon after having a baby. It affects around one in 1,000 mothers after giving birth (NHS, 2023). As a paramedic, you may be called to a patient suffering from this, where the husband/partner/carer is very concerned about the mother's behaviour to others or towards the baby (Comer and Comer, 2021).

Personality disorder

Another disorder that you may identify in a patient/client is personality disorder (see Box 8.9). Personality disorder is defined by instability and intensity in personal relationships as well as turbulent and impulsive behaviour. In Britain, the prevalence of personality disorder ranges from 2–6 per cent, according to different studies.

Box 8.9 Personality disorder

All personality disorders have some things in common:

- long-standing – begin at a relatively early age;
- chronic – continue over time;
- pervasive – occur in most contexts.

The behaviour, thoughts and feelings seen in personality disorder are:

- inflexible – resistant to change and are applied in a rigid manner;
- maladaptive – they do not enable the person to get what they expect/want.

Sufferers of personality disorder will generally consider their behaviour perfectly normal and will blame others for the behaviour shown. Consequently, this may lead to treatment issues. It is always wise to consider your own safety as well as that of your patient in difficult situations (Comer and Comer, 2021).

The DSM-5 (APA, 2022) describes the main disorders and their traits. There are 10 personality disorders that form three clusters:

Cluster A – the odd and eccentric cluster

- paranoid – suspicious, distrustful, makes hostile attributions;
- schizoid – interpersonally and emotionally cut off, unresponsive to others, a 'loner';
- schizotypal – odd thoughts, behaviours, experiences, poor interpersonal functioning.

Cluster B – the dramatic and erratic cluster

- histrionic – dramatic, craves attention, emotionally shallow;
- narcissistic – inflated sense of self-importance, will feel entitled, low empathy, hidden vulnerability;
- anti-social – behaviours that disregard laws, norms, rights of others; lacking in empathy – commonly men;
- borderline – instability in thoughts, feelings, behaviour and sense of self – commonly women.

Cluster C – the fearful and avoidant cluster

- obsessive-compulsive – rigid, controlled, perfectionist;
- avoidant – fears negative evaluation, rejection and abandonment;
- dependent – submissive, dependent on others for self-esteem.

Personality disorders are long-term patterns of emotional functioning. Each of the 10 disorders has a low prevalence in the general population. Most people with personality disorders do not seek, want or comply with treatment; consequently, treatment is not always effective (Comer and Comer, 2021).

Reflection: points to consider

Consider the three clusters and think about how you would manage a person expressing these symptoms towards you, who may require immediate treatment and who may be resistant.

Now consider asking yourself these three questions to assess immediate risk:

- Are they at risk to themselves?
- Are there risks to others?
- Is there someone else to support them?

Psychoses

Psychosis is a collection of signs that constitutes a current mental state and may indicate the presence of a physical cause or a 'functional' disorder, such as schizophrenia or bipolar affective disorder. It is not a diagnosis in itself. Psychoses and functional psychoses are disorders that produce disturbances in thinking and perception that are severe enough to distort the person's perception of the world and the relationship of events in it. Psychoses are normally divided into two groups:

1. *Organic psychoses*, such as dementia and Alzheimer's.
2. *Functional psychoses*, which mainly cover schizophrenia and bipolar depression (although 'functional psychosis' does not necessarily have to belong to either one of these two diagnoses and can exist as a diagnosis in itself).

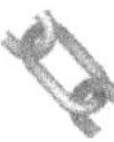 **Chapter 15** for information on caring for people with dementia.

Schizophrenia

The diagnostic label in ICD-11 and DSM-5 aligns schizophrenia with a group of psychotic disorders whereby personality seems to disintegrate; there is withdrawal from reality; thought and perception are distorted; and emotions are blunted. When considering schizophrenia, people often think of 'madness' or 'insanity'. Schizophrenia is a complex and puzzling illness (see Box 8.10); experts in the field are not exactly sure what causes it.

Box 8.10 Schizophrenia

Presentation of positive, negative and disorganised symptoms:

- perceiving things that are not there – auditory hallucinations, may also be visual and tactile;
- paranoid delusions – believing things that are not true, delusions of grandeur, delusions of persecution;
- using bizarre language, 'word salad' (jumbled words);
- their behaviour may be reported by others as seriously disordered or irrational;
- lack of demonstrating emotions facially, inappropriate laughing, crying and anger.

Behaviour disturbances can be grouped into four areas:

- repetitive movements and mannerisms;
- significant lack of motivation – this is termed 'avolition';
- struggle to take care of themselves with 'basic' care such as washing or dressing;
- social withdrawal, poor social skills and strained relationships with others.

This is a common and often severe mental illness. It may present acutely with severe change in behaviour or insidiously as a slow but progressive change over a period of time. Some physicians think that the brain may not be able to process information correctly. Genetic factors appear to play a role, as people who have family members with schizophrenia are at greater risk of inheriting the disease themselves (Field and Cartwright-Hatton, 2015). While prevalence rates are the same for men and women, age and gender together form an important factor: one study shows incidence for men aged 15–24 years is twice that for women, whereas for those aged 24–35 years, it is higher among females. This reflects a common late onset of the illness for females (Comer and Comer, 2021).

Positive symptoms describe unusual occurrences, such as hallucinations, delusions and odd speech. Negative symptoms describe the lack of behaviour that is normal for the rest of society, including good social skills, motivation, expression of emotion and being able to look after oneself (see Box 8.10).

Paramedics should be aware that some of the features of schizophrenia can occur alongside the presence of physical disease, intoxication with legal or illicitly obtained substances, or being under the influence of psychotropic drugs. It is important that the paramedic attempts to ascertain what the person may have taken in the form of drugs or substances in order to report it and, at the same time, identify risk factors to the patient/client and to themselves.

LEGISLATIVE POWERS AND MENTAL HEALTH

This chapter has provided the reader with a brief overview of mental ill health, including a consideration of the relatively common mental health problems/disorders that paramedics are likely to encounter in children, young people and adults during their working practice. This section will look at the legislative powers related to mental health.

The Mental Health Act 2007 and Mental Capacity Act 2005

The Mental Health Act 2007 (Legislation.gov.uk, 2007) was passed in July of that year, and updated the previous Act of 1983. There were seven major amendments to the 1983 Act and a further eighth amendment, updating the Mental Capacity Act 2005 (Legislation.gov.uk, 2005; Amblum, 2014). See AACE/JRCALC (2022) for detailed information on the Mental Capacity Act 2005. The amendments provide better safeguards for mental health service users, new rights to advocacy, a say in who their nearest relative is and the right to refuse electroconvulsive therapy and other treatments.

The Mental Health Act 2007 is still in place for practitioners; however, in 2022, the government published a draft Mental Health Bill (GOV.UK, 2022b) to make changes to the current Act, which are still under consideration.

Criteria for application for admission under the Mental Health Act 2007

A person suffering from a mental illness, who is either a danger to themselves or to the public, may be removed from a public place or their home to a place of safety (usually a police station or hospital) by a police officer.

As a paramedic, you would usually be empowered by the appropriate approved mental health professional (AMHP) or family member to convey the patient compulsorily under a Section Order to hospital or a mental health facility. You may have to call on the services of a police officer to aid with the escort of the patient, especially in the presence or threat of violence. It is vitally important that a bed has been secured for the patient, if required. However, in reality, it may be some time before a bed is available and the hospital may enlist the help of a psychiatric nurse while the patient remains in the emergency department, until he or she has been fully assessed and a decision made. Where there is an AMHP on scene to identify the legislation required, the services of the police may not be required, as the AMHP may have the powers to issue a Section Order (Legislation.gov.uk, 2007).

Reflection: points to consider

- In your practice area, do AMPHs work alongside paramedics regularly?
- Do you know their jurisdiction?
- Consider the value of their expertise and write down some points that highlight the importance of the AMPH role alongside that of the paramedic.

The Mental Health Act 2007 was designed to protect the individual from potential abuses to their freedom, while protecting the public and the patient from any consequences of the mental illness. AMHPs, GPs and specialist approved doctors (psychiatrists) are usually involved in assessing the patient for a Section Order. This multidisciplinary approach to invoking the Section Order is designed to protect the patient from unnecessary admission and removal of human rights.

There are a variety of sections within the Act that may be used to secure a patient's admission (see Box 8.11).

Box 8.11 Sections of the Mental Health Act 2007 relevant to the paramedic

- *Section 2 (Admission for assessment)*: Admission for up to a period of 28 days. Two doctors make a recommendation for admission, one of whom must be approved. Assessment from both doctors must occur within a period of five days of each other.
- *Section 3 (Admission for treatment)*: Admission for up to a period of six months, renewable for periods of up to one year at a time for severe mental illness/impairment/disorder, which requires treatment in hospital (Amblum, 2014).
- *Section 4 (Admission for assessment in an emergency)*: Admission for a period of up to 72 hours (the patient can be placed under Section 2 or 3 after examination) for urgent assessment.
- *Section 131 (Informal admission)*: The patient voluntarily agrees to be admitted but can change their mind and refuse. There is no time limit.
- *Section 135 (Place of safety order – private)*: Admission for a period of up to 72 hours. A person suffering from mental illness can be removed from a private dwelling to a place of safety for assessment. The patient should not be removed directly to hospital under Section 135 unless an AMHP/ approved social worker or GP has attended.
- *Section 136 (Place of safety order – public)*: Admission for a period of up to 72 hours. A person suffering from a mental illness can be removed from a public place to a place of safety (usually a police station or possibly a hospital) by a police officer or an AMHP/approved social worker.

Under the 2007 Act, both Sections 135 and 136 have been amended to allow transfers between places of safety, within the 72-hour detention period. Transfer during the 72-hour detention period was not allowed under the 1983 Act. Paramedics may be asked to provide safe transfer of patients under these sections.

For further reading, see: AACE/JRCALC (2022); Legislation.gov.uk (2007); GOV.UK (2022a).

CONCLUSION

As a paramedic, you will come across people with psychological problems in your working life. It is essential that you have an understanding of the theoretical underpinnings of your practice in order that you can assess and care for these patients, both holistically and competently. It is important that your approach to these patients be calm, and you should take your time to communicate during assessment.

This chapter has attempted to provide the reader with an understanding of some of the psychological problems that a child, young person or adult can face along with the relevant legislation when caring for the patient. The patterns of functioning associated with atypical psychology include:

- dysfunctional (interfering with the person's ability to conduct daily activities in a constructive way);
- deviant (different, extreme, unusual, perhaps even bizarre);
- distressful (unpleasant and upsetting for the sufferer and significant others);
- dangerous (to themselves or to others, hostile and careless).

However, we should be clear that these criteria are often vague and subjective and not all sufferers will show all behaviours. It is also important to mention that, despite popular misconceptions, most sufferers with anxiety, depression and even 'bizarre' thinking and behaviour pose no immediate danger to themselves or to others. However, as a paramedic, you should always assess your personal safety when approaching an upset, disorientated, agitated or threatening patient. If you think you are at considerable risk, you may need to call the police who are better trained for these situations (AACE/JRCALC, 2022). It may be wise to regularly refresh your knowledge of conflict resolution training/education to aid your care of patients.

 **Reflection: points to consider**

The mnemonic **GASPIPES** was developed to aid understanding when thinking through the assessment of a patient/client's mental state. Ask yourself and the patient whether the patient is experiencing any of the following:

Guilt and self-reproach
Appetite is disturbed

Sleep disturbance, suffering insomnia
Paying attention to your questions or not, orientation to time, place
 and person
Interest in things is lacking, such as eating, television, getting dressed
Psychomotor disturbance – slow, agitated, pacing, mood, hallucinations
Energy – loss, tired, slowed down
Suicidal – expressed thoughts of not wanting to live

Adapted from Whitnell (2012).

When caring for any patient, do not rush, because a distressed or agitated person may react negatively to being hurried. It is most important that you are always honest regarding what is going to happen to help gain their confidence and trust in your care.

Chapter key points:

- The paramedic requires knowledge and understanding of the mental ill health of children, young people and adults.
- The paramedic requires an awareness of the signs and symptoms of potential mental ill health.
- The paramedic needs to understand the relevant legislation, national guidelines and local Trust policy, to assess a patient's condition correctly and instigate appropriate treatment or obtain specialist assistance (AACE/JRCALC, 2022).
- Paramedics should always be aware of their personal safety as well as that of the patient.

REFERENCES AND SUGGESTED READING

Achenbach, T.M. (2013a) *Assess Adaptive and Maladaptive Functioning: Achenbach System of Empirically Based Assessment (ASEBA)*. London: Harcourt Press.

Achenbach, T.M. (2013b) *DSM-Orientated Guide for the Achenbach System of Empirically Based Assessment (ASEBA)*. Burlington, VT: University of Vermont Research Centre for Children, Youth and Families. Available at: www. aseba.org/research/ aseba-dsm-5-orientated-scales/ (accessed 7 April 2024).

Amblum, J. (2014) A critical appraisal of the impact of Section 3 of the Mental Capacity Act 2005, *Journal of Paramedic Practice*, 6 (8): 422–28.

American Psychiatric Association (APA) (2013) *Diagnostic and Statistical Manual of Mental Disorders*, DSM-V. Philadelphia, PA: APA.

American Psychiatric Association (APA) (2022) *Diagnostic and Statistical Manual of Mental Disorders*, DSM-5-TR, 5th edition, text revision. Philadelphia, PA: APA. Available at: www.dsm.psychiatryonline.org/doi/book/10.1176/appi.books.9780890425596 (accessed 9 April 2024).

Association of Ambulance Chief Executives/Joint Royal Colleges Ambulance Liaison Committee (AACE/JRCALC) (2022) *JRCALC Clinical Guidelines*. Bridgwater: Class Publishing. Available at: www.jrcalc.org (accessed 9 April 2024).

Baker, C. and Kirk-Wade, E. (2023) *Mental health statistics: Prevalence, services and funding in England*. London: House of Commons Library. Available at: https://researchbriefings.files.parliament.uk/documents/SN06988/SN06988.pdf (accessed 7 April 2024).

Berger, K.S. (2021) *The Developing Person through Childhood and Adolescence*, 12th edition. New York: Worth Publishers.

Comer, R.J. and Comer, J.S. (2021) *Abnormal Psychology*, 11th edition. New York: Worth Publishers.

Culbert, K.M., Racine, S.E. and Klump, K. (2015) Research review: What we have learned about the causes of eating disorders: a synthesis of sociocultural, psychological, and biological research, *Journal of Child Psychology and Psychiatry*, 56 (11): 1141–64.

Dogra, N., Parkin, A., Gale, F. and Frake, C. (2017) *A Multidisciplinary Handbook of Child and Adolescent Mental Health for Front-Line Professionals*, 3rd edition. London: Jessica Kingsley.

Field, M. and Cartwright-Hatton, S. (2015) *Essential Atypical and Clinical Psychology*. London: Sage.

Gerrig, R.J., Zimbardo, P.G., Svartdal, F., Brennen, T. et al. (2013) *Psychology and Life*. Harlow: Pearson Education.

GOV.UK (2022a) *Draft Mental Health Bill 2022*. Available at: https://www.gov.uk/government/publications/draft-mental-health-bill-2022 (accessed 7 April 2024).

GOV.UK (2022b) Children and young people, in *Covid-19 mental health and wellbeing surveillance report*. Available at: https://www.gov.uk/government/publications/covid-19-mental-health-and-wellbeing-surveillance-report/7-children-and-young-people#references (accessed 7 April 2024).

Jones, S., Williams, B. and Monteith, P. (2014) Decision making for refusals of treatment: a framework to consider, *Journal of Paramedic Practice*, 6 (4): 180–86.

Kalat, J.H. (2023) *Biological Psychology*, 14th edition. Belmont, CA: Wadsworth.

Kerrig, P.K., Ludlow, A. and Wenar, C. (2012) *Developmental Psychopathology: From Infancy through Adolescence*, 6th edition. Maidenhead: Open University Press.

Kessler, R.C., McLaughlin, K.A., Green, J.G., Gruber, M.J. et al. (2010) Childhood adversities and adult psychopathology in the WHO World Mental Health Surveys, *British Journal of Psychiatry*, 197 (5): 378–85.

King's College London (2022) *How has COVID-19 impacted children and young people?* Available at: https://www.kcl.ac.uk/an-isolated-generation-the-impact-of-covid-19-on-children-and-young-people (accessed 5 April 2024).

Laver-Bradbury, C., Thompson, M.J.J., Gale, C. and Hooper, C.M. (2021) *Child and Adolescent Mental Health: Theory and Practice*, 3rd edition. London: Routledge.

Legislation.gov.uk (2005) *Mental Capacity Act 2005*. Available at: https://www.legislation.gov.uk/ukpga/2005/9/contents.

Legislation.gov.uk (2007) *Mental Health Act 2007*. Available at: https://www.legislation.gov.uk/ukpga/2007/12/contents.

Levine, P.A. and Kline, M. (2018) *Trauma through a Child's Eyes: Awakening the Ordinary Miracle of Healing*. Berkeley, CA: North Atlantic Books.

Marks, D.F., Murray, M., and Estacio, E.V. (2021) *Health Psychology: Theory, Research and Practice*. London: Sage.

Mental Health Foundation (MHF) (2018) *Statistics*. Available at: https://www.mentalhealth.org.uk/explore-mental-health/statistics (accessed 2 April 2024).

Mental Health Foundation (MHF) (2020) *Mental Health Foundation Strategy 2020–2025: Making prevention happen*. Available at: https://www.mentalhealth.org.uk/about-us/strategy (accessed 1 April 2024).

MIND (2024a) *Bipolar disorder*. Available at: https://www.mind.org.uk/information-support/types-of-mental-health-problems/bipolar-disorder/about-bipolar-disorder/ (accessed 6 August 2024).

MIND (2024b) *Mental health facts and statistics*. Available at: https://www.mind.org.uk/information-support/types-of-mental-health-problems/mental-health-facts-and-statistics/ (accessed 6 August 2024).

National Health Service (NHS) (2023) *Mental health conditions: Postpartum psychosis*. Available at: https://www.nhs.uk/mental-health/conditions/post-partum-psychosis/ (accessed 2 April 2024).

National Health Service Confederation (2016) *Mental Health Network factsheet: Key facts and trends in mental health*. Available at: https://www.mentalhealth.org.uk/sites/default/files/2022-06/The-Fundamental-facts-about-mental-health-2016.pdf (accessed 2 April 2024).

National Institute for Health and Care Excellence (NICE) (2018) *Post-traumatic stress disorder*, NICE guideline NG116. Available at: https://www.nice.org.uk/guidance/ng116 (accessed 1 April 2024).

NHS England (2018) *Mental health of children and young people in England, 2017*. Available at: https://digital.nhs.uk/data-and-information/publications/statistical/mental-health-of-children-and-young-people-in-england/2017/2017 (accessed 2 April 2024).

NHS England (2020) *Mental health of children and young people in England, 2020 – wave 1 follow up to the 2017 survey*. Available at: https://digital.nhs.uk/data-and-information/publications/statistical/mental-health-of-children-and-young-people-in-england/2020-wave-1-follow-up (accessed 2 April 2024).

NHS England (2021) *Mental health of children and young people in England, 2021 – wave 2 follow up to the 2017 survey*. Available at: https://digital.nhs.uk/data-and-information/publications/statistical/mental-health-of-children-and-young-people-in-england/2021-follow-up-to-the-2017-survey (accessed 2 April 2024).

NHS England (2022) *Mental health of children and young people in England, 2022 – wave 3 follow up to the 2017 survey*. Available at: https://digital.nhs.uk/data-and-information/publications/statistical/mental-health-of-children-and-young-people-in-england/2022-follow-up-to-the-2017-survey (accessed 2 April 2024).

Office for National Statistics (ONS) (2017) *Suicide by occupation, England: 2011 to 2015*. Available at: https://www.ons.gov.uk/peoplepopulationandcommunity/birthsdeathsandmarriages/deaths/articles/suicidebyoccupation/england2011to2015#:~:text=Main%20points,the%20time%20of%20death%20registration (accessed 6 August 2024).

Office for National Statistics (ONS) (2023a) *Mental health of children and young people in England, 2023 – wave 4 follow up to the 2017 survey*. Available at: https://digital.nhs.uk/data-and-information/publications/statistical/mental-health-of-children-and-young-people-in-england/2023-wave-4-follow-up (accessed 6 August 2024).

Office for National Statistics (ONS) (2023b) *Suicides in England and Wales: 2022 registrations. Registered deaths in England and Wales from suicide analysed by sex, age, area of usual residence of the deceased, and suicide method*. Available at: https://www.ons.gov.uk/peoplepopulationandcommunity/birthsdeathsandmarriages/deaths/bulletins/suicidesintheunitedkingdom/2022registrations#suicides-in-england-and-wales (accessed 6 August 2024).

Office for National Statistics (ONS) (2024) *Suicide by occupation in England: 2020–2022*. Available at: https://www.ons.gov.uk/peoplepopulationandcommunity/birthsdeathsandmarriages/deaths/adhocs/2028suicidebyoccupationinengland2020to2022 (accessed 6 August 2024).

Palmer, A. (2011) Improving the assessment and referral of mental health patients, *Journal of Paramedic Practice*, 3 (9): 496–503.

Rees, N., Rapport, F. and Snooks, H. (2015) Perceptions of paramedic and emergency staff about the care they provide to people who self-harm: constructivist metasynthesis of the qualitative literature, *Journal of Psychosomatic Research*, 78 (6): 529–35.

Royal College of Psychiatrists (RCP) (2022) *Depression in children and young people*. Available at: https://www.rcpsych.ac.uk/mental-health/parents-and-young-people/depression-in-young-people (accessed 2 April 2024).

Suleman, M., Sonthalia, S., Webb, C., Tinson, A. et al. (2021) *Unequal pandemic, fairer recovery: The COVID-19 impact inquiry report*. London: The Health Foundation. Available at: https://www.health.org.uk/publications/reports/unequal-pandemic-fairer-recovery (accessed 9 April 2024).

Whitnell, J. (2012) Child and adolescent mental health, *Early Years Educator*, 13 (11): 38–44.

Whitnell, J. (2019) Mental health: children, young people and adults, in A.Y. Blaber (ed.) *Blaber's Foundations for Paramedic Practice: A Theoretical Perspective*, 3rd edition. London: Open University Press.

Wilmshurst, L. (2017) *Child and Adolescent Psychopathology: A Casebook*, 4th edition. London: Sage.

World Health Organization (WHO) (2022) *ICD-11 International Classification of Diseases, 11th Revision. The global standard for diagnostic health information*. Geneva: WHO. Available at: https://icd.who.int/en (accessed 6 August 2024).

Young Minds (2021) *Coronavirus: Impact on young people with mental health needs*. Available at: https://www.youngminds.org.uk/about-us/reports-and-impact/coronavirus-impact-on-young-people-with-mental-health-needs/#main-content (accessed 9 April 2024).

USEFUL WEBSITES

BEAT, the UK's Eating Disorder Charity: www.beateatingdisorders.org.uk
Mental Health First Aid (MHFA) – for useful statistics by topic: https://mhfaengland.org/mhfa-centre/research-and-evaluation/mental-health-statistics/ (accessed 9 April 2024)
The Mental Health Foundation: https://www.mentalhealth.org.uk/
MIND: www.mind.org.uk
Sane: www.sane.org.uk
Young Minds: https://www.youngminds.org.uk/

Introduction to sociology, social factors and social policy

Amanda Y. Blaber and Chris Storey

In this chapter:

- Introduction
- Why is this relevant?
- Introduction to sociology
- Review of classical sociology theorists
- Socialisation
- Social stratification
- Case studies and associated theory
- Introduction to social policy
- Conclusion
- Chapter key points
- References and suggested reading
- Useful websites

INTRODUCTION

This chapter will introduce you to some key classical sociologists whose work is important to healthcare professionals. To gain a more in-depth understanding, you will need to read some 'pure' sociology textbooks. Student paramedics come to their undergraduate studies having studied a variety of academic subjects, and sociology may or may not have been one. There are, however, other areas of our lives where contemporary sociologists have focused their work, such as social aspects of health and illness and the changing role of families. Whatever is happening within our society is of interest to sociologists, and their subsequent research and theories reflect the dynamic nature of the society we live in now.

This chapter will use a case-study approach to explore a few of the main factors that affect all of our lives and how we function within society. All the factors discussed will no doubt be familiar and probably are areas you may not have thought much about previously, taking things for granted, such as age and culture. The third edition of the *Foundations* text (Blaber, 2019) contains more theoretical information on these and other areas, as do sociology textbooks. Finally, the chapter closes with an introduction to the importance of social policy and its relevance to paramedic practice.

WHY IS THIS RELEVANT?

All professionals working in the NHS have contact with members of the public. So why do paramedics require an understanding of sociology and its key concepts? Paramedics and other healthcare community workers are unique in the sense that they see people in their own social world – in their homes, with family and friends, and in their neighbourhood. Hospital-based workers do not see people functioning in their own environments because the fact of being hospitalised brings them into the hospital organisation, with its own culture. If paramedics have a wider understanding of why people talk and act, respond to illness and operate within society in the way that they do, clinicians may be able to adjust their own behaviour accordingly, when dealing with patients. This would obviously improve the experience for both clinician and patient and may enhance the overall quality of care provided.

As well as introducing some new concepts/theories, this chapter will invite you to question areas of your life that you may take for granted and have grown up with. Although brief (in comparison with sociology texts), the chapter hopes to raise the student's awareness of sociology and how it can assist us in understanding ourselves and others. Readers are invited to explore their thoughts on certain areas of social life. Many areas will require further reading in order to avoid 'skimming the surface' of a subject.

INTRODUCTION TO SOCIOLOGY

Many people find the study of sociology frustrating because it does not have concrete answers and is sometimes the cause of disagreement between clinicians and academics. The study of anatomy and physiology is very different: you know it or you don't and there is little ambiguity about the facts. To embrace sociology requires students to open their minds and eyes, be curious, ask questions about the world around them and think about and discuss their own ideas and beliefs.

There are many key theorists who have done just that, have become eminent in their field and have created concepts that can still be applied to our
social world today. This is perhaps a good starting point for students who
have not studied sociology before, as it provides concepts to explore and
discuss in relation to the twenty-first century.

Every one of your actions results in a reaction from the person you are
caring for, their families, your colleagues and other social and healthcare
practitioners; sociology may assist you in experiencing positive rather than
negative reactions on a daily basis (Blaber and Storey, 2019). This chapter
asks you to challenge the obvious, think about things you take for granted,
and be curious to try and understand (a little more) about people and the
society that we are part of. Students may also learn something about themselves. Self-awareness is essential when caring for others.

REVIEW OF CLASSICAL SOCIOLOGY THEORISTS

Table 9.1 summarises the lives and work of three classical sociologists –
Emile Durkheim, Karl Marx and Max Weber – and their theories that have
relevance to society today. Although at first glance, this may not be immediately obvious, many of the contemporary theories draw upon the seminal
works of these sociological 'masters'. If you are not familiar with the work
of the classical sociologists, then please delve further into 'pure' sociology
textbooks for more detail.

Emile Durkheim

The three classical sociologists whose work originates in the eighteenth
century still have relevance today. Durkheim developed the concept of
'social solidarity' to explain the various ways in which societies can be
integrated. Durkheim also explained other types of solidarity, such as
mechanical solidarity, where individuals identify with each other, usually
because they have similar lives. Durkheim applied this to pre-modern
societies, with respect to clans and tribes. Regarding modern societies,
Durkheim identified that no individual or section of society could function without engaging in interaction with others; he termed this organic
solidarity. Durkheim states that a complete society is reliant on the close
interrelationship between individuals and sections of society. Where individuals act independently (or outside) of commonly recognised norms
of behaviour or social standards, Durkheim used the term 'anomie' to
explain their behaviour. He believed societies were at greater risk of social
disintegration because of the growth of individualism and self-importance –
with these come the increase of divergence of experiences and values for
members of society.

Table 9.1 Summary of classical sociologists and their key theories

	Key moments that may have influenced their work	Key theories
Emile Durkheim (born France 1858, died 1917)	1860–71 Franco-Prussian War – France defeated by Prussia 1914–18 First World War Brought up as Orthodox Jew Father was a Rabbi Converted to Catholicism in adulthood	Explores the nature of societies Develops the concept of 'social solidarity' Mechanical solidarity Organic solidarity Anomie Functionalism Suicide
Karl Marx (born Germany 1818, died 1883)	At university became more radicalised politically Lived in Paris Worked as a journalist Visited Germany during the 1848 revolution Exiled in London from 1849	Examined dynamics of society and changes over time Evolution of capitalism Conflict in society 'Mode of production' Power relations
Max Weber (born Germany 1864, died 1920)	Huge changes in Germany's industrial status during his lifetime Worked as an academic in economics and political economy Suffered with depression: nervous breakdown after his father's death	Explored becoming a modern society 'Rational-legal' authority 'Social action' Protestant work ethic

Functionalism assumes that society works as a social system and is not just made up of social facts. The ways we think and live are established in a culture and can be called institutionalised behaviour and beliefs, in sociological terms. The integration, solidarity and balance of a society are maintained by institutions such as the family, the political system, the education system and the legal system, each performing their functions properly and interdependently. For students who prefer human biology, think of our society as a human body: there are organs that perform necessary functions to keep a human healthy. This is, in essence, the basis of a functionalist approach.

Suicide was a subject that Durkheim studied in terms of social causes, rather than explaining it in terms of individual or psychological factors. Durkheim believed suicide was the result of social factors more than anything else.

Reflection: points to consider

You may or may not have had experience of suicide. Perhaps someone you know personally has taken or attempted to take their own life, or someone famous reported in the media. Reflecting upon this, do you agree with Durkheim that social factors are more likely to influence a person's decision to end their life, more than other factors? Social causes such as bullying, unemployment, debt or substance misuse may well have played a part, but is Durkheim right to suggest it is the *main* cause of suicide?

Karl Marx

Like Durkheim, Karl Marx was interested in the dynamics of societies and the changes that take place in societies over time. Marx wanted to explain the evolution of capitalism and how this, he believed, would eventually lead to a communist system. He was concerned with exploring conflict in society. One of Marx's concepts, the mode of production, describes ways in which the production of goods, necessary for individuals to survive and prosper, was organised in society. Marx argued that in capitalist societies, the motivation for the production of goods is to make a profit. Workers generate wealth for their employers but only get to keep a small percentage of it, a case of the rich getting richer at the expense of the poor. This is still the case in capitalist societies today.

After visiting Germany during the 1848 revolution, Marx was exiled in London from 1849 until his death. During this time, Marx tried to build a workers' party while analysing capitalism, as he believed political power is closely linked to economic power. He adopted class analysis as one of his central themes: he saw power as being unequally distributed across societies and believed that economic power is the basis for other forms of power. Two distinct forms of Marxism have developed since Marx's death: (1) structural Marxism, concerned with class exploitation and the importance of economics; and (2) humanist Marxism, focused upon the alienation of the human spirit due to capitalism.

Max Weber

Max Weber's work expresses his own fears and anxieties about modernity (becoming a modern society), which he believed was irreversible. Weber believed that an individual's needs would not be fulfilled by the material gain, increased power and economic dependence that modernity brings. One of Weber's central themes was that rules, regulations and laws naturally accompany capitalist modernity and that society would become dependent on this organised structure. Weber believed 'rational-legal' authority characterised modern society. He believed this is based upon impersonal rules that have been rationally formalised and organised without emotion or intuition and have created bureaucracy. Weber introduced the concept of 'social action' and called on sociologists to examine the consequences of individuals (or as he termed them, 'social actors'); these may not always be intended or anticipated (Punch et al., 2013; Giddens and Sutton, 2021).

Reflection: points to consider

How many rules and regulations are there in your university and clinical placement provider? We accept these and take these for granted, but are they all necessary? Are they impersonal? Is there too much bureaucracy? These are the points Weber was trying to make.

The classical theorists' work still has resonance in the twenty-first century. Other sociologists have developed their thinking and theories based upon these classical sociologists' concepts. There are key areas of our lives that influence 'who we are', such as our social class, our family, our education and our work. Some of these areas will be examined in terms of sociological theory, in order that students can link theory to their own lives and the lives of patients.

SOCIALISATION

Socialisation is an important sociological term and is perhaps an appropriate starting point for students to begin to question why they are who they are. This process commences at birth. Denny et al. (2016: 9) define socialisation as 'processes by which individuals acquire the roles, norms and cultures of society'.

The initial stages of a child's development are primarily with parents and members of the family and are face-to-face. As a child grows up, other influences, such as school and friends, become involved in the child's development; this is when formal social rules are predominantly learnt. Charles Cooley (1864–1929) was a US sociologist who developed his theory of symbolic interactionism in the 1920s and 1930s. Another writer in this area is George Mead, who linked social behaviour with social psychology. Cooley (1909, cited in Ritzer 1996) describes the initial face-to-face socialisation as being undertaken by a primary group and the latter stages as secondary group socialisation. It is when children enter other social institutions, such as school, that they realise they form part of a 'larger picture' and are, perhaps for the first time, judged by society's rules and standards. This is described as Cooley's 'primary group' theory. Another of Cooley's concepts (1902, cited in Kornblum 1997) was the 'looking-glass self', where we judge ourselves as we imagine others view us.

There are three steps to this concept:

1. We imagine how we present ourselves to others – for example, are we smart, caring, tall, funny?
2. Then we interpret how people react to us – for instance, do they see us as we see ourselves, or do they see something else?
3. We then use interpretations of others' reactions to us to develop our sense of self. If we sense that people are at odds with our perception of ourselves, then our 'self-concept' becomes diminished, and we may change our behaviour. If, on the other hand, we believe that others see us as we see ourselves, our self-concept will become stronger.

Cooley's approach is described as symbolic interaction.

Reflection: points to consider

Think about yourself. Who would you say constituted your primary group during your socialisation? Who constituted your secondary group? Does this process ever stop? Has your paramedic education socialised you in a different way? Think about the ambulance station 'crew room' – how might this (and the conversations that take place here) shape you and condition you into the 'norms' of ambulance culture? Is this a good thing? When might it be positive and when might it be negative?

During socialisation with both primary and secondary groups, an individual forms an identity. Sociologists suggest that identity formation is a combination of the physical, the personal and the social. During the process of growing up, the individual does not take on all influences, but reflects, negotiates and incorporates (or rejects) them.

Erving Goffman (1922–1982), another important US sociologist, considered all individuals to 'act' for their audiences in everyday life. His approach is interactionist. Goffman argued that our behaviour follows patterns and that individuals follow a set of instructions that influence and determine behaviour.

The interactions between ourselves and the world we live in help establish our identity. Sociologists such as Cooley (1902, cited in Kornblum 1997; and 1909, cited in Ritzer 1996), Mead ([1934] 1967) and Goffman (1963) believe our identities are subject to change and not assigned at birth. Most of us have a variety of identities that we adopt according to our varying roles in society, such as parent, colleague, paramedic, student (Goffman, 1963; Cohen, 1994).

Punch et al. (2013) suggest that as our socialisation with the secondary group increases, we will influence others' views of us through the use of dress and language. For example, consider the influence (either positive or negative) of your paramedic uniform (see case study 9.4). To challenge your own first impressions, you should take time to discover as much as possible about the person you are treating. Obviously in out-of-hospital care, this is unrealistic; as paramedics you make informed guesses or predictions about others, based on your own socialisation and your own experiences. Being aware of how we are socialised into society should enable you to appreciate the influences on development of identity and challenge your first impressions of members of society (see case studies 9.1 and 9.2).

Reflection: points to consider

What factors influence the first impressions you have when you arrive at the scene of an incident?

SOCIAL STRATIFICATION

Having briefly explored how we develop our own identities, it is logical to explore our position in society and introduce some sociological concepts/ approaches.

Inequality

The effects of not being able to escape poverty can clearly be seen in towns and cities across the UK, but the effect poverty can have on children's educational attainment may not be so obvious. Even before they reach school age, some children from poorer backgrounds are already at a substantial disadvantage. Children from financially less well-off backgrounds have significantly lower language skills, compared with children from financially better off backgrounds, by the time they commence school. There is a link between annual income and the time spent reading to children in the home. There is also a relationship between reading at home, language development and the finances of the family during the pre-school years (Punch et al., 2013; Denny et al., 2016; Giddens and Sutton, 2021).

Paramedics are faced with the consequences of financial inequalities daily, manifesting in the wide variety of homes that are visited. Inequalities are also demonstrable in the types of illness people succumb to, some of which are indicative of the person's living conditions, for example, childhood asthma will worsen in damp living conditions.

Crompton (2008) suggests that inequality leads to social stratification – members of society being ranked in a hierarchical manner. This ranking system depends on factors such as income, wealth, age, power, status and gender. The importance of inequality must not be underestimated; it has been the subject of much research and profoundly affects a person's quality of life and can specifically affect the length of life (Giddens and Sutton, 2021).

A term that students may be more familiar with is that of social class. Prior to industrialisation, societies were relatively closed. This refers to people not really moving far from where they were born and not having any other prospects, other than those associated with the social group they were born into. With industrialisation, a more open system developed, due to competition and more opportunity for social mobility (Punch et al., 2013; Giddens and Sutton, 2021). It is commonly accepted by sociologists that modern societies are stratified on the basis of social class (Crompton, 2008).

Reflection: points to consider

Would you consider yourself as being from the same social class as your ancestors?

With a stratified approach to society, it is important that we can all identify where we are in the hierarchy. The Office for National Statistics (ONS, 2021a) classification has not changed significantly since 2010 and remains the current recognised system of occupational class hierarchy (see Box 9.1).

Box 9.1 National Statistics Socio-Economic Classification (NS-SEC) analytic classes, operational categories and subcategories

Analytic classes	Operational categories and subcategories
1.1	L1 Employers in large establishments
	L2 Higher managerial and administrative occupations
1.2	L3 Higher professional occupations
	L3.1 'Traditional' employees
	L3.2 'New' employees
	L3.3 'Traditional' self-employed
	L3.4 'New' self-employed
2	L4 Lower professional and higher technical occupations
	L4.1 'Traditional' employees
	L4.2 'New' employees
	L4.3 'Traditional' self-employed
	L4.4 'New' self-employed
	L5 Lower managerial and administrative occupations
	L6 Higher supervisory occupations

3	L7	Intermediate occupations
		L7.1 Intermediate clerical and administrative occupations
		L7.2 Intermediate sales and service occupations
		L7.3 Intermediate technical and auxiliary occupations
		L7.4 Intermediate engineering occupations
4	L8	Employers in small organisations
		L8.1 Employers in small establishments in industry, commerce, services, etc.
		L8.2 Employers in small establishments in agriculture
	L9	Own account workers
		L9.1 Own account workers (non-professional)
		L9.2 Own account workers (agriculture)
5	L10	Lower supervisory occupations
	L11	Lower technical operations
		L11.1 Lower technical craft occupations
		L11.2 Lower technical process operative occupations
6	L12	Semi-routine operations
		L12.1 Semi-routine sales occupations
		L12.2 Semi-routine service occupations
		L12.3 Semi-routine technical occupations
		L12.4 Semi-routine operative occupations
		L12.5 Semi-routine agricultural occupations
		L12.6 Semi-routine clerical occupations
		L12.7 Semi routine childcare occupations
7	L13	Routine occupations
		L13.1 Routine sales and service occupations
		L13.2 Routine production occupations
		L13.3 Routine technical occupations
		L13.4 Routine operative occupations
		L13.5 Routine agricultural occupations
8	L14	Never worked and long-term unemployed
		L14.1 Never worked
		L14.2 Long-term unemployed
*	L15	Full-time students
*	L16	Occupations not stated or inadequately described
*	L17	Not classifiable for other reasons

Source: ONS (2021a).

Classification systems are rarely perfect and Punch et al. (2013) highlight some criticisms of this eight-class scale. Marxist writer Coser (1977) believes a scale does not reflect the relationship between each class and therefore negates the importance of division, conflict and dynamics of class struggle. Other criticisms of a class scale are that variations between occupations are not taken into account. Despite being in the same category, for example, a consultant doctor and a junior doctor do very different jobs and have different standards of living. The scale is based on the working population, so how are retired people and housewives represented? Crompton (2008) criticises the scale, as the occupation of the male head of household dictates the category. The terms upper, middle and working classes are still commonly used within society, but are they valid sociological concepts in twenty-first-century Britain?

There is no argument that social class affects opportunities and lifestyle. It is a common perception that we are all able to move up the social class 'ladder', if we have the right conditions to do so (education and employment opportunities, for example). This is commonly referred to as social mobility. One would assume that in twenty-first-century Britain, people have the opportunities to change and shape their lives; however, inequalities still exist.

CASE STUDIES AND ASSOCIATED THEORY

There are many inextricably linked aspects of our lives that sociologists have been researching, observing and commenting on for many years. Within the scope of this text, it is not possible to explore all of them, but the following have been chosen as being most relevant for paramedics to have a sociological appreciation of and will be accompanied by a case study and questions.

Age

Our social world is structured and ordered by age. At times, we may not be able to do something because of our age, such as enter a pub alone under the age of 18 years; or it is more acceptable to behave in a certain way because of our age – a child having a tantrum, for example. We can be both enabled and constrained by our age. Age can be classified into three types: chronological age, biological age and social age. Our chronological or numerical age results in us being able to access certain privileges and may be linked to laws, such as being able to drink alcohol legally in pubs. Biological age and chronological age are linked. Biological age is linked to physical appearance. One of the reasons why we are so concerned with our biological age and appearance is centred on society's response to biological age. It is about how you look and the way people respond to the way you look. How a person feels in relation to their age group and life experiences is termed social age. A 70-year-old may biologically look older, but may feel socially 'young' and no different to when they were

40 years of age. Society expects people to act and look their age – hence comments like 'mutton dressed as lamb' when an individual acts outside the social norm.

'Age stratification' as a sociological concept refers to the 'unequal distribution of social resources, including wealth, power and status, which are accorded to people on the basis of their age' (Punch et al., 2013: 301). Childhood, youth, young adulthood, mid-life and old age are key groupings. Some sociologists also refer to the 'old old' as an additional stratified group. Care must be taken not to apply groupings to people without considering them as individuals. People's life chances, education, family upbringing and employment will all have an impact on how they experience older age. Talking about age 'groupings' is only useful to describe people's chronological age (e.g. 'the retired'). Paramedics will also be interested in the physiological changes that happen over the lifespan. But it is also important to take time to understand an individual's experience of the life course. This will be dependent upon where the individual is at a particular point in time when they require your assistance (Denny et al., 2016). Old age and childhood are prime examples in British society where we ascribe less status and value to those age groups compared with others. Just the titles of some organisations indicate this to be true. Why is there a *National* Society for Prevention of Cruelty to Children (NSPCC) and a *Royal* Society for the Protection of Cruelty to Animals (RSPCA)?

In addition to having fun and socialising during our older years, communication technology has a major part to play in many older people's lives and can be an enriching experience. We must be mindful that this also has the potential to isolate and exclude older people who do not have access to the internet, especially if we take its use for granted. Increasingly, to be an active member of society, a person now has to own and be fluent in the use of a smart phone. For example, most car parks now require a person to have a parking app to use them, as machines taking cash have been removed. The person who does not own a smart phone, or does not wish to use one, finds themselves marginalised or even excluded from society as a result. Older people can be led to believe that they are at fault for this and that society doesn't regard them as valued members of the whole. Healthcare professionals need to think about their communications with older people and suggest appropriate advice for the 'age' and circumstance (people/families in poverty may not have internet access) in respect of technology and using it to support health care, such as re-ordering prescriptions, checking symptoms via the NHS website before making an appointment with your GP and so on.

 **Reflection: points to consider**

When was the last time you heard a paramedic give advice that required the individual to access information or appointments online? Was their advice 'age and circumstance appropriate'? Think before you fall into the same trap, it is not good 'customer care'.

Case study 9.1

Norman is a 90-year-old man who lives alone in a small bungalow. Due to his frailty, he struggles to clean his home or do any repairs needed. As a result, he lives in very unkempt conditions. Norman also struggles with personal care. He washes his face and hands every day (he cannot get in or out of a bath or shower) and he always wears a shirt and tie (though his clothes are rarely washed). He has several medical conditions, including chronic obstructive pulmonary disease (though he gave up smoking 30 years ago), atrial fibrillation and Type 2 diabetes for which he is on medications (including a blood thinner). Norman has frequent falls due to decreasing mobility. After a spate of falls, he was seen by the falls service team who fitted his home with 'grab' rails and boosters for his chair and toilet, and gave him a walking frame to aid his mobility. Norman now also has carers who come in twice a day: the morning to get him up and give him his breakfast and medications, and then again in the evening to put him to bed. Norman has two grown-up children who live several miles away and he does not see them very often.

Address the following questions and then reflect upon your answers:

- How does society view Norman?
- What is Norman's place in society now that he no longer works or contributes through his taxes or through raising his children?
- Is Norman a 'problem' for society/the NHS?
- How has Norman's role within the family changed over the years?
- How do employment, age and family role affect our view of one another?
- How might the paramedics who attend Norman reinforce a negative social view of him or challenge it, presenting a more positive one?
- Though Norman has carers, he is just one of the clients they have to see each day. How might this impact Norman's life? For example, the time he wants to go to bed or get up in the morning?

Common perceptions of what constitutes 'old age' are being challenged by older people themselves, and paramedics should be questioning their own beliefs and stereotypes of the older generation, as Case study 9.1 highlights.

In addition to being a biological process, age is also socially constructed and our experiences of age depend on society at large. As with gender, ethnicity and class, age is a social variable. There can also be social divisions associated with age; for example, the experience of ageing for a working-class woman will be very different from that of an older middle-class man (Giddens and Sutton, 2021).

Before 1990, the sociology of childhood was mainly concerned with a child's future worth as an adult. This changed in the 1990s to focus on children's present-day lives, not their future as adults. Now sociology takes children's views seriously and considers them to be able to shape their own lives, within certain constraints. There is a dichotomy in society about how children are viewed. On the one hand, they are seen as vulnerable and innocent, in need of protection from the adult world. On the other, they are vulnerable and corruptible and in need of control. Children are subject to many age-based institutions – which clearly shows the different statuses afforded to children and adults – where they learn about power and authority, including playgroups, nurseries, Cubs/Brownies and youth clubs. These experiences and membership of age-related groups enable children to understand the way society is structured through age. Our perceptions of the very young and very old are shaped by society. The influences on our perceptions are also interrelated factors: social, political and historical context, language, ideologies and media (Punch et al., 2013; Giddens and Sutton, 2021). The policies and politics associated with a particular age group also influence our thinking, which may change over time. For example, the concept of retirement is generally thought to be positive and associated with enjoyment but many older people find retirement frustrating and boring.

Case study 9.2

During concurrent 12-hour shifts where the youngest patient I had cared for was in their early eighties and where every patient had a number of age-related conditions, I had cause to reflect.

The frailty of age along with the cruelty of chronic illness started to negatively affect my thoughts about the ageing process and my view of elderly people. I started to look at some patients I went to and thought, 'I don't ever want to end up like that'. This soon became, 'I don't want to live beyond 80 years old!'

I was then called to an elderly lady (over 80 years old) who had 'difficulty breathing'. It transpired that this was a diagnosed chest infection and was being treated with antibiotics. Her reason for calling had been more to do with anxiety, which my crewmate and I were able to address by reassuring her.

As part of our assessment, I took her blood pressure, which was 120/80. 'Wow, that's Olympic standard blood pressure!', I told her. She giggled, lent forward and whispered in my ear: 'I competed in three Olympic Games'. In that moment, I suddenly stopped seeing her as some 'generic old lady' whose 'presenting complaint' I needed to address before moving on to the next 'elderly patient'. I saw her with a value I had not considered her to have before, due to the negative opinion of ageing I had allowed myself to adopt. She then showed me photos of herself at each of the Olympics she had attended along with her GB Team blazer and other Commonwealth Games medals she had won. Attending her as a patient transformed her from being a pressure into a privilege.

During that visit, I had reassured an elderly lady over her anxiety, but she had changed my view of every elderly person I have met since. Now I love meeting the old fighter pilots, Bletchley Park code breakers and athletes who ran a hundred marathons who now need my arm to lean on as they walk to their chair. Now I feel that we all have an enduring value which outlasts our 'finest hour' when we might have done something society would count as productive. We do not stop being 'productive' but we sometimes need a change of perspective to see it.

The paramedic experience of elderly people is not a normal one. The vast majority of elderly people we see are not well at all. We do not spend time with the 80-year-olds who are improving their handicap on the golf course or heading off for their weekly Pilates class – they are not the ones who call for an ambulance. This can cloud our judgement about ageing if we're not careful, which in turn could affect our attitude towards patients.

I'd like to live to be over 80 now – though I'll probably never make the Olympics!

Address the following questions and then reflect upon your answers:

- What is your view of the ageing process: is it fatalistic or hopeful?
- Have you found yourself viewing different sections of society negatively due to your exposure to them in emergency situations? In what way is this realistic or representative of these groups as a whole?
- How could you as a paramedic ensure you do not let 'the job' cloud your opinion of people?
- How could you as a paramedic act to change any negative opinion of diverse social groups you encounter in your role?

People can be 'stereotyped' within social groups and this can prevent paramedics from exploring the wide diversity of experiences or knowledge that individuals may have. All retired people had a 'life' before retirement, in addition to their retired 'life', as can be seen in case study 9.2. Do you ever ask what they did before retiring? It may provide valuable insight into their decision-making and illness behaviour. People's lives, in any age grouping, will vary according to many variables, including class, gender, ethnicity and disability. This stereotyping is reflected in the terminology and language used in society today: older people are sometimes referred to as that 'little old lady', the 'old boy' or 'old biddy' (Blaber and Storey, 2019).

In addition, women are more likely to live in poverty because their pension tends to be less than that of men. Women also tend to live longer than men, meaning they are more likely to end up living alone in later life (Denny et al., 2016). Exploring the social construction of age and ageing may assist clinicians to question their own practice, language and general approach to people.

Culture

The term 'race' is often used to describe a person's heritage, ancestry or biological differences, whereas 'culture' tends to link people to particular religious beliefs, social customs and social norms (Giddens and Sutton, 2021).

Society and culture are so closely linked that one could not exist in any 'meaningful' way one without the other. Punch et al. (2013) remind us that what is regarded as normal and acceptable behaviour by one society or cultural group may be punished as a crime in another part of the world. We all have a set of values and beliefs which shape the way we view the world;

the opinions we hold and the judgements we make about others. Our world view has its foundations in our upbringing, through the people who shaped our early development – parents, extended family and teachers – but also it develops through our own experiences, both positive and negative. Socialisation alone in a child's early years is not sufficient for physical, intellectual, emotional and social development. The quality of children's cultural experience is crucial for their development, as exhibited by cases of physical child abuse and neglect. Sociologists believe cultural deprivation can help explain differences in patterns of criminal behaviour and educational achievement between the various social groups (Giddens and Sutton, 2021).

Historical events, including the making and relinquishing of empire, globalisation, world wars, internal conflicts and the resulting mass movements of people, have resulted in people from across the world with different world views living side by side as neighbours. The potential for individuals from one culture, holding one world view, to offend or come into conflict with those of a different culture and world view is high. The potential for the paramedic to contribute negatively or positively to this situation is also high.

Sometimes, youth within a culture break away from their 'parents' culture' (Hebdige, 1979) to form 'subcultures', holding their own unique world views that are often in conflict with their parents' culture – Punks and Skinheads, Goths and Emos, for example. Most youth subcultures within British society have formed in reaction to, and often in opposition to, their parents' culture, defining themselves and their world view around norms of fashion and musical taste. It is often the case that anyone who is not regarded as being part of one's group will be considered of less value and/or as someone to be suspicious of (Williams, 2024).

Reflection: points to consider

How might ambulance service personnel contribute to or diffuse such mistrust among members of subcultures they interact with?

In many ways, paramedics themselves are part of a 'subculture' – they have a group identity that involves a uniform, a set of customs and practices, and opinions about other members of society. Students and new graduate paramedics can quickly be 'normalised' into an ambulance culture that views some calls from the public as being less 'worthy' than others, as case study 9.3 will explore.

Case study 9.3

We were called to a 24-year-old male with knee pain. En route, my crewmate and I were less than impressed, pre-judging the situation and questioning whether this job warranted a 999 call, as often happens among weary ambulance crews. Opinions about the resilience of the younger generation and their ability to manage day-to day life were expressed. On arrival, we put on our 'professional face' and walked into the patient's house to find a young man who was a quadruple amputee (having lost both arms below the elbow and both legs below the knee after developing sepsis from an infection). That day, while adjusting one of his prosthetic legs he had lost his balance and landed on the stump of his knee, causing him excruciating pain. When the pain was not managed with his normal analgesia, he had reluctantly called NHS111 for advice, and an ambulance was dispatched. Feeling very ashamed, my crewmate and I hastily adjusted our attitude and tended to our patient. We learned a valuable lesson from that job: not to let a culture of cynicism towards certain calls affect our preparation prior to arrival.

A few years later, my own son (who was 23 at the time) suffered a stroke following a traumatic neck injury. The ambulance crew who came to him (following his call to NHS111) treated him as *'a 23-year-old with a headache'*. They asked him how much he'd had to drink and if he'd taken any recreational drugs. They did not conduct a FAST test because *'23-year-olds don't have strokes'*. They eventually took him to the emergency department (ED) because he appeared to be deteriorating. In ED, the doctor suggested the cause of his headache and ataxia was stomach flu. Eventually, following his insistence on a second opinion, a CT scan revealed he was having a posterior stroke. I reflected on the fact that we are all biased towards others in society – elderly people 'are all cantankerous', a young person with a headache must be 'hungover' ... 'paramedics are all cynics'. The lesson I learnt was that sometimes what you are faced with is not what your bias assumes it is – and that if you stop and think for a minute, you could be the paramedic your patient needs you to be, rather than a person who just sees a stereotype and responds accordingly.

Address the following questions and then reflect upon your answers:

- What cultural differences have you noticed in the area where you live/work?
- Have they led to segregation or integration of people in that area?

- What initiatives and activities reach across cultural back-grounds and bring people together here? Is the ambulance service represented/active in these initiatives?
- Have you recognised that there is an 'ambulance culture'? How does this shape your thinking about patients, incidents, and other emergency services or areas of the NHS?

Each of us has varying views on the importance of one area of our social lives over another (such as family and work), but there can be no argument that culture is one of the areas of our lives that has an impact on subsequent education and employment opportunities (Punch et al., 2013; Giddens and Sutton, 2021).

Religion

The role of religion in society is as old as society itself. As such, it is recognised in the UK as one of nine 'protected characteristics' that it is illegal to discriminate against. The vast majority of the world's population holds to a world view that includes the existence of a deity or Supreme Being. In the UK, an 'atheistic' view (non-belief in God) or 'agnostic' view (the belief that there is not enough evidence to decide either way as to whether God exists) has grown steadily since the middle of the twentieth century. However, although the proportion of people in England and Wales stating they have no affiliation to any religion has grown from 25.2 per cent in 2011 to 37.2 per cent in 2021, 62.8 per cent of the population still identify with some form of religion (ONS, 2021b).

Although in the majority of cases, religious beliefs may not affect the assessment or treatment a patient is willing to accept, there are times when they do – and the paramedic needs to approach such occasions with sensitivity and professionalism. A patient's view may differ from your own but the back of the ambulance is not the place to debate the issue. However strong a paramedic's own belief on the subject of faith, they should be aware that when in uniform they represent the Ambulance Service, which has no formal affiliation to any particular religion, belief or non-belief system. While some patients may find comfort and reassurance in talking about faith with ambulance personnel during a traumatic event, this needs to be handled with sensitivity, compassion and professionalism. Lazarsfeld-Jensen and O'Meara (2013) suggest that student paramedics find it easier to discuss (in classroom situations) religion than more abstract sociological concepts. Discussing religion may enable students to examine their own fundamental values and may lead to discussion about inclusiveness, prejudice and tolerance, consent and patient choice. Examination of the students' own beliefs and values can also lead to more complex sociological debate, using religion as a 'vehicle' initially. This may translate to the students becoming more sociologically aware and confident to discuss complex issues while in the practice arena. If it helps the patient, talking about faith is not 'off limits'; however, if it does not help, do not do so. Let the patient bring the subject up if they wish, as the paramedic should not initiate such a conversation.

Emergency services personnel hold a unique position in society in that their uniform and the meaning, respect and value society places upon those who wear it grant them permission to act in ways that a culture, religion or custom might not afford others (Blaber and Storey, 2019), as case study 9.4 explores.

Case study 9.4

We were dispatched to care for a female patient whose family were devout followers of a particular faith. The husband of the patient was initially concerned that as two male paramedics, my crewmate and I should not examine his wife to assess her condition. We explained that we could request a female paramedic to attend if he and the patient would prefer, but this might take time and his wife needed urgent assessment.

The husband pointed to the ambulance crest on our shirts and said, 'Forgive me, you are medical professionals and my wife needs your help, please do all you can'. Later, as we discussed what medications the patient was taking, I was told I would find a prescription in the top drawer of a bureau in the couple's bedroom. While retrieving the prescription, it struck me how our uniform (and the importance society places in it) enable us to walk into strangers' houses, carry out sensitive observations on them, and look into cupboards and rooms in search of medications without objection. This is a privileged position to be in and should never be taken for granted, as it provides the opportunity to either build or break public trust in the service.

Many areas of our social lives are interrelated. This chapter has addressed a few of these areas; others are explored in the second edition of *Foundations* (see Blaber, 2012). To develop a deeper insight and greater understanding of sociology, we encourage you to read more widely on the subject. In addition to sociological awareness, paramedics' working lives are dictated by government policy, which is constantly changing and evolving, according to political pressures and agendas. This results in ambulance services and other NHS organisations having to respond, change practices and adhere to current social policies. Paramedics require an understanding of how social policy develops in order to appreciate the 'bigger picture' of working within a 'national' health service.

INTRODUCTION TO SOCIAL POLICY

The rate of change in government and local policy means that it is more appropriate to signpost the reader to websites that are regularly updated. The speed of change means that this chapter will likely be out of date by the time it is published!

The everyday practice of any healthcare professional is guided by social policy. An awareness of social policy is fundamental to ensuring contemporary practitioners are up to date with policy developments and 'move with the times' in their specific profession. Paramedics have a choice: to let policy be published and subsequent changes be implemented by their Trust without consultation; or be aware of proposals being made about future services, ensure they have a chance to comment as professional practitioners and individually secure their future as paramedics ahead of the game, and be aware of how policy shapes practice. Paramedics who work in this manner are often able to foresee changes before they happen; this in itself will put them in a much stronger position professionally (Blaber and Storey, 2019).

The Department of Health issues guidance on priorities for service development and circulars on a range of topics, explaining national policy that NHS bodies are expected to follow. Therefore, an awareness of the Department of Health and NHS, organisational structures and functions is useful. Their web addresses are as follows:

DH: https://www.gov.uk/government/organisations/department-of-health-and-social-care/about

NHS: https://www.england.nhs.uk/long-read/structure-of-the-nhs/

Once you are familiar with the organisational structure, you will need to know how to access the plethora of publications that are produced by the Department of Health on a regular basis. To find all their publications listed in date order, in addition to being able to filter and undertake a keyword search, go to:

https://www.gov.uk/search/all?keywords=publications+department+of+health&order=relevance.

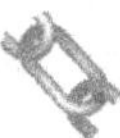

Chapter 5 for more information about successful searching techniques.

Some of the many health circulars are prescriptive and others are advisory in nature. The Department publishes Green Papers, which enable NHS bodies and other interested parties to influence the final definitive White Paper (see Box 9.2).

Box 9.2 Definition of Green and White Papers

Consultative documents can also be termed 'Green Papers'. These are published in order that comments can be submitted by members of the public and/or the professionals concerned. This is available prior to the final decisions made about service provision.

Future government policy is presented in White Papers. Some of these may go on to become Acts of Parliament.

The rate of policy production will mean that paramedics will be required to update themselves on a regular basis. During your education, you will be required to examine many of the key policy documents relating to ambulance services, emergency and out-of-hospital care.

Reflection: points to consider

What do you know about recent policy documents? Can you name some? What implications do they have for your work on a daily basis?

NHS services work differently in the four devolved areas of the UK. Please see the following websites for the structure and function of the NHS where you work:

England: http://www.nhs.uk/nhsengland/thenhs/about/pages/nhs-structure.aspx

Wales: http://www.wales.nhs.uk/nhswalesaboutus/structure

Scotland: http://www.scot.nhs.uk/about-nhs-scotland/

Northern Ireland: http://online.hscni.net/home/hsc-structure/

You will find an extensive amount of information on the websites listed in this chapter. As a current professional paramedic, you have a duty to understand how the system you are working within works, from the highest level to your more local level. Most of the ways you are asked to work (e.g. meeting targets) have come from a policy document that has its origins in the Department of Health. Many paramedics work with the Department of Health in order to influence policy and help shape your working practices.

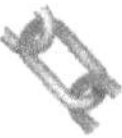 **Chapter 21** for your professional continuing professional development responsibilities.

CONCLUSION

We hope that your awareness of the importance of each of the areas mentioned in this chapter has widened your view of your own world and that of others. This chapter has asked that you reflect upon your own personal and working lives, in an attempt to make the theory more relevant to practice. It has introduced you to various sociological theorists and demonstrated the value of understanding how theory can impact practice.

An awareness of the structure of the Department of Health is a step towards understanding the process of policy development. An awareness of social policy proposals means that there is an opportunity to comment in a professional or personal capacity at the discussion stage. Being up to date with current social policy in relation to out-of-hospital care implies that paramedics are aware of what this may mean for them and colleagues in the future shape of ambulance services, and has the potential to highlight areas of personal development and career opportunities.

Chapter key points:

- The work of the classical sociologists still has resonance today.
- Our own lives and the lives of others can be explored and understood through sociological theory linked to case studies.
- Many areas of our lives can be examined from a sociological perspective, and you are encouraged to examine your own beliefs, judgements and behaviour.
- Most areas of our lives can be examined in sociological terms. There are areas that we cannot easily change and have 'grown up' with, such as culture, age and religion.

- All of these aspects of our lives are interdependent and inextricably linked.
- Sociology should encourage us to question and discover our own self and explore the world around us.
- The importance of government and local offices is explored.
- Signposting is provided to key websites.
- The importance of keeping up to date with policies is highlighted.

REFERENCES AND SUGGESTED READING

Blaber, A.Y. (2012) Social factors, in A.Y. Blaber (ed.) *Foundations for Paramedic Practice: A Theoretical Perspective*, 2nd edition. Maidenhead: Open University Press.

Blaber, A.Y. (ed.) (2019) *Blaber's Foundations for Paramedic Practice: A Theoretical Perspective*, 3rd edition. London: Open University Press.

Blaber, A.Y. and Storey, C. (2019) An introduction to sociology, social factors and social policy, in A.Y. Blaber (ed.) *Blaber's Foundations for Paramedic Practice: A Theoretical Perspective*, 3rd edition. London: Open University Press.

Cohen, R. (1994) *Frontiers of Identity: The British and the Others*. London: Longman.

Coser, L.A. (1977) *Masters of Sociological Thought: Ideas in Historical and Social Context*. New York: Harcourt Brace.

Crompton, R. (2008) *Class and Stratification*, 3rd edition. Cambridge: Polity Press.

Denny, E., Earle, S. and Hewison A. (2016) *Sociology for Nurses*, 3rd edition. Cambridge: Polity Press.

Durkheim, E. (1956) *Education and Sociology*. New York: Free Press.

Giddens, A. and Sutton, P.W. (2021) *Sociology*, 9th edition. Cambridge: Polity Press.

Goffman, E. (1963) *Stigma: Notes on the Management of Spoiled Identity*. New York: Prentice-Hall.

Hebdige, D. (1979) *Subculture: The Meaning of Style*. London: Routledge.

Kornblum, W. (1997) *Sociology in a Changing World*. New York: Harcourt Brace.

Lazarsfeld-Jensen, A. and O'Meara, P. (2013) Sources of wellbeing: sharpening a sociological tool for diverse populations, *Journal of Paramedic Practice*, 5 (4): 206–10.

McLellan, D. (ed.) (2000) *Karl Marx: Selected Writings*. Oxford: Oxford University Press.

Mead, G.H. ([1934] 1967) *Mind, Self and Society: Works of George Herbert Mead, 1934, from the Standpoint of a Social Behaviourist*. Edited and with an introduction by Charles W. Morris. Chicago, IL: University of Chicago Press.

NHS Confederation (2017) *Key Statistics on the NHS*. London: NHS Confederation.

NHS Employers (2017) *Gender in the NHS*. London: NHS Employers. Available at: http://www.nhsemployers.org/~/media/Employers/Publications/Gender%20in%20the%20NHS (accessed 9 August 2017).

Office for National Statistics (ONS) (2021a) *Census 2021. The National Statistics Socio-Economic Classification (NS-SEC)*. Available at: https://www.ons.gov.uk/methodology/classificationsandstandards/otherclassifications/thenationalstatisticssocioeconom-icclassificationnssecrebasedonsoc2010 (accessed 14 April 2024).

Office for National Statistics (ONS) (2021b) *Religion in England and Wales 2011*. Available at: https://www.ons.gov.uk/peoplepopulationandcommunity/culturali-dentity/religion/articles/religioninenglandandwales2011/2012-12-11 (accessed 14 April 2024).

Punch, S., Harden, J., Marsh, I. and Keating, M. (2013) *Sociology: Making Sense of Society*, 5th edition. London: Pearson Education/Prentice-Hall.

Ritzer, G. (1996) *Sociological Theory*. New York: McGraw-Hill.

Williams, P.J. (2024) *Interpreting Subcultures: Approaching, Contextualizing, and Embodying Sense-Making Practices in Alternative Cultures* (Interpretive Lenses in Sociology). Bristol: Bristol University Press.

USEFUL WEBSITES

Age Concern: www.ageuk.org.uk

Department of Health: https://www.gov.uk/government/organisations/department-of-health

Inequality resources: www.inequality.org (organisations with inequality-related agendas)

Office for National Statistics: www.statistics.gov

The Equality Trust: www.equalitytrust.org.uk (the Trust works to improve the quality of life in the UK by reducing economic inequality)

The Joseph Rowntree Foundation: https://www.jrf.org.uk/ (an independent organisation that works to inspire social change through research, policy and practice)

10

Introduction to the psycho-social aspects of health and illness

Amanda Y. Blaber and Chris Storey

In this chapter:

- Introduction
- Why is this relevant?
- Models of health
- Medicalisation
- Power of the health professions
- Stigma
- The sick role
- Chronic illness and disability
- Decision-making to access health care
- Inequalities in health care
- The postcode lottery of health care
- Social media and health care
- Conclusion
- Chapter key points
- References and suggested reading
- Useful websites

INTRODUCTION

Having briefly discussed some of the areas that affect our socialisation, experience of life and society in Chapter 9, it is important to look at our experience of health and illness in the twenty-first century. Everyone's (including your own) experience of ill health and access to healthcare services shapes and may dictate their views, feelings and behaviour when accessing these services again. A positive experience will enhance trust, belief and thanks. A negative experience may result in trepidation, fear that the same will happen again, delay in accessing services and a negative attitude towards caregivers (even if they are totally professional and doing their best), as this is a coping mechanism, a form of defence against being let down again. Interaction with health services usually occurs when a person or family is vulnerable. Our words/actions/reactions/omissions will be long remembered during a time of such heightened emotion. We will quickly move onto the next person in need, but the importance of every interaction should not be underestimated.

WHY IS THIS RELEVANT?

This chapter aims to introduce how sociologists and psychologists perceive what should be the paramedic's area of *business* – ill health. This chapter assumes that the reader is familiar with definitions and meaning of health; if not, see Chapter 10 in the second edition of *Foundations* (Blaber, 2012).

MODELS OF HEALTH

Paramedics are often taught to 'assess, treat, manage and refer'. This approach to patient care can be described as a 'medical' approach and sits squarely in the medical model of health care. This approach is one that has been described by sociologists and is a phrase used to describe the ways doctors practised in the past.

In an attempt to address more social issues/causes of ill health, the term 'biopsychosocial' was advocated, as a way to be more holistic and treat the 'whole' patient. There remains an underlying assumption, and sometimes a bias, that the physical body takes precedence over the mental, emotional or psychological body. This can lead to health inequalities in the way people are treated, the care they receive and the priority their illness is given.

 **Reflection: points to consider**

Think about a call you attended where the reason for the call was more for mental ill health than physical illness. Before you arrived, how was the person's illness prioritised? Reflect on the attitude of your colleagues to receiving this call to attend. Was a medical approach adopted, or was the approach taken more of a biopsychosocial one? Would you change anything when attending a similar call in the future?

In the UK, communities and families are more fragmented now than ever before. As a result, family support is diminished. The emergency and social services and voluntary community groups are called upon to try and fulfill individual and family needs. Rather than advocate the medical model over the social approaches, it is worth considering the merits of a continuum of care.

Reflection: points to consider

Think about your own family. Try and identify where members of your family lived three generations ago. Are your family members more widely spread across the UK/world now than they were three generations ago?

Paramedics expect, quite rightly, to be sent to the scene of an emergency. Therefore, in an emergency situation the medical model is wholly appropriate. For calls where an initial assessment has been conducted and it is clear that the situation is more social in nature, the paramedic will need to be competent and confident to focus on more social issues and provide more of a holistic approach. Paramedics aim to provide holistic care for all patients; sometimes, this is more medical, sometimes more social, depending on the situation they encounter. A proposed continuum of health models is given in Figure 10.1.

Of course, the focus of the paramedic is multifaceted and will depend on the following:

- professionalism;
- how they perceive their role;
- their ability to understand the patient's condition/situation;
- empathy;
- caring ability;
- level of humanity;
- own educational role preparation.

This list is not exhaustive and you may be able to add to it.

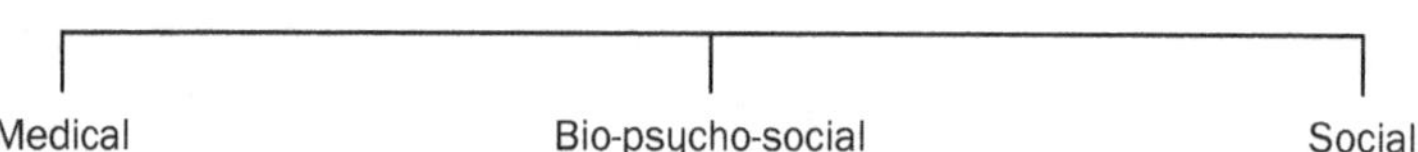

Figure 10.1   Continuum of health models used in everyday paramedic practice

Reflection: points to consider

Do you focus more on the physical health of patients or are you equally interested in their mental, emotional and psychological wellbeing?

We all have our strengths and areas that we can develop both personally and professionally. By being more self-aware of your 'comfort zone', it may highlight areas of your practice where you could develop your expertise.

MEDICALISATION

The medicalisation of health was most notably of interest to the sociologist Ivan Illich. The fact that the medical profession had extended its scope of practice to normal processes, such as birth, interested Illich. This extension of role also meant further development of the power of the medical profession over 'healthy' people and the power to define what is a natural process. Illich developed his thoughts and proposed that medicalisation also posed a risk to people who were at risk of 'doctor-generated illness' or the effects of medical treatment, which he called 'iatrogenesis'. Illich (1975) proposed three types of iatrogenesis:

- **Clinical iatrogenesis:** unwanted side effects of medications, malpractice, neglect or ignorance – e.g. diarrhoea from antibiotics; severe sickness from chemotherapy.
- **Social (spiritual) iatrogenesis:** medicine encourages people to be health consumers and seek curative, preventative medicine – e.g. visiting the doctor for the common cold; going to the emergency department for sunburn; taking vitamin supplements. Spiritually, healthcare professionals are commonly asked for advice and provide guidance on more social issues (see case study 10.1).
- **Cultural iatrogenesis:** societies weaken due to over-medicalisation, as people expect medicine to be able to cure and treat all illnesses successfully, so people's responses to suffering, impairment and death are more profound, as they feel they have been 'let down' by medicine.

Case study 10.1

James is a 47-year-old who was referred to us from NHS111. He had phoned his GP but was advised that as it was the weekend, no one was available to see him. He had been feeling depressed and ill for a number of weeks and had mentioned to the call taker that he wondered whether it would be better if he was dead.

After assessing James' physical and mental state and listening to him describing how he felt, it became obvious that his issues stemmed from his belief that his life 'was going nowhere'. He had split up with his long-term girlfriend two months earlier, had not got the promotion at work that he had hoped for and found his time out of work had become mundane and repetitive (cooking, washing and ironing, watching television, and working on his car). While talking with him and assessing his mental state, it also became clear that though 'not being here' had been something he wondered about, he had not seriously contemplated suicide.

Since the reason for James's call was more of a social issue, we listened and talked with him about how he was feeling and the support and help that might be available to him. While one of these was 'to make an appointment with his GP' (for an assessment of whether any medication was appropriate), we were also able to advise him of 'talking therapies' in the local area which might help and suggest ways he could bring variety and new experiences into his free time. By the end of our conversation, James felt a lot better. He had decided to see his GP the following Monday and planned to contact an old friend for a 'catch-up'. Just listening and encouraging our 'patient' had changed his outlook that day. Some people just want someone to listen to them for a while, and it can make a huge difference.

In relation to case study 10.1, Pink et al. suggest that 'the spiritual role that used to be the domain of the priest has been thrust into the medical sphere' (2007: 841). This has repercussions for paramedics as well as GPs, as increasingly, paramedics are acting as filters to GP services and accident and emergency units within the community. The issues of life which people face – loneliness, relationship problems, feeling unfulfilled – are still very much present in society; however, with the decline in church attendance and the rise of scientism, people have to look to alternative sources for advice and help with their issues other than the church ministers who previously took this role. Increasingly, the healthcare professional is seen as the person to provide such answers and, it seems, is also willing to undertake the role, or at least to acknowledge society's expectation that they will.

Illich persistently argued that medicine made people sick and sometimes did more harm than good. Medicalisation is one reason why paramedics get called to imminent births. Society is reliant on the medical profession, and by association, midwives and paramedics. Natural processes, such as births, would have been managed without medical assistance in years gone by across the world.

POWER OF THE HEALTH PROFESSIONS

Before discussing power, it is useful to explore the notion of what a 'profession' is. The first group of workers to use the term 'profession' were doctors within the medical profession. The superiority of the medical profession within the sphere of health care has been explored by sociologists and psychologists. They agree that a professional has distinct characteristics:

- a specialised body of knowledge;
- a monopoly of practice;
- autonomy to define the boundaries and the nature of their work;
- a code of ethics that regulates relationships both between professionals and between professionals and their clients.

Although this distinctly refers to the medical profession, some of these characteristics are common to all healthcare professions, including paramedicine. Professions have tried to distinguish themselves from this medical ideal and create their own definitions, specific to their profession or semi-profession, a term some sociologists have used for professions other than medicine within health care. The intention was not to be derogatory, but to stand alone and independent from the medical profession.

Goffman (1971) suggested that in a patient–doctor relationship, the doctor was the 'expert' and the patient the 'object' of treatment. He assumed that as the medical model understands the human body scientifically, the focus is on 'fixing it', much as you would a broken-down car. Given that Goffman's (1968b) interest was mental health, it is easier to see how restrictive, and in some cases inappropriate, a purely medical model approach would seem. History has shown us that in the large Victorian asylums, residents were subjected to inhuman and experimental brain surgery to 'cure' conditions like depression. This is just one example of an extreme, severe form of power and abuse perpetrated on vulnerable adults. As health professionals, we all have the potential to exert power over patients and families in our care. Your title and uniform have a large part to play here.

Reflection: points to consider

Think about entering a patient's home. Are you invited in? And do family members trust you in general when attending to their relative, especially when it is a child?

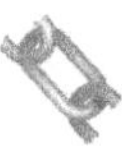

Chapter 9 and read case study 9.4.

We all work towards a positive outcome for patients, advocating for the best possible standards of care and striving to provide the most appropriate and timely care at all times. We each, however, bring our prejudices, stereotypes and preconceived ideas with us to any patient encounter. It is a 'professional' who can 'park' these and approach each patient encounter with an open mind and fresh approach. Unfortunately, some professionals will abuse their position of power with some patients.

Reflection: points to consider

- Have you ever witnessed a colleague potentially abuse their position in a given situation?
- What did you do about it?
- If it happened again, would you do anything differently?
- Refresh your understanding of the *Standards of Proficiency* (HCPC, 2023) and *Standards of Conduct, Performance and Ethics* (HCPC, 2024).

Abuse of power does not need to be abusive or overt. It can be as simple as adopting a posture that says, 'I am not interested in caring for you'; hands in pockets are a prime example of the message you are potentially sending.

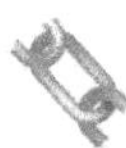

Chapter 1 for more on communication and posture and **Chapter 4** on law and ethics.

STIGMA

Pre-existing medical or psychological conditions carry with them a 'stigma' or negativity that can form deep-seated personal opinions or beliefs. Some of these can be societal in nature.

You may have witnessed your colleagues display prejudice towards a patient. Unfortunately, some medical and psychological conditions cause the person to experience stigma from society, where they may feel different or excluded, and experience inequality in life in general, not just in health-related issues.

Goffman (1968a) identified three kinds of stigma:

- The first he terms 'discrediting' or visually obvious physical deformities, such as loss of a limb or use of a wheelchair. Stigmas challenge our expectations of 'normal' social interaction and the stigmatised person is unsure of how they will be treated and how they will manage any interaction with a 'normal' person.
- Discreditable stigmas or blemishes of individual character: the stigma is not visually obvious, but may become disruptive if discovered, for example history of mental health problems, epilepsy or crime.
- Tribal stigma of race, nation and religion.

People who are considered to have a stigma very often find that it becomes dominant in their life and social role, so no matter what their other responsibilities (partner, parent, employee), they become defined by their stigmatised role, such as 'a wheelchair user' or 'an epileptic'. The use of derogatory language by healthcare professionals sometimes reinforces a person's stigma – 'the stroke patient' or 'the alcoholic', for example. It is important to be aware that attributes that result in stigma in some situations may not be the same in other situations; for example, being a single mother in some cultures or subcultures may be discreditable but is the norm in others, so may not result in stigma. It is also important to acknowledge that people with obvious stigmas may pose difficulty for the paramedic, especially if they have little experience of dealing with the general public and are new to health care. It is vital that interpersonal communication skills are practised and that difficult situations are reflected upon, in order that student paramedics can improve their interpersonal skills and approach to members of the public in a non-judgemental, confident and professional manner. Goffman (1968a) identified 'stigma' as being a social concept. This is interesting to discuss, while remembering Talcott Parsons' concept of classifying illness as a 'deviance' (1951).

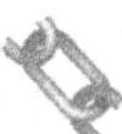

Chapter 1 for more on interpersonal communication and **Chapter 4** for ethical considerations concerning paramedic practice.

THE SICK ROLE

Parsons (1951) explored the behaviour of ill people and professional responses to it as a social phenomenon, rather than a biological cause. He assumed two things: (1) that the 'patient-doctor relationship is a social system', based on appropriate behaviour and concerned with norms; and (2) that 'illness is a deviance and is potentially disruptive to social order'. Coming from a functionalist perspective, Parsons viewed illness as disrupting the functioning of society, but was intrigued to explore the role of health care in maintaining society's wellbeing. People cannot contribute to society if they are ill – health is needed to fulfill all of our normal social roles, as a parent or worker, for instance. Having looked at this macro perspective, Parsons examined how individuals respond to illness (Giddens and Sutton, 2021).

Reflection: points to consider

Although there have been many critiques of Parsons' theory, you still have to visit your GP to be signed off as 'sick' for more than a short period. For any type of recompense – for example, holiday insurance or government benefit – you require documents to be completed and signed by your GP to validate your claim.

The term 'sick role' was coined by Parsons (1951) to describe the way individuals and social institutions concerned with medical care (hospitals, general practitioners) socially sanctioned being ill. Parsons believed that individuals had two rights and two obligations when in the sick role:

- The two rights are: sick people are allowed to give up their normal activities (going to work, school), and they cannot be blamed for their incapacity.
- The two obligations are: to get well as quickly as possible, and to seek competent care and cooperate with medical help.

Parsons makes a clear distinction between illness and other types of deviance (crime), as the person is not held responsible.

Contemporary sociologists (Allan et al., 2016; Nettleton, 2020; Giddens and Sutton, 2021) balance the discussion by noting limitations to Parsons' theory. Long-term health problems, such as diabetes or arthritis, do not *fit* Parsons' ideology, as these illnesses have no cure and the individual cannot be obligated to *get well*. However, as can be seen in case study 10.2, situations are often complex and frustrating, both for the individual concerned and the professional. The concept of power is also important when discussing the sick role, as doctors act in a social sense to sanction the sick role and also have legal obligations concerning long-term sick leave or controlling access to financial benefits, on behalf of the government. It seems that many individuals crave legitimisation of their illness; doctors and paramedics may be involved in the process.

Case study 10.2

Craig is a frequent caller to the ambulance call centre. He has chronic obstruction pulmonary disorder (COPD), is very overweight and is alcohol-dependent. He lives alone but has a friend who sees him daily and acts as his carer. Craig lives in a very unkempt flat but he likes it that way. He does not want 'official' carers and he does not want interference from anybody.

However, Craig often slips out of his chair and cannot get up off the floor. He also regularly feels short of breath due to his COPD. If either of these situations occurs, he or his friend call 999. Craig has been offered the help of support services for his conditions and situation several times but chooses not to access them. Craig is not following the 'rules' of the sick role and this leads to frustration among the healthcare professionals (HCPs) who answer his calls. Some HCPs who know Craig feel resentment towards him and speak about 'abuse of NHS services'. Craig says everyone will be happy when he is dead.

What do you think might change things more positively for both Craig and those attending any calls that Craig might make to the ambulance service in the future?

Parsons (1951) viewed illness as a deviance. This has been criticised as being too simple in its explanation of what can be a complex process in terms of accessing assistance, coming to terms with a diagnosis and complying with treatment. If your views are similar to those of Parsons, then some illnesses will be classified as more 'deviant' than others. In the sick role and stigma sections of this chapter, we have discussed the role of institutions.

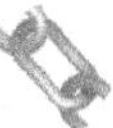 For more historical and sociological information on institutions, see **Chapter 10** in the second edition of *Foundations for Paramedic Practice: A Theoretical Perspective* (Blaber, 2012).

CHRONIC ILLNESS AND DISABILITY

Chronic illness is a feature of twenty-first-century Britain, as people are living longer. Many people experience the symptoms of chronic conditions. These vary widely but Giddens and Sutton (2021) suggest that chronic diseases share certain features:

- they present long-term health problems;
- they often present multiple health problems;
- there is usually no 'cure', only treatment for symptoms;
- there may be uncertainty about how illness will progress and when;
- they can potentially cause major disruption to the lives of sufferers and their families.

Charmaz (1983) describes a *loss of self* as being a central feature of people who experience chronic conditions. An individual's confidence and self-worth are affected. The stigma associated with their chronic condition may mean they distance themselves from social interaction, leading to a negative vicious circle. In describing the sick role, Parsons (1951) considered the individual to be passive and seeking medical help, but many individuals with chronic illness will be 'experts' concerning their condition and a valuable source of information and learning for the paramedic. It is crucial that the paramedic respects and values the individual's expertise and utilises that knowledge to learn from the patient and provide quality care for them. It must also be remembered that people living with chronic illness often have to 'juggle' relationships with health professionals, family and friends, requiring many adaptations and adjustments. It has been argued that in Britain,

> [i]mpairment acts as a reminder of the fragility and vulnerability of the body ... Most disabled people experience their actual physical impairment as the least of their problems, it is the attitudes and reactions of others to the impairment which are felt to cause the most frustration, hurt and pain. (Wilson 2006: 177)

Case study 10.3

Many disabled patients I have attended express the feeling that they are not wholly part of society. They felt accepted in certain circumstances (e.g. disabled sporting events) and when viewed as 'brave victims'. But when it came to looking round the shops on a Saturday afternoon, they 'got under people's feet' or 'clogged up the high street'. One young man, who is a wheelchair user, was applauded and praised for winning a bronze medal for Great Britain but the following day no one would help him get on a bus. 'The real kick in the teeth', he told me, 'is that the bus stop is right outside my house; I see it every day, but the step up onto the bus is too high and no one is willing to give me a hand. My legs don't work but that's not what makes me disabled ... it's society that disables me every day'.

When discussing disability, sociologists advocate a move away from a medical model, where the focus is to cure or care, and return the individual to *normal* – an example of the biomedical model. Disability is not a function of the physical incapacities of the individual but is socially created, as highlighted in case study 10.3. The focus should be on moving towards a social model, where restrictions within society that disable the individual – for example, lack of access to buildings and public transport – are addressed. The social model encourages society to enable people with a disability to participate in society and reduce oppression via appropriate social policies.

 ## Reflection: points to consider

The Paralympic movement has done much to reduce the stigma surrounding physical disability. Is this the experience of disability that people you care for have?

The vast majority of people who are physically disabled have an extremely difficult time negotiating everyday tasks such as getting to a shop, let alone shopping, due to the society and environment we have created for the able-bodied. As such, society discriminates against the disabled, when the able-bodied are capable of making adjustments. Have you ever asked yourself why door handles are not at wheelchair height? Able-bodied people have the ability to bend down to reach a door handle, something a wheelchair-dependent person cannot do.

DECISION-MAKING TO ACCESS HEALTH CARE

Sociologists have considered how and when people make the decision to seek professional help. Kasl and Cobb (1966) reviewed the literature, finding that the severity of symptoms plays only a small part in people's decision-making. There are many other factors that an individual considers before seeking help, as shown in Figure 10.2. There are other examples of such models, such as Kasl and Cobb's model, created in 1966. A person's past experience of health care is a crucial aspect of their decision-making. This is an area where healthcare professionals have the opportunity to make a difference. Every interaction that a person has with healthcare services, whether that be emergency or routine, will to varying extents affect their future decision-making. All of us need to be aware of this and take it seriously. The individuals and their situations described in case studies 10.1 and 10.2 are a case in point, where attitudes and judgements made by healthcare professionals may affect future decision-making.

If we know and understand how people make decisions and recognise that our own behaviour may have a large part to play, we can seek to modify our behaviour and image, as appropriate. If you recognise a behaviour that might have affected a person's past experience of paramedics, you are in a position to alter your public image and improve the client's view and experience of the out-of-hospital care service (Blaber and Storey, 2019).

INEQUALITIES IN HEALTH CARE

The Office for National Statistics regularly produces statistical data on a vast array of issues, one of them being inequality. Box 10.1 details life expectancy data for 2017–22 (ONS, 2024).

The data presented in Box 10.1 clearly highlights the impact that deprivation has on health and subsequently on life expectancy in different parts of the UK (ONS, 2024). Box 10.2 presents data related to the number of years that individuals can expect to live in 'good' health or have healthy life expectancy, 2017–22 (ONS, 2022). Healthy life expectancy (HLE) at birth in the UK showed no significant change between 2015–17 and 2018–20.

Box 10.2 highlights the disability-free life expectancy, which refers to the 'years of life spent free from disability'. Disability-free life expectancy (DFLE) at birth in the UK decreased significantly for both males and females between 2015 to 2017 and 2018 to 2020; this change was driven by decreases in England and Scotland. DFLE at age 65 years showed no significant change in the UK and its constituent countries between 2015 to

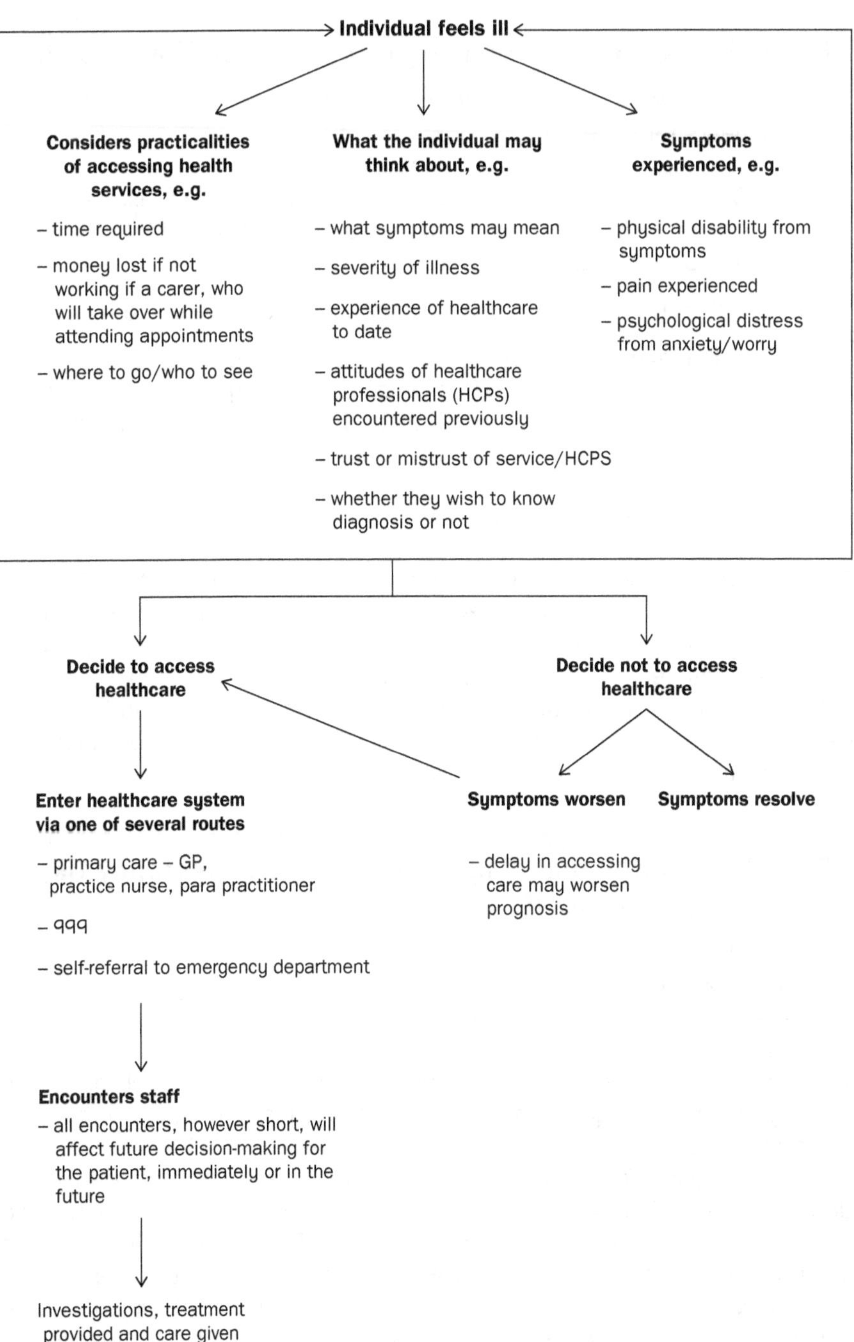

Figure 10.2 An example of a model of illness behaviour

Box 10.1 Life expectancy inequality, 2017–22 (ONS, 2024)

- Life expectancy at birth in the UK in 2020 to 2022 was 78.6 years for males.
- Life expectancy at birth for females was 82.6 years.
- Compared with 2017 to 2019, life expectancy had fallen by 38 weeks from 79.3 years for males and by 23 weeks from 83.0 years for females.

Life expectancy at birth in 2020 to 2022 was estimated to be:

- in England, 78.8 years for males and 82.8 years for females;
- in Scotland, 76.5 years for males and 80.7 years for females;
- in Wales, 77.9 years for males and 81.8 years for females;
- in Northern Ireland, 78.4 years for males and 82.3 years for females.

2017 and 2018 to 2020. It must be mentioned that figures in the ONS publications relate to the period 2018 to 2020 and therefore include mortality and health state prevalence data collected in 2020 during the coronavirus (COVID-19) pandemic. The ONS also provides regional and gender-specific statistical data for those of you who are interested in exploring inequality data in more detail. The data presented in Boxes 10.1 and 10.2 highlight the consistent health inequalities that exist in the UK.

Box 10.2 Healthy and disability-free life expectancy UK, 2018–20 (ONS, 2022)

- Males – 62 years
- Females – 60.7 years

There are many areas of life where inequalities exist and affect the health of the population. Inequalities in health and premature death have become a feature of sociologists' and psychologists' work both before and after the Black Report (Townsend et al., 1988), which suggested that inequalities were real and, in some areas, widening. Successive governments have attempted to develop social policy to try and reduce inequalities, but as inequalities are inextricably linked with other areas of social life, this is proving exceedingly difficult and economically expensive. Sociologists and psychologists have explored the prerequisites of good health (access to jobs, education and quality housing) and their impact on health. Racism affects the access to, and quality of, service received. Gender, as a social construction, affects what we expect of men and women in terms of health. The list goes on. If you wish to read more widely, the following texts provide a comprehensive overview: Allan et al. (2016), Nettleton (2020) and Giddens and Sutton (2021).

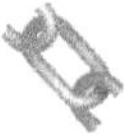 **Chapter 9** for more information relating to social factors affecting our lives.

It is not only age and disability that are affected by inequality. Indeed, all areas of our lives are inextricably linked, both in health and in our experience of and predisposition to illness. This serves as a brief introduction to the concept of inequality; see the suggested reading for dedicated books and websites on each of the subjects.

THE POSTCODE LOTTERY OF HEALTH CARE

NHS England regularly releases data on the performance of Clinical Commissioning Groups (CCGs). The government encourages patients to examine the data on their local services in the key areas of cancer, dementia, diabetes, mental health, learning disability and maternity services. Some areas have better records of access to health care than others, so this is called the 'postcode lottery of health care'. There is extensive data published by the NHS (https://www.nhs.uk/mynhs/health-wellbeing.html). One thing to consider is whether the government is contributing to health inequality by relying on website use. What about the older generation or poorer members of society who may not own computers or have internet access?

 **Reflection: points to consider**

Do you always consider a person's age/ability/financial situation when you discuss advice or recommend technology to access information?

Medication rationing

The continuing and competing demands placed upon the NHS are infinite and resources are limited. This gives rise to a basic economic problem – demand is outstripping supply. Of course, each individual patient would like the most expensive option for treatment if it promises to make the difference between them living or dying. In doing so, the cost of their individual treatment narrows the options for others, as resources are not infinite and a line must be drawn somewhere. The same can be said for doctors when they seek the best treatment for their patients, as this means fewer resources for other patients. When they choose expensive options for some, you could argue that others suffer. So, what is at play here is 'cost versus benefit'. What the NHS strives to achieve is an efficient resource allocation. Of course, if it is you or a family member who are 'denied' a treatment option or expensive medication, it is not easy to accept.

In order to prevent these decisions being subjective and arbitrary, the National Institute for Care and Clinical Excellence (NICE) has been tasked with attempting to tackle these difficult financial and ethical issues. NICE publishes guidance about whether pharmaceuticals and other technologies should be provided by the NHS. NICE provides guidance to the NHS in England and Wales when requested to do so by the Department of Health (DH) and the Welsh Assembly. The guidance indicates whether a particular technology or medication, based on the balance of the current evidence, should be recommended as the most cost-effective use of NHS resources. Since 2017, any medications that are likely to cost the NHS £20 million per year or more have been subject to further cost-benefit analysis as part of government reviews of spending in the NHS (NICE, 2024). For more information about the role of NICE and its processes, see NICE (2012).

SOCIAL MEDIA AND HEALTH CARE

You should all be familiar with the guidance from the HCPC (2020) and College of Paramedics (2019) regarding your personal and professional use of social media. If you are not, then you need to be as disciplinary cases have been brought against paramedics and other health professionals for inappropriate and unprofessional use of social media. This section of the chapter intends to examine the rise of social media in society and its use in health care from a sociological perspective.

There are huge benefits – and associated risks – of the relatively rapid rise in 'connectedness' as a result of the social media 'boom'. There are risks that we all need to be mindful of in respect of our reliance on technology.

Every social connection we make personally on platforms such as Facebook or Twitter is logged and scrutinised and we are then targeted for products and services. Your social platforms are also often monitored by employers and potential employers who wish to examine the profile of employees or job candidates. The use of social media can be personally and professionally risky if you are not clear on your boundaries and professional guidance, but there are some positive aspects.

Reflection: points to consider

- When you attend a patient, do you automatically set about connecting them to technology, such as lifepacks? Or do you take your time and actually 'look' at the patient first?
- Have you considered how your organisation would work if your computers were hacked and how you would be allocated to calls? Do you know the 'back-up' plan for your organisation?
- If you use electronic patient care records, what is the plan if the system fails?

There are intelligent uses, such as building virtual communities that link like-minded people across diverse geographical areas and in other parts of the world. These connections are devoid of limitations of time and place and, as such, may prove to be a useful means of support and solidarity, especially for shift and lone workers. Of course, this comes with risk. What may previously have been said in a mess room but shared in private, if put on social media, has the potential to be eavesdropped on by the public. Professionalism and codes of conduct are of major importance and boundaries need to be clear in the paramedic's mind. However, used appropriately and as a means of education, sharing ideas and developing the profession, social media is a powerful tool (Allan et al., 2016; Nettleton, 2020).

Remember that the use of social media within our professional role has the potential to create inequalities. For example, some older people may not be knowledgeable about social media or computer 'savvy' and therefore may even find it more difficult to book an appointment with their GP; they may lose out while relying on the telephone during office hours, while others can book appointments via the internet 24/7.

Reflection: points to consider

Think about one of your shifts. Did you give advice, treatment or refer a patient that required the use of the internet? Did you take for granted that the person you cared for had access to the internet via a computer or mobile phone? If you had thought about this, what could you have done differently?

In May 2017, the NHS suffered the most widespread hacking incident to date. This caused chaos across the country and personal misery for many patients, as operations were cancelled, ambulances diverted and departments shut down (*The Independent*, 2017). More recently in 2023, a university cyberattack led to a million NHS patients' details being compromised (*The Independent*, 2023). It is likely that such incidents will become more commonplace. These incidents emphasise the importance of having a 'back-up plan' in all areas of health care and being able to revert to basic, non-technologically reliant care.

There is a growing area of medical sociology that focuses purely on medical technology in health care. As you would expect, there is much debate on this subject, ranging from those who see technologies as discrete, inert tools to be used, abused or neglected to those who see technologies as forming part of patients' lives forever more. Nettleton (2020) provides a concise summary, if you are interested in reading further. It is beyond this chapter's scope to provide a discussion about the expensive technological equipment that is being used within the NHS. As with medications, the purchase of expensive equipment requires careful consideration and NICE is at the forefront of the appraisal of technology (for technology appraisal guidance and processes, see NICE, 2024).

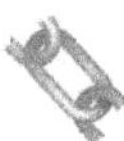 **Chapter 19** for more on digital health, telehealth and remote decision-making

CONCLUSION

The area of health and illness is complex and subject to many sociological and psychological views/perspectives. This chapter has introduced some of the issues, but it is no substitute for further reading and investigation. We envisage that students will gain an understanding of psychology and sociology and sociological/psychological principles from this discussion and hope it will act as a catalyst for further enquiry.

Chapter key points:
- We explored some models of health, the sick role and stigma.
- People react in a variety of ways to acute illness and chronic ill health.
- People's reactions and behaviour in respect of decision-making were discussed.

- Consider your communication skills, demeanour and attitude. Consider the impact you may have on a person's future health-care decision-making – are you making it easier or harder for them?
- All of the above are considered in terms of some sociological and psychological theories and theorists.

REFERENCES AND SUGGESTED READING

Allan, H., Traynor, M., Kelly, D. and Smith, P. (2016) *Understanding Sociology in Nursing*. London: Sage.

Blaber, A.Y. (2012) Psycho-social aspects of health and illness: an introduction, in A.Y. Blaber (ed.) *Foundations for Paramedic Practice: A Theoretical Perspective*, 2nd edition. Maidenhead: Open University Press.

Blaber, A.Y. and Storey, C. (2019) Psycho-social aspects of health and illness: an introduction, in A.Y. Blaber (ed.) *Foundations for Paramedic Practice: A Theoretical Perspective*, 3rd edition. London: Open University Press.

Charmaz, K. (1983) Loss of self: a fundamental form of suffering in the chronically ill, *Sociology of Health and Illness*, 5 (2): 168–95.

College of Paramedics (CoP) (2019) *Social media guidance.* Bridgwater: College of Paramedics. Available at: https://collegeofparamedics.co.uk/COP/Professional_development/Social_Media_Guidance/COP/ProfessionalDevelopment/social_media_guidance.aspx?hkey=9424140f-ca5e-444d-bb9a-2b7126bd876f (accessed (accessed 9 April 2024).

Giddens, A. and Sutton, P. (2021) *Sociology*, 9th edition. Cambridge: Polity Press.

Goffman, E. (1968a) *Stigma: Notes on the Management of Spoiled Identity*. New York: Prentice-Hall.

Goffman, E. (1968b) *Asylums: Essays on the Social Situation of Mental Patients and Other Inmates*. Harmondsworth: Penguin.

Goffman, E. (1971) *The Presentation of Self in Everyday Life*. Harmondsworth: Penguin.

Health and Care Professions Council (HCPC) (2020) *Guidance on the use of social media*. Available at: https://www.hcpc-uk.org/standards/meeting-our-standards/communication-and-using-social-media/guidance-on-use-of-social-media/ (accessed 9 April 2024).

Health and Care Professions Council (HCPC) (2023) *Standards of Proficiency for Paramedics*. Available at: https://www.hcpc-uk.org/standards/standards-of-proficiency/paramedics/ (accessed 9 April 2024).

Health and Care Professions Council (HCPC) (2024) *Standards of Conduct, Performance and Ethics*. Available at: https://www.hcpc-uk.org/standards/standards-of-conduct-performance-and-ethics/ (accessed 9 April 2024).

Illich, I. (1975) *Medical Nemesis*. London: Calder & Boyars.

Kasl, S.V. and Cobb, S. (1966) Health behaviour, illness behaviour and sick role behaviour, *Archives of Environmental Health*, 12 (2): 246–66.

Nettleton, S. (2020) *The Sociology of Health and Illness*, 4th edition. Cambridge: Polity Press.

National Institute for Care and Clinical Excellence (NICE) (2012) *The guidelines manual. NICE Process and Methods, PMG6*. Available at: https://www.nice.org.uk/process/pmg6/chapter/introduction (accessed 10 April 2024).

National Institute for Care and Clinical Excellence (NICE) (2024) *Technology appraisal guidance*. Available at: https://www.nice.org.uk/About/What-we-do/Our-Programmes/NICE-guidance/NICE-technology-appraisal-guidance (accessed 9 April 2024).

Office for National Statistics (ONS) (2022) *Health state life expectancies, UK: 2018 to 2020*. Available at: https://www.ons.gov.uk/peoplepopulationandcommunity/healthandsocialcare/healthandlifeexpectancies/bulletins/healthstatelifeexpectanciesuk/2018to2020 (accessed 10 April 2024).

Office for National Statistics (ONS) (2024) *National life expectancy tables 2020–2022*. Available at: https://www.ons.gov.uk/peoplepopulationandcommunity/birthsdeathsandmarriages/lifeexpectancies/bulletins/nationallifetablesunitedkingdom/2020to2022#main-points (accessed 10 April 2024).

Parsons, T. (1951) *The Social System*. London: Routledge & Kegan Paul.

Pink, J., Jacobson, L. and Pritchard, M. (2007) The 21st century GP: physician and priest?, *British Journal of General Practice*, 57 (543): 840–42.

The Independent (2017) NHS cyber-attack. Available at: http://www.independent.co.uk/news/uk/home-news/nhs-cyber-attack-hospitals-hack-england-emergency-patients-divert-shutdown-a7732816.html (accessed 9 April 2024).

The Independent (2023) More than a million NHS patients' details compromised after cyberattack. Available at: https://www.independent.co.uk/news/health/nhs-patient-data-attack-b2364202.html (accessed 9 April 2024).

Townsend, P., Davidson, N. and Whitehead, P. (1988) *Inequalities in Health (The Black Report)*. Harmondsworth: Pelican.

Wilson, S. (2006) To be or not to be disabled: the perception of disability as eternal transition, *Psychodynamic Practice*, 12 (2): 177–91.

USEFUL WEBSITES

NHS data on Health and Wellbeing. https://nhs.uk/mynhs/health-wellbeing.html

Office for National Statistics – specifically disability-free life expectancy by region: https://www.ons.gov.uk/peoplepopulationandcommunity/healthandsocialcare/healthandlifeexpectancies/bulletins/disabilityfreelifeexpectancybyuppertierlocalauthorityengland/2014-07-24

Safeguarding children

Gwenan Jones-Parry, Mike Brady
and Nikki Harvey

In this chapter:

- Introduction
- Why is this relevant?
- UK legislation and guidance
- Who is at risk?
- Harm, abuse and neglect
- Types of abuse
- Reporting safeguarding concerns
- Professional concerns
- Case study
- Conclusion
- Chapter key points
- References and suggested reading

INTRODUCTION

Safeguarding is an umbrella term for child protection and the promotion of children/young people's health and wellbeing. Professionals have the responsibility to recognise situations where harm has not yet been caused, and to see the early warning signs that if something does not change, children would be at risk of harm. Reporting concerns early can prevent the harm from happening.

Safeguarding has always been a paramedic's responsibility; however, it has not always been considered a high priority in education compared with, for example, trauma and resuscitation. All organisations working with children must have safeguarding procedures in place to ensure children are protected from harm. Safeguarding protects children from harm (abuse or maltreatment) and promotes their welfare; it includes the child/young person's health, growth, development and what can be done to support them to reach their full potential. Safeguarding policies must include child protection, which is the system/actions taken to respond to children who have already been harmed (NSPCC, 2023d).

Revelations and lessons learned from child protection cases, including historical sexual abuse and child deaths, as well as the current socioeconomic climate, have reiterated the need for all healthcare professionals (HCPs) to be proactive regarding child safeguarding and maintain their safeguarding knowledge. This chapter provides the reader with a basic understanding of the theory of safeguarding children and young people, which can be applied to everyday paramedic practice in a range of settings.

WHY IS THIS RELEVANT?

Safeguarding children is relevant to paramedic practice, professionally, legally and ethically – child protection is everyone's responsibility. In relation to safeguarding, a child is an individual under the age of 18 (CPS, 2023). Whether the young person is over 16 years, in full-time education or work, living in supported living, living independently or is known to the local authority, they are still classed as a child up to their eighteenth birthday in relation to safeguarding (CPS, 2023). Child safeguarding is relevant to paramedic practice not only because of the deleterious effects such experiences can have on a child's later life – emotional difficulties, drug and alcohol addictions, and poor educational attainment (NSPCC, 2024b) – but also because in many cases, such abuse can be recognised by HCPs and prevented.

Paramedics often encounter and treat children and families who are at risk of abuse/neglect, and need to be able to competently identify and respond to these concerns. Paramedics are often invited into family homes when social workers, police officers and health visitors are not; they need to understand how best to use this advantage to gather information to support the reporting of identified concerns (Brady, 2018).

The guidelines of the Joint Royal Colleges Ambulance Liaison Committee (JRCALC Plus, 2024) have a safeguarding children section which outlines a paramedic's responsibilities. The welfare and safety of the child is paramount; there is a duty to report concerns in a timely manner and inform police of any immediate risk.

The Health and Care Professions Council (HCPC) asserts that registrants should take appropriate action to protect the rights of children and ensure that the wellbeing of service users is always safeguarded (HCPC, 2023). For paramedics to meet their professional obligations, they require an understanding of child protection theory which they can link to practice effectively. Furthermore, to be able to practise lawfully, as expected by the *Standards of Proficiency for Paramedics* (HCPC, 2023), paramedics require a basic understanding of the specific Acts applicable to their practice.

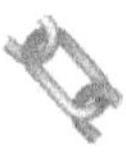

Chapter 4 for more on ethics and law.

Paramedics are often in a prime position to identify and thus prevent abuse and neglect (Brady, 2018). Quality education and training is essential for paramedics to effectively safeguard. Safeguarding children is part of many health and social care organisations' annual mandatory training and there are safeguarding training opportunities. Recent guidance has included updated safeguarding terminology (e.g. safeguarding reports have replaced safeguarding referrals). This change has originated from the fact that professionals have a *duty to report* safeguarding concerns. Table 11.1 is a list of updated terminology; these terms are interchangeable.

Table 11.1 Safeguarding Terminology

Previous term/wording	Updated term/wording
Vulnerabilities	Needs for care and support
Child protection	Child at risk
Safeguarding referral	Safeguarding report

UK LEGISLATION AND GUIDANCE

There is a long history of child safeguarding in the UK (NSPCC, 2023a). Various pieces of legislation underpin many guidance documents to help support HCPs to carry out their legal and professional responsibilities to protect children and young people. The UK has multiple Acts of Parliament that cover child safeguarding, and there are also Acts specific to each of the home nations. Paramedics should ensure they are knowledgeable of the legislation where they practise and are apprised of their employers' safeguarding policies and reporting mechanisms.

Paramedics should understand the overarching safeguarding theories and realise that legislation supports and often mandates reporting concerns. The agencies receiving safeguarding concerns will decide which piece of legislation an act/omission contravenes.

Although not an exhaustive list, Box 11.1 captures the main elements of UK legislation currently influencing child safeguarding practice.

Every Child Matters, the Children Act, Working Together to Safeguard Children and the Munro Review

Following Victoria Climbié's death in 2000, the UK government launched the initiative Every Child Matters (GOV.UK, 2003) and passed the Children Act 2004. Every Child Matters set out a range of measures to dramatically reform and improve children's care, including proposals to support parents/carers, provide early intervention, ensure accountability and propose workforce reform. Early intervention and effective prevention are key responsibilities of paramedics. The Children Act 2004 provides a legal framework for multiple guidance documents and provides a legislative duty on 'relevant partners' to cooperate, collaborate, collect data and share information (Welsh Government, 2021). Such duties include the need for professionals, including paramedics, to report their concerns appropriately, sometimes to multiple agencies (Welsh Government, 2021).

This emphasis on expanding and including all potential partners in safeguarding is reiterated in a later government initiative, *Working Together to Safeguard Children* (WTSC), first published in 2006, most recently revised in 2023 (GOV.UK, 2023c). WTSC sets out how organisations and individuals should work together to safeguard and promote the welfare of children and young people in accordance with the Children Acts (1989/2004).

In 2010, the Munro Review made recommendations to all those working in child protection and further afield, such as education and health care. The review mentions frontline practitioners within the community, and its findings are applicable to paramedic practice. Support and development recommendations include:

- regular up-to-date training and education;
- access to senior clinical support and advice 24/7;
- regular feedback or audit of their child safeguarding reports;
- access to safeguarding polices and guidance via portable tablet;
- the ability to submit electronic safeguarding reports.

There is a relative paucity of research related to paramedics' involvement in child protection, and more is needed to understand both their involvement in and the barriers they face when recognising children at risk.

Box 11.1 UK Legislation

- Care Act 2014 (Legislation.gov.uk, 2014a)
- Children (Abolishment of Defence of Reasonable Punishment) (Wales) Act 2022 (Legislation.gov.uk, 2020a)
- Children Act 1989 (Legislation.gov.uk, 1989)
- Children Act 2004 (Legislation.gov.uk, 2004)
- Children and Education (Amendment) (Jersey) Law 2020 (Jersey Legal Information Board, 2020)
- Children and Families Act 2014 (Legislation.gov.uk, 2014c)
- Children (Scotland Act) 2020 (Legislation.gov.uk, 2020b)
- Children and Social Work Act 2017 (Legislation.gov.uk, 2017)
- Children and Young Persons Act 2008 (Legislation.gov.uk, 2008)
- Children (Equal Protection from Assault) (Scotland) Act 2019 (Legislation.gov.uk, 2019)
- Counter-Terrorism and Security Act 2015 (Legislation.gov.uk, 2015a)
- Data Protection Act 2018 (Legislation.gov.uk, 2018a)
- Domestic Abuse Act 2021 (Legislation.gov.uk, 2021a)
- Domestic Abuse and Civil Proceedings Act (Northern Ireland) 2021 (Legislation.gov.uk, 2021b)
- Domestic Abuse (Scotland) Act 2018 (Legislation.gov.uk, 2018b)
- Education Act 2011 (Legislation.gov.uk, 2011)
- Female Genital Mutilation Act 2003 (Legislation.gov.uk, 2003a)
- Female Genital Mutilation (Protection and Guidance) (Scotland) Act 2020 (Legislation.gov.uk, 2020c)
- Health and Care Act 2022 (Legislation.gov.uk, 2022)
- Modern Slavery Act 2015 (Legislation.gov.uk, 2015b)
- Protection of Freedoms Act 2012 (Legislation.gov.uk, 2012)
- Safeguarding Vulnerable Groups Act 2006 (Legislation.gov.uk, 2006)
- Serious Crime Act 2015 (Legislation.gov.uk, 2015c)
- Sexual Offences Act 2003 (Legislation.gov.uk, 2003b)
- Social Services and Well-being (Wales) Act 2014 (Legislation.gov.uk, 2014b)
- Violence Against Women, Domestic Abuse and Sexual Violence (Wales) Act 2015 (Legislation.gov.uk, 2015d)
- Wales Safeguarding Procedures 2019 (Social Care Wales, 2019)

The Serious Crime Act

The Serious Crime Act 2015 builds upon current criminal and civil law to ensure that enforcement agencies can continue to disrupt, pursue and prosecute serious and organised criminals effectively and relentlessly. While it may appear to be an Act which predominantly focuses upon the management of crime, it has implications for how paramedics carry out their work, including the management of female genital mutilation (FGM) and domestic violence incidents.

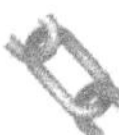

Chapter 4 for differences between criminal and civil law and **Chapter 14** for more detail on adult safeguarding.

Introduction of this Act made it a mandatory legal obligation for HCPs to report evidence, disclosures or suspicions of FGM. This bolstered the position of HCPs to report concerns without consent where needed but made paramedics among many professionals legally accountable. It is important paramedics can recognise the signs, symptoms and causal factors of FGM (for further details, see Box 11.8).

Section 76 of the Serious Crime Act created a new offence of 'controlling or coercive behaviour in an intimate or family relationship', which closed the gap in previous existing law regarding psychological and emotional abuse (Home Office, 2022). Prohibited behaviours include:

- enforcing rules and activity which humiliate, degrade or dehumanise;
- proliferating themes of family 'dishonour';
- depriving someone of their basic needs;
- threats to harm a child.

Such behaviours affect children and young people who witness domestic violence, suffer emotional abuse, sexual abuse or exploitation. Paramedics are in a prime position within the community to recognise these behaviours as they enter houses and gather information (Brady, 2018; Robinson, 2020).

Arthur Labinjo-Hughes and Star Hobson

In 2020, Arthur (6 years) and Star (16 months) were both murdered following abuse and neglect by their caregivers. Child safeguarding practice reviews were undertaken, and similarities identified in the two cases. Both involved close family members as perpetrators and concerns reported by extended family members being disregarded. The issues identified included a lack of multi-agency working, robust critical thinking and professional curiosity. It highlighted the need for sharper specialist child protection skills/expertise. These issues are not new and sadly are often seen in case reviews. One of the published key findings was the requirement for organisations to have robust information sharing protocols in place when there are child safeguarding concerns (Child Safeguarding Practice Review Panel, 2022).

Domestic abuse acts

England, Scotland, Wales and Northern Ireland have their own domestic abuse acts and importantly now recognise that children are victims of domestic abuse in their own right. With these changes in legislation, it is imperative that professionals report concerns of domestic abuse/violence when there are children at the property they are visiting. Bartlett et al. (2022) state that in Australia, few paramedics respond appropriately to children living in domestic abuse households. There are many reasons for this, including concerns about breaching the boundaries of family privacy, limited on-scene time and uncertainty regarding the responsibility to report (Bartlett et al., 2022). With the introduction of the new domestic abuse acts across the UK, it is crucial paramedics are aware of the expectation to report when domestic abuse is suspected and children involved. Moritz et al. (2020) and Bartlett et al. (2022) recommend the development of policies which clearly explain a paramedic's role in recognising children living with domestic abuse.

Ending child physical punishment

Physical punishment is when a child is punished using physical force, examples of which are shaking, slapping, smacking or hitting (Welsh Government, 2022). Laws have been changed in recent years to remove the 'defence of reasonable punishment'; these laws apply to everyone. Physically punishing a child has been illegal in Wales since 21 March 2022, after the introduction of the Children (Abolishment of Defence of Reasonable Punishment) (Wales) Act 2022. Child physical punishment has also been made illegal in Jersey (Children and Education (Amendment) (Jersey) Law 2020) and Scotland (Children (Equal Protection from Assault) (Scotland) Act 2019).

WHO IS AT RISK?

Any child can be at risk of abuse or neglect at some point during their lifetime. Perpetrators can be anyone from any background, gender, profession, race or religion, and could be a stranger, friend, family member, carer or peer (NSPCC, 2023b; JRCALC Plus, 2024). Starns (2019) states that an opportunity to take advantage is all a perpetrator needs to cause harm. Paramedics should keep safeguarding in mind during every interaction with service users as understanding risk factors can help support HCPs in safeguarding children.

There has been a lot of research on adverse childhood experiences (ACEs) in recent years. ACE is the term used for anything traumatic experienced during childhood, including harm that is caused directly (e.g. abuse/neglect) and indirectly (e.g. losing a parent as a result of divorce, incarceration or death). Long-term harm can result from chronic stress in childhood. Research has shown that children who suffered four or more ACEs in childhood were 20 times more likely to be incarcerated during their lifetime, 4 times more likely to be a high-risk drinker and 15 times more likely to have been violent towards someone in the previous twelve months (WAST, 2019). The most common contributing factor to children developing resilience in childhood is to have at least one positive relationship with an adult. To break the ACE cycle, recognition and early support are paramount (WAST, 2019).

Box 11.2 outlines some of the possible exacerbating factors that may increase the likelihood of abuse/neglect/exploitation and should raise paramedics' suspicions. These factors are for awareness/consideration but context is key to safeguarding (e.g. a family living in poverty are not necessarily neglectful, and a parent who abused themselves in childhood does not always go on to abuse their own children).

Box II.2 Possible exacerbating factors

Parent/carer/guardian

- Stress
- Aggression
- Low self-esteem
- Alcohol/substance misuse
- Mental health issues
- Lack of parenting skills
- Poor coping mechanisms
- Isolation and lack of support
- Domestic abuse/violence
- Normalised self-injurious behaviour

- Unrealistic expectations of children
- Physical and/or emotional dependence on others
- Poor communication

The environment/location

- Overcrowding
- Geographical isolation
- Other children with challenging behaviour
- Poor/insecure living conditions, homelessness

Relationships

- Financial difficulties
- Self-gain (sexual exploitation)
- Unequal power dynamic/relationships
- Challenging behaviour the carer finds intolerable/stressful
- Isolation due to the demands of caring – lack of practical/emotional support
- History of abuse in the family

There are many variables relating to physical punishment, including conscious thoughts and unconscious motives of parents (Holden, 2020). Abuse is often the result of a poor understanding and unrealistic expectations of what a child can and cannot do. For example, bed wetting and poor toilet use are viewed by some parents as a sign of insolence as opposed to normal development, and a child failing to pass an exam or win a competition can be put down to laziness or disobedience. In addition to this perception of challenging behaviour, children often display behaviours that are challenging to manage, which may lead to parental impotence and then anger. Such displays of poor coping mechanisms and inadequate parenting styles often lead to emotional and/or physical abuse/neglect. Often situations can be exacerbated by poor parental mental health, learning difficulties or intellectual limitations (JRCALC Plus, 2024).

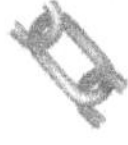

Chapter 7 and **Chapter 8** for more detail on child development, and children and young people's mental health.

Although historically, abuse was perpetrated predominantly within private dwellings, it is important to remember children and young people can be at risk anywhere. Harm can be caused within vehicles, public places, educational establishments, and health and social care settings – all a perpetrator requires is an opportunity.

It is important for paramedics to understand the risk factors to children and young people being abused or neglected. It may heighten awareness and contribute to clinical decision-making. Knowledge of such risk factors needs to be used alongside knowledge of the different types of abuse, neglect and social concerns.

 **Reflection: points to consider**

You do not need proof that a child is being abused or neglected, just reasonable grounds to suspect. If in doubt, seek specialist support or complete a safeguarding report.

HARM, ABUSE AND NEGLECT

Child safeguarding encompasses all possible forms of harm, including abuse, neglect and exploitation. Some professionals refer to abuse as the maltreatment of a child (CPS, 2023). The National Society for the Prevention of Cruelty to Children (NSPCC) defines child abuse as when a child is intentionally harmed by another (the abuser can be an adult or another child), whereas maltreatment is the cruel or violent treatment of another.

The OED offers several different definitions of abuse (formerly immoral behaviour/defilement): misuse, inflicting harm or damage (emotional, physical or sexual). Exploitation is when someone is unfairly (or unethically) taken advantage of (*Oxford English Dictionary*, 2023). It is impossible to provide definitions of child abuse and neglect that would be accepted throughout the world, given differences in race, religion, culture and gender emphasis.

Neglect is the failure to complete parenting tasks required to meet child development needs (Social Care Wales, 2019). The NSPCC (2023d) summarises neglect as a lack of love, care and attention. It is important to understand that while both abuse and neglect can be carried out purposely and with malicious intent, neglect can also result from socioeconomic deprivation or an inability to cope for various reasons. Recognising these differences is important for those working with children and young people, as the emphasis can be either one of protection or one of guidance, support and financial assistance. This highlights how complex safeguarding can be, and further highlights how paramedics should remain open-minded to possible causes, while still reporting all their concerns.

TYPES OF ABUSE

There are many ways to cause harm to children, and this section will discuss some of the main categories and their possible indicators (signs/symptoms). Paramedicine is a developing discipline, with many paramedics now working in a range of remote clinical capacities. This means not all paramedics will physically walk through front doors but will instead be working remotely. Some of the following indicators may not apply to remote working, but it is surprising how much information can be gleaned remotely.

Physical abuse

Physical abuse is defined as deliberately hurting and causing physical harm (NSPCC, 2023c). It may involve hitting, shaking, throwing, poisoning, burning/scalding, drowning, suffocating, the deliberate induction of illness or otherwise causing physical harm to a child. When paramedics assess injured children, the possibility of non-accidental injury must be considered. Even if the thought of deliberate harm is quickly dismissed, it is an integral part of assessment (JRCALC Plus, 2024). Skin discoloration (e.g. bruising) found on a non-mobile baby must be seen by a paediatrician.

Box 11.3 Indicators of physical abuse

- Extensive injuries
- Withdrawal from physical contact
- Anxious when other children cry
- Fear of returning home/history of running away
- Wearing inappropriate clothing for the weather, e.g. long sleeves in summer
- Aggressive towards others
- Parents unable to proffer reasonable explanations for injuries
- Changing explanation for mechanism of injury
- Repeated burns

Source: JRCALC Plus (2024).

Emotional/psychological abuse

Emotional abuse, also known as psychological abuse, is the persistent emotional maltreatment of a child such that it causes severe and persistent adverse effects on the child's emotional development. It includes coercive control, humiliation, threats of abandonment, threats of harm and isolation (Social Care Wales, 2019). It may involve conveying that the child is worthless/unloved, inadequate or valued only as far as they meet the needs of another person. Living in a domestic abuse household and witnessing abuse of others is emotional abuse and should always be reported to the local authority.

Box 11.4 Indicators of emotional/psychological abuse

- Low self-esteem, lack of confidence, poor personal hygiene
- Extremes of aggression or passivity
- Self-harm
- Lying, stealing (hoping to get caught)
- Poor social relationships/inability to have fun/inability to understand others
- Poor language skills/developmental delay/poor educational attainment

Sources: JRCALC Plus (2024), NSPCC (2023b).

Sexual abuse

Sexual abuse involves forcing or enticing a child/young person to take part in penetrative or non-penetrative sexual activities, whether or not they are aware of what is happening. Sexual abuse can be contact or non-contact and may involve digital aspects (e.g. the production of images/videos). Perpetrators can be of any gender, race, age, background or religion. Social media are a significant risk factor as they present perpetrators with opportunities from a distance (Quayle, 2020).

Box 11.5 Indicators of sexual abuse

- Injuries to genital areas, chest, abdomen or neck
- Blood-stained clothing/underclothing
- Soreness/discomfort around mouth or genitals
- Swollen/infected penis or vaginal discharge (consider sexually transmitted diseases and repeated thrush/urinary infections)
- Child may display inappropriate sexual behaviour/knowledge for their age/development
- Child may cry hysterically when underclothing removed
- Child may regress interpersonally, low self-esteem
- Nightmares, bed wetting, insomnia
- Talk about a 'friend' being abused
- Have large amounts of money/products of monetary value (presents) beyond their means (child sexual exploitation)

Source: BHSCP (2019).

Financial abuse

Financial abuse is now a recognised category of abuse in children, although there is limited research in this area. Financial abuse seldom occurs in isolation, but is instead seen together with other abusive behaviours (GOV.UK, 2023b). Paramedics must be aware of 'child financial exploitation', when a child or young person's bank account is used to store/move/place illegally sourced money (Fearless, 2023).

Box 11.6 Indicators of financial abuse

- Parent/guardian consistently takes child's gifted or earned money
- Child's possessions being sold to pay for parental alcohol/ substances
- Child punished for spending or has no access to their own money
- One young person in a relationship has to ask partner to use their own money
- A young person's partner does not allow them to work
- A child with a credit report is a concern for possible identity theft

Source: (EndCAN) (2021).

Neglect

Neglect is a failure to meet basic needs, or an act of omission that will impact a child's health and wellbeing (Social Care Wales, 2019). The failure to protect a child from danger is also considered neglect (e.g. a child unsupervised crossing the road being hit by a vehicle). Neglect has historically been the most common reason for children being placed on the child protection register.

Box 11.7 Indicators of child neglect

Physical neglect

- Nappy rash/poor personal hygiene (the smell of urine, unbrushed hair)
- Underweight/obese for their age
- Always hungry (stealing/scavenging food)

- Unwell often – no GP involvement
- Underdressed for the time of year/clothes do not fit
- Clingy to other parental figures
- Poor hygiene/dirty clothes

Emotional neglect

- Developmental delay/poor educational attainment
- Inability to express emotions
- Signs of stress/pressure
- Fear of new social situations/environments
- Lack of confidence/low self-esteem
- Parents may have uncaring/abrasive attitude

Source: NSPCC (2024a).

Domestic abuse

Domestic abuse is any incident or pattern of incidents of controlling, coercive or threatening behaviour (including violence or abuse) between those aged 16 or over, who are, or have been, intimate partners or family members (regardless of gender or sexuality). Domestic abuse does not need to involve physical violence; victims/survivors often say that the abuse is emotional in nature, including coercive controlling behaviours. Children are just as affected as adults by domestic abuse and are now recognised as victims. It can leave children feeling trapped, confused and afraid, and living constrained lives (Katz et al., 2020; Home Office, 2022). Coercive controlling behaviours can disadvantage children and young people educationally, emotionally, socially and physically (Katz et al., 2020).

Youth intimate partner/dating violence is defined as physical, sexual, psychological or emotional violence within a dating relationship, including stalking. It can occur in person or electronically and might involve a current or former dating partner.

Contextual safeguarding

Young people have a number of experiences outside their home environment where they can be subjected to harm; understanding and responding to concerns outside the home environment is known as 'contextual safeguarding' (formerly known as systems theory). This is an approach to looking at the wider picture; a child/young person should not be viewed in isolation from the environments in which they find themselves. Young people create different relationships within schools, neighbourhoods and increasingly on online forums, and these are not always healthy relationships. Family relationships can be greatly affected by these relationships and parents/carers/guardians often have little influence.

Child sexual exploitation

Child sexual exploitation includes relationships where a young person receives 'something' (e.g. food, alcohol) as a result of performing, and/or others performing on them, sexual activities. This is a transactional relationship, 'quid pro quo'. There is often a power imbalance between partners as one person has power over the other by virtue of their age, gender, intellect, physical strength and/or economic standing (resources) (JRCALC Plus, 2024).

Forced marriage

Forced marriage is when someone faces physical pressure to marry (e.g. threats, physical violence or sexual violence) or emotional and psychological pressure (e.g. family dishonour), and is illegal in the UK. An arranged marriage involves the consent of both parties, whereas forced marriage is not consensual.

Fabricated (induced) illness

Fabricated illness is a rare condition in which a parent or carer fabricates or induces illness/injury in others. The victim is most commonly a child and there is often no obvious motive or gain. Recognising/identifying fabricated illness is challenging and may require clinicians to suspend their disbelief and use their professional curiosity, as the child's welfare is paramount. Professional curiosity means questioning something further and not making assumptions or accepting information at face value (Leeds Safeguarding Children Partnership, 2021).

Female genital mutilation

Female genital mutilation (FGM) is also known as female genital cutting, sewing or female circumcision. This procedure is illegal in the UK (Female Genital Mutilation Act 2003) and includes any partial or total removal of the external female genitalia or injury to the female genital organs for non-medical reasons. FGM is predominantly practised worldwide on females between infancy and the age of 15. The assaults are often completed by untrained community leaders and are a breach of a woman's human rights. Although FGM may be performed anywhere in the world, the countries with the highest reported occurrences include Somalia, Egypt and Sudan (UNICEF, 2023).

Peate (2014) states that paramedics as frontline HCPs are well placed to identify girls/women needing treatment as a consequences of FGM, and to identify and protect those at risk. The introduction of the Serious Crime Act saw a legal obligation for HCPs, such as paramedics, to report actual or suspicions of FGM in children. It is important for paramedics to understand the risk factors and indicators of FGM (see Box 11.8).

Box 11.8 Indicators of female genital mutilation

- Taken out of the country, without other siblings or parent
- Taken to a high-risk country without sufficient explanation
- Difficulty urinating or frequent incontinence or urinary infections
- Menstrual problems or kidney failure/cysts/abscesses
- Relatives who are FGM victims
- Lone young females in the company of older unfamiliar, unrelated leader (the cutter)

Source: Home Office (2019).

Child trafficking

The definition of human trafficking is the

> *recruitment, transportation, transfer, harbouring or receipt of persons whether by force or other forms of coercion, of abduction, of fraud, of deception, of abuse of power or of a position of vulnerability or of the giving or receiving of payments or benefits to achieve the consent of a person having control of another person, for the purpose of exploitation. (CPS, 2023)*

There is a misconception that child trafficking means the movement of a child or young person from one *country* to another. However, trafficking applies to the movement of a child or young person from any one *location* to another, including from house to house or town to town (Barnardo's, 2024).

When children are trafficked, it can be for organ harvesting, domestic servitude, criminal/sexual exploitation or forced labour. Many children are conned, persuaded or even forced to leave their homes, as traffickers use grooming, coercion and exploitative techniques to gain trust or as a means of debt collection. Children unaccompanied when fleeing danger or moving away, child refugees and runaway or missing children are at increased risk (Barnardo's, 2024; JRCALC Plus, 2024). Children often do not recognise what is happening to them and HCPs must recognise the indicators (Barnardo's, 2024).

Box II.9 Indicators of child trafficking

- Spend a lot of time doing household chores and have no time for play
- Living apart from their family, in unregulated private foster care
- Unsure which country, city or town they are in
- Unable or reluctant to give personal details
- Not registered with a school or a GP practice
- No access to their parents or guardians
- Seen in inappropriate places such as brothels or factories
- Injuries from workplace accidents
- Have rehearsed story, similar to stories given by other children

Source: Barnardo's (2024).

Child radicalisation

Child radicalisation is a complex and multifaceted safeguarding concern and can, itself, be indicative of neglect and abuse. Radicalisation can be caused by many factors, including high unemployment, reactions to terror attacks, disillusion, disengagement from mainstream society or grooming.

The UK Prevent Strategy aims to prevent people from being drawn into terrorism and ensure that they are given appropriate advice and support. The aim is to help people make better choices and stay safe, stopping susceptible individuals from becoming involved in terrorism (GOV.UK, 2023a).

The internet makes it simpler for groups to promote radicalising content and target individuals (GOV.UK, 2023a). Adolescents as they begin to engage within their communities without their parents can be at high risk (JRCALC Plus, 2024). The age group most investigated in relation to terrorist-related behaviours is 15–17 years. Of the children younger than 15 who were investigated, many had additional needs (GOV.UK, 2023a). Of the referrals submitted by Prevent in 2021/22, 1 per cent were incel-related, 2 per cent involved school massacres concerns, 11 per cent concerned Islamist radicalisation, 19 per cent were extreme right-wing related and 37 per cent involved individuals with vulnerabilities but no ideology and no current counter-terrorism risk (Home Office, 2023a).

Through their everyday practice, paramedics will encounter children and young people who may be susceptible to radicalisation. There is a statutory responsibility under the Counter-Terrorism and Security Act 2015 to identify those at risk from radicalisation, and report to appropriate agencies. Paramedics should know their local Prevent referral mechanism as they are expected to complete referrals when they have reasonable suspicions/ concerns (no proof or evidence is required).

Box 11.10 Child radicalisation indicators

- Individuals who present as feeling marginalised, invisible or insignificant
- Reading/reviewing extremist material online
- Publicly promoting specific ideology
- Public comments regarding hate and division
- Adoption of symbols/icons of certain groups
- Plans to travel to an area of conflict

Source: Home Office (2023b).

REPORTING SAFEGUARDING CONCERNS

Organisations have reporting processes in place for when their employees have child safeguarding concerns. It is a paramedic's responsibility to ensure they are aware of these reporting mechanisms (whether digitally using tablets or over the phone). The *Standards of Proficiency for Paramedics* (HCPC, 2023) include in Standard 6.3 the expectation of responding in a timely manner when there are safeguarding concerns (both children and adults).

There may be occasions when paramedics decide there are immediate safeguarding concerns, such as when a child may have been abused by a parent/guardian; this would require making direct contact with the local authority emergency duty team and/or police. When an emergency duty team is contacted, any concern must also be submitted in writing. If paramedics suspect a crime, they need to contact the police.

One barrier to effective child protection for paramedics is a misconception that definitive proof of maltreatment is required before reporting can occur (Brady, 2018). It is the responsibility of paramedics to use their professional curiosity to identify risk and report those concerns to enable investigations by the local authority/police (JRCALC Plus, 2024).

Paramedics are in a privileged position to:

- observe if a child's needs are being met;
- observe interactions between children and carers;
- observe if a child is being adequately safeguarded from harm at home;
- gather information on the home environment.

Best practice dictates that children and families should be made aware of any safeguarding report – and ideally, they would provide permission. This is often not practical (or safe) in clinical practice, as *the safety and welfare of the child is paramount*. Paramedics can share information without the consent of the parent/guardian/child (or share it against their wishes) when there is an overriding public interest in the disclosure; when a young person does not have the maturity/understanding to decide; or disclosure is required by law. Consideration needs to be given to when and how information is shared; it must be necessary, proportionate and relevant, and shared in a timely, secure manner (Data Protection Act, 2018).

Trust between a paramedic and child cannot be emphasised enough, and the child must be treated with dignity, respect and honesty. *Any allegation of abuse by a child is a serious matter, and it is imperative they are listened to and reassured.* If a child does not have English as their first language, a family member must not be asked to interpret in cases of suspected abuse. Care must be taken not to directly accuse parents/carers/guardians, as it will make immediate communication and cooperation, and ultimately patient care and safety, more difficult.

If a paramedic is working alone, they can ask for support from their senior clinical advisor, or seek advice from the emergency duty social team (or children's emergency department). When transporting the child, paramedics must conduct a verbal handover to the receiving HCP, documenting the details of the discussion and with whom they spoke (JRCALC Plus, 2024). See Box 11.11 for things to include/cover in a safeguarding report.

Box 11.11 Factors to address in a safeguarding report

Child's developmental needs

- Health
- Education
- Emotional and behavioural development
- Identity
- Family and social relationships
- Social presentation

Family and environmental factors

- Housing and environment
- Income
- Employment
- Family history and functioning

Parenting capacity

- Basic care
- Ensuring safety
- Emotional warmth
- Stimulation
- Guidance and boundaries
- Stability

Reflection: points to consider

You cannot rely on someone else completing a safeguarding report. If you do not do it, no one will and there is a **duty to report**.

PROFESSIONAL CONCERNS

Paramedics have a statutory obligation to report safeguarding concerns they have regarding colleagues (employed or voluntary). There is a responsibility to put the safety and wellbeing of service users first. The HCPC is clear that employers should encourage a culture that positively supports practitioners reporting their concerns (HCPC, 2016). The reporting method varies depending on who the concern involves. A concern relating to a fellow HCP can be raised with their employer and if they are on the HCPC register, it can also be reported to the HCPC. Organisations should have internal policies which provide further bespoke guidance. There are regulatory bodies within the UK; any concerns regarding the management or practices of a health or social care service can be reported to the relevant responsible body. Paramedics need to be aware that HCPs in the UK have been prosecuted for abuse.

CASE STUDY

Read case study 11.1 to help you reflect on some of the main points covered in this chapter.

Case study II.I

At 0300 hours, you are called to the home of Angela, a 46-year-old female who has intentionally overdosed. You enter Angela's home and find her house to have little furniture, with no food visible in the kitchen and sections of carpet missing in the living room. As you assess Angela, her eight-year-old son Tom appears in pyjamas. There is no one else at the property. Tom appears well, but is quiet and stays to the side of the room while you treat Angela. Tom is reticent to interact with you and there is little evidence of children's paraphernalia in the home. Angela requires transportation to hospital.

1. Is there a possible problem here?
2. What would you do immediately?
3. Would you record the event, and if so where?
4. Do you need permission to report your concerns?
5. From whom could you take further advice?

Having read case study 11.1 and thought about questions 1–5, look at the reflection box below. Were your thoughts about potential action at all similar?

Reflection: points to consider

1   Yes – Angela appears to be struggling with her mental health and has taken an intentional overdose while being the sole carer for her eight-year-old son. There is also evidence Angela is

struggling to provide for the family as there is little food present and you have concerns about the home environment for Tom.

2   Discuss with Angela whether there is anyone who could come and stay with Tom while she is assessed in hospital. Contact the on-call duty team to inform them of your concerns and to let them know Angela is being taken to hospital and Tom is either at home with a family member or at the hospital with his mum (depending on discussion outcome).

3   Yes – document you have safeguarding concerns on your patient clinical record and complete a child at risk report in accordance with your employer's reporting process. Complete the report, specifying you have already spoken to the on-call emergency duty team.

4   No – it is best practice to speak to Angela, but it would be understandable (if you deemed appropriate) based on her presentation not to distress her further at this time and you could complete a report without consent.

5   You can call your operational manager, clinical support desk or duty social team for advice and support. Remember that you do not need proof to report your concerns. Share your decision with others and document the discussions/actions taken.

NOTE: It could be that Angela is struggling with mental health and finances and is currently unable to provide for Tom as she would like and requires some support. This case could also be intentional neglect. There is no expectation that paramedics know for sure what is happening; it is not for them to investigate, but to report concerns to the relevant local authority to enable them to complete enquiries.

CONCLUSION

Paramedics obviously have a key role to play in child safeguarding. Paramedics have the chance to fundamentally change the lives of the children and young people with whom they come into contact. Embedded within the community, they are called on in times of emergency and have access to children's and young persons' home environments.

Individual paramedics and the organisations for whom they work must ensure that training is of good quality, support is effective and accessible, reflection is completed and learning is embedded. Paramedics, legally, professionally and morally, have a duty of care, not to undertake in-depth investigations but to support children, young people and their families by recognising and reporting safeguarding concerns.

Paramedicine continues to evolve and there may be new career pathways for paramedics in the future (Eastwood et al., 2023). It is imperative that all paramedics, no matter where they practise, understand that they must always safeguard children.

Chapter key points:

- Paramedics have an integral part to play in safeguarding children.
- Paramedics are in a unique position within the community to identify children and young people at risk of harm.
- Paramedics are legally and professionally obligated to protect children and young people.
- Paramedics are expected to identify and report possible child abuse/neglect.
- Paramedics must maintain their safeguarding knowledge and competently report safeguarding concerns.

REFERENCES AND SUGGESTED READING

Barnardo's (2024) *Child trafficking*. Available at: https://www.barnardos.org.uk/get-support/support-for-parents-and-carers/child-abuse-and-harm/child-trafficking#:~:text=If%20you%20suspect%20a%20child,referral%20to%20your%20local%20authority (accessed 9 April 2024).

Bartlett, S., Mathews, B. and Tippett, V. (2022) Paramedics encounters with children exposed to domestic violence: identifying and overcoming barriers to sound responses, *International Journal on Child Maltreatment: Research, Policy and Practice*, 5 (1): 31–56.

Brady, M. (2018) UK paramedics' confidence in identifying child sexual abuse: a mixed-methods investigation, *Journal of Child Sexual Abuse*, 27 (4): 439–58.

Brighton and Hove Safeguarding Children Partnership (BHSCP) (2019) *Signs of sexual abuse*. Available at: https://www.bhscp.org.uk/preventing-abuse-and-neglect/spotting-the-signs/signs-of-sexual-abuse/#:~:text=Signs%20that%20a%20child%20is,infections%20or%20sexually%20transmitted%20infections (accessed 9 April 2024).

Child Safeguarding Practice Review Panel (2022) *National review into the murders of Arthur Labinjo-Hughes and Star Hobson*. Available at: https://www.gov.uk/government/publications/national-review-into-the-murders-of-arthur-labinjo-hughes-and-star-hobson (accessed 9 April 2024).

Crown Prosecution Service (CPS) (2023) *Modern slavery and human trafficking: Offences and defences, including the section 45 defence*. Available at: https://www.cps.gov.uk/legal-guidance/modern-slavery-and-human-trafficking-offences-and-defences-including-section-45 (accessed 25 April 2024).

Eastwood, K., Johnson, M., Williams, J., Batt, A.M. et al. (2023) Paramedicine: an evolving identity, *Paramedicine*, 20 (6): 177–80.

Fearless (2023) *Child financial exploitation (CFE)*. Available at: https://crimestoppers-uk.org/fearless/professionals/crime-types-explained/child-financial-exploitation-cfe (accessed 7 April 2024).

GOV.UK (2003) *Every Child Matters*. Available at: https://www.gov.uk/government/publications/every-child-matters (accessed 9 April 2024).

GOV.UK (2023a) *CONTEST: The United Kingdom's strategy for countering terrorism 2023*. Available at: https://www.gov.uk/government/publications/counter-terrorism-strategy-contest-2023 (accessed 27 April 2024).

GOV.UK (2023b) *Economic abuse toolkit*. Available at: https://www.gov.uk/government/publications/public-sector-toolkits/economic-abuse-toolkit-html (accessed 27 April 2024).

GOV.UK (2023c) *Working Together to Safeguard Children*. Available at: https://www.gov.uk/government/publications/working-together-to-safeguard-children–2 (accessed 9 April 2024).

Health and Care Professions Council (HCPC) (2016) *Standards of Conduct, Performance and Ethics*. Available at: https://www.hcpc-uk.org/standards/standards-of-conduct-performance-and-ethics/ (accessed 27 April 2024).

Health and Care Professions Council (HCPC) (2023) *Standards of Proficiency for Paramedics*. Available at: https://www.hcpc-uk.org/standards/standards-of-proficiency/paramedics/ (accessed 9 April 2024).

Holden, G.W. (2020) Why do parents hit their children? From cultural to unconscious determinants, *Psychoanalytic Study of the Child*, 73 (1): 10–29.

Home Office (2019) *Female genital mutilation: The facts*. Available at: https://www.gov.uk/government/publications/female-genital-mutilation-leaflet/female-genital-mutilation-the-facts-accessible-version (accessed 26 April 2024).

Home Office (2022) *Controlling or coercive behaviour: Statutory guidance framework*. Available at: https://www.gov.uk/government/publications/controlling-or-coercive-behaviour-statutory-guidance-framework (accessed 7 April 2024).

Home Office (2023a) *Prevent and channel factsheet – 2023*, Home Office in the media. Available at: https://homeofficemedia.blog.gov.uk/2023/09/07/prevent-and-channel-factsheet-2023/ (accessed 9 April 2024).

Home Office (2023b) *Prevent duty training*. Available at: https://www.gov.uk/guidance/prevent-duty-training (accessed 27 April 2024).

Jersey Legal Information Board (2020) *Children and Education (Amendment) (Jersey) Law 2020*. Available at: https://www.jerseylaw.je/laws/enacted/Pages/L-03-2020.aspx (accessed 7 April 2024).

Joint Royal Colleges Ambulance Liaison Committee Plus (JRCALC Plus) (2024) *Joint Royal Colleges Ambulance Liaison Committee Plus*. Available at: https://jrcalcplusweb.co.uk/ (accessed 14 April 2024).

Katz, E., Nikupeteri, A. and Laitinen, M. (2020) When coercive control continues to harm children: Post-separation fathering, stalking and domestic violence, *Child Abuse Review*, 29 (4): 310–24.

Leeds Safeguarding Children Partnership (2021) *Professional curiosity*. Available at: https://www.leedsscp.org.uk/practitioners/improving-practice/professional-curiosity (accessed 27 April 2024).

Legislation.gov.uk (1989) *Children Act 1989*. Available at: https://www.legislation.gov.uk/ukpga/1989/41/contents (accessed 9 April 2024).

Legislation.gov.uk (2003a) *Female Genital Mutilation Act 2003*. Available at: https://www.legislation.gov.uk/ukpga/2003/31/contents (accessed 26 April 2024).

Legislation.gov.uk (2003b) *Sexual Offences Act 2003*. Available at: https://www.legislation.gov.uk/ukpga/2003/42/contents (accessed 27 April 2024).

Legislation.gov.uk (2004) *Children Act 2004*. Available at: https://www.legislation.gov.uk/ukpga/2004/31/contents (accessed 9 April 2024).

Legislation.gov.uk (2006) *Safeguarding Vulnerable Groups Act 2006*. Available at: https://www.legislation.gov.uk/ukpga/2006/47/contents (accessed 7 April 2024).

Legislation.gov.uk (2008) *Children and Young Persons Act 2008*. Available at: https://www.legislation.gov.uk/ukpga/2008/23/contents (accessed 9 April 2024).

Legislation.gov.uk (2011) *Education Act 2011*. Available at: https://www.legislation.gov.uk/ukpga/2011/21/contents (accessed 7 April 2024).

Legislation.gov.uk (2012) *Protection of Freedoms Act 2012*. Available at: https://www.legislation.gov.uk/ukpga/2012/9/contents (accessed 7 April 2024).

Legislation.gov.uk (2014a) *Care Act 2014*. Available at: https://www.legislation.gov.uk/ukpga/2014/23/contents (accessed 9 April 2024).

Legislation.gov.uk (2014b) *Social Services and Well-being (Wales) Act 2014*. Available at: https://www.legislation.gov.uk/anaw/2014/4/contents (accessed 27 April 2024).

Legislation.gov.uk (2014c) *Children and Families Act 2014*. Available at: https://www.legislation.gov.uk/ukpga/2014/6/contents (accessed 9 April 2024).

Legislation.gov.uk (2015a) *Counter-Terrorism and Security Act 2015*. Available at: https://www.legislation.gov.uk/ukpga/2015/6/contents (accessed 9 April 2024).

Legislation.gov.uk (2015b) *Modern Slavery Act 2015*. Available at: https://www.legislation.gov.uk/ukpga/2015/30/contents/enacted (accessed 27 April 2024).

Legislation.gov.uk (2015c) *Serious Crime Act 2015*. Available at: https://www.legislation.gov.uk/ukpga/2015/9/contents (accessed 7 April 2024).

Legislation.gov.uk (2015d) *Violence Against Women, Domestic Abuse and Sexual Violence (Wales) Act 2015*. Available at: https://www.legislation.gov.uk/anaw/2015/3/contents (accessed 9 April 2024).

Legislation.gov.uk (2017) *Children and Social Work Act 2017*. Available at: https://www.legislation.gov.uk/ukpga/2017/16/contents (accessed 9 April 2024).

Legislation.gov.uk (2018a) *Data Protection Act 2018*. Available at: https://www.legislation.gov.uk/ukpga/2018/12/schedule/8/crossheading/safeguarding-of-children-and-of-individuals-at-risk (accessed 7 April 2024).

Legislation.gov.uk (2018b) *Domestic Abuse (Scotland) Act 2018*. Available at: https://www.legislation.gov.uk/asp/2018/5/contents/enacted (accessed 7 April 2024).

Legislation.gov.uk (2019) *Children (Equal Protection from Assault) (Scotland) Act 2019*. Available at: https://www.legislation.gov.uk/asp/2019/16/contents (accessed 9 April 2024).

Legislation.gov.uk (2020a) *Children (Abolition of Defence of Reasonable Punishment) (Wales) Act 2020*. Available at: https://www.legislation.gov.uk/anaw/2020/3 (accessed 9 April 2024).

Legislation.gov.uk (2020b) *Children (Scotland) Act 2020*. Available at: https://www.legislation.gov.uk/asp/2020/16/contents (accessed 9 April 2024).

Legislation.gov.uk (2020c) *Female Genital Mutilation (Protection and Guidance) (Scotland) Act 2020*. Available at: Available at: https://www.legislation.gov.uk/asp/2020/9/contents (accessed 26 April 2024).

Legislation.gov.uk (2021a) *Domestic Abuse Act 2021*. Available at: https://www.legislation.gov.uk/ukpga/2021/17/contents/enacted (accessed 7 April 2024).

Legislation.gov.uk (2021b) *Domestic Abuse and Civil Proceedings Act (Northern Ireland) 2021*. Available at: https://www.legislation.gov.uk/nia/2021/2/enacted (accessed 7 April 2024).

Legislation.gov.uk (2022) *Health and Care Act 2022*. Available at: https://www.legislation.gov.uk/ukpga/2022/31/contents (accessed 27 April 2024).

McCoy, M.L. and Keen, S.M. (2022) *Child Abuse and Neglect*. New York: Routledge.

Moritz, D., Ebbs, P. and Carver, H. (2020) Paramedic ethics, capacity and the treatment of vulnerable patients, *Journal of Paramedic Practice*, 12 (12): 1–7.

Munro, E. (2010) *The Munro Review of Child Protection: Final Report*, Cm 8062. London: TSO.

National Foundation to End Child Abuse and Neglect (EndCAN) (2021) *What is financial child abuse*. Available at: https://endcan.org/2021/10/21/3-forms-of-financial-child-abuse/ (accessed 7 April 2024).

National Society for the Prevention of Cruelty to Children (NSPCC) (2023a) *History of child protection in the UK*, NSPCC Learning. Available at: https://learning.nspcc.org.uk/child-protection-system/history-of-child-protection-in-the-uk (accessed 26 April 2024).

National Society for the Prevention of Cruelty to Children (NSPCC) (2023b) *Preventing emotional abuse*, NSPCC Learning. Available at: https://learning.nspcc.org.uk/child-abuse-and-neglect/emotional-abuse (accessed 25 April 2024).

National Society for the Prevention of Cruelty to Children (NSPCC) (2023c) *Protecting children from physical abuse*, NSPCC Learning. Available at: https://learning.nspcc.org.uk/child-abuse-and-neglect/physical-abuse (accessed 7 April 2024).

National Society for the Prevention of Cruelty to Children (NSPCC) (2023d) *Safeguarding children and child protection*, NSPCC Learning. Available at: https://learning.nspcc.org.uk/safeguarding-child-protection (accessed 18 April 2024).

National Society for the Prevention of Cruelty to Children (NSPCC) (2024a) *Neglect*. Available at: https://www.nspcc.org.uk/what-is-child-abuse/types-of-abuse/neglect/ (accessed 9 April 2024).

National Society for the Prevention of Cruelty to Children (NSPCC) (2024b) *Signs, symptoms and effects of child abuse and neglect*. Available at: https://www.nspcc.org.uk/what-is-child-abuse/effects-of-child-abuse/ (accessed 7 August 2024).

Oxford English Dictionary (2023) Available at: https://www.oed.com/ (accessed 7 April 2024).

Peate, I. (2014) FGM: the role of front-line staff, *Journal of Paramedic Practice*, 6 (5): 221.

Quayle, E. (2020) Prevention, disruption and deterrence of online child sexual exploitation and abuse, *ERA Forum*, 21 (3): 429–47.

Robinson, S. (2020) Child public health part 4: paramedics at the forefront of child protection, *Journal of Paramedic Practice*, 12 (11): 456–58.

Social Care Wales (2019) *Wales Safeguarding Procedures*, Safeguarding Wales. Available at: https://safeguarding.wales/en/ (accessed 27 April 2024).

Starns, B. (2019) *Safeguarding Adults Together Under the CARE Act 2014: A Multi-agency Practice Guide*. St Albans: Critical Publishing.

United Nations Children's Fund (UNICEF) (2023) *Female genital mutilation country profiles*, UNICEF Data. Available at: https://data.unicef.org/resources/fgm-country-profiles/ (accessed 6 April 2024).

Welsh Ambulance Services NHS Trust (WAST) (2019) *Adverse childhood experiences (ACEs): A guide for emergency services practitioners*. Swansea.

Welsh Government (2021) *Safeguarding*, Law Wales. Available at: https://law.gov.wales/safeguarding (accessed 26 April 2024).

Welsh Government (2022) *Ending physical punishment in Wales: Information for the healthcare sector*. Available at: https://www.gov.wales/sites/default/files/publications/2022-10/healthcare-sector-factsheet.pdf (accessed 9 April 2024).

Welsh Parliament (2020) *Children (Abolition of Defence of Reasonable Punishment) (Wales) Act 2020*. Available at: https://business.senedd.wales/mgIssueHistoryHome.aspx?Ild=24674 (accessed 7 April 2024).

12

Public health from a paramedic perspective

Madeleine Cole

In this chapter:

- Introduction
- Why is this relevant?
- Public health development
- Wider determinants of health and health inequalities
- The impact of COVID-19
- The paramedic's role in public health
- Conclusion
- Chapter key points
- References and suggested reading
- Useful websites

INTRODUCTION

As life expectancy continues to rise and individuals are living longer with chronic health conditions and co-morbidities, public health and health promotion are now arguably more prevalent features of the paramedic skill set than ever before. With the advancement of the paramedic profession, paramedics are now more exposed to the complexities of health and social care requirements and their underlying influences. Paramedics can now find employment in a variety of healthcare settings, not only providing 24-hour front-line emergency care to those with acute care needs, but also working within urgent treatment centres, GP practices and hospices, to name just a few. This increased exposure to different patient groups therefore requires a wider understanding of the meaning of public health and how this relates to the role of the paramedic within their chosen area of health care.

Though specified in the Health and Care Professions Council (HCPC, 2023) *Standards of Proficiency for Paramedics* as an element which should be incorporated into practice, the nuances of health promotion go further than encouraging individuals to take control of their own health and wellbeing. Some public health goals, such as participation in early detection cancer screening programmes and cardiovascular disease prevention, are usually conducted in a primary care setting; however, front-line paramedics specifically are in a privileged position to provide first contact and subsequent health promotion to those individuals who are unable to engage with the wider healthcare system. Though patient choice can be a factor in the uptake of services, access to healthcare services can be limited for other reasons, including the disparity in health care between socioeconomic groupings and within ethnic minority groups. Public health is, therefore, multifaceted and requires a tailored approach according to different patient needs and healthcare settings. For example, a 15-minute consultation in a GP practice may not provide adequate time to discuss health education or promotion regarding the progression of frailty unless directly related to the patient's care needs. However, a paramedic making a home visit may be granted more scope to open discussions around the holistic nature of an individual's wellbeing. This tailored approach not only applies to healthcare settings, but also to the needs of the patient and their families and/or caregivers.

The ultimate aim of public health is to prevent disease and promote good health to enable the population to live well for longer. This has evolved over recent years, with the focus shifting to reducing the inequalities in health care, ensuring health policies are person-focused and developing the role of the public workforce to ensure the health of 'the many'. As the role of the public health workforce develops, the role of the paramedic must therefore develop with it, to ensure that health risks are identified and acted on early, and opportunities for health promotion are sought out. Therefore, it is essential that both student and qualified paramedics have the underpinning knowledge and tools to understand what public health means, how it is adopted throughout communities and how, specifically, paramedics can help improve public health and reduce preventable ill health and mortality.

WHY IS THIS RELEVANT?

This drive to facilitate change in how public health is managed in recent years initially came about during the COVID-19 pandemic with the introduction of test and trace and the reorganisation of Public Health England into, what is now, the Office for Health Improvement and Disparities and the UK Health Security Agency. Not only did the public health workforce have to adapt the way in which health care was being delivered, health education and the awareness of public health became an integral part of patient care. Throughout this time, ambulance clinicians were still providing vital emergency care in society and interacting with patient groups who may not have experienced acute health needs previously. Therefore, the opportunity to adopt the preventative approach to public health broadened, and this continues post-pandemic.

Paramedics engage with the population and their health needs in a range of settings and have a unique insight into an individual's overall circumstances, allowing them to assess the patient from a holistic perspective. This allows paramedics to identify the needs of the patient and areas in which the individual may benefit from support or services that can improve their overall health. There are a multitude of preventable risk factors which can cause ill health, such as tobacco and alcohol consumption, social issues such as isolation and loneliness in the elderly, socioeconomic status and the cost-of-living crisis, mental health issues, obesity and substance misuse. Although some of these issues will require further input than what a paramedic can provide, having an awareness of them and being able to access support available can make a difference to an individual's health and wellbeing. Societal health can be improved through various public health initiatives, together with early recognition and risk prevention on the part of healthcare providers.

Reflection: points to consider

Have you ever come away from an incident wishing you could have done more? Wondering what impact your actions may have had? Or simply wondering if anything will change? Think of some prominent public health initiatives and campaigns and consider how your interactions with a patient may have been related to these and worked towards improving the health and wellbeing of the population.

PUBLIC HEALTH DEVELOPMENT

Although public health initiatives specifically did not emerge until the 1800s, various aspects of and attempts at controlling disease through public action have been documented throughout history. Even though the understanding was limited, the isolation and quarantine of the unwell occurred as far back as the 1700s through the implementation of laws in port cities to help reduce the transmission of diseases such as smallpox. With advancements in scientific and medical knowledge, the effect of public action on the epidemic spread of disease became more apparent and quarantine became common practice.

The first great advancement in public health which questioned the conceptualisation of disease and outbreak, however, was not until the 1848 Public Health Act. Though mainly economic in nature, the initial driver behind the reform was to reduce the amount of people seeking poor relief – a relief in 'aid of wages' such as money, food and clothing. The surge in the amount of people claiming poor relief, as much of this was given to the families of men who had died from infectious diseases, led to social reformer Edwin Chadwick reviewing the ways in which the health of the poor could be improved. If the health of the poor improved, the number of families claiming the relief would decline, thus reducing the costs to local parishes. His main idea to improve the overall health of the public was to overhaul the sanitation system, or lack thereof. This was due to the appalling unsanitary conditions in working-class areas and, as a result, an unprecedented level of infectious diseases, such as cholera and typhoid, leading to very poor life expectancy. Despite efforts at quarantine, the over-population of these areas meant that attempts at controlling any outbreak were futile. The industrial revolution and urbanisation meant that the class divide no longer provided protection to the wealthy and the spread of infectious disease across all classes was unavoidable. The previous notion that disease only affected the impoverished or those of poor moral standing was dismissed, and the common goal became the cleanliness of the shared environment and improvement in living and working conditions. This more 'holistic' approach also included a change in the treatment of mental health issues and an understanding that there were several compounding factors which led to a diagnosis.

Part of Chadwick's reform was to introduce a National Board of Health and local district boards that would oversee the implementation of the infrastructure needed to achieve improvements in sanitation. Even with the introduction of the Public Health Act 1848, and Chadwick's controversial proposals, it was not until 1871 and three further outbreaks of cholera later, that these local boards were given formal powers to protect the public from disease. This led to advancements in providing access to clean water and sewage systems, waste disposal, and improvements to city landscapes and environments. With sanitation reform and an understanding that disease was a societal problem and therefore public health also needed to be viewed in this manner, the notion of protecting the health of the many became viewed as public activity. This change in mindset paved the way for further developments in public health (UK Parliament, no date; Hamlin, 2010).

Now that epidemiology had begun to be explored and scientific understanding of disease and bacteria had developed, the focus became proactive care in the form of vaccinations and antibiotics. Variolation and inoculation date back hundreds of years and were key elements in the eradication of smallpox. Practices from Asia and parts of Africa were documented to show that exposing others to small doses of the disease could help develop immunity. These practices were built upon, leading to the first successful vaccine against smallpox in 1796. Extensive testing showed that the vaccine was successful in preventing smallpox and eventually vaccines became mandatory in some parts of the world. In 1980, following worldwide vaccination programmes, smallpox was officially declared eradicated. Significant developments in vaccines progressed over the course of the next two centuries with notable advancements in the 1900s against diseases such as yellow fever, influenza, polio and the MMR vaccine. More recently, the development of the COVID-19 vaccination was an integral part of reducing the severity of the disease and lowering mortality rates.

With the use of antibiotics and vaccines, the leading causes of deaths changed over time from transmissible diseases to non-communicable diseases such as cancer, cardiovascular disease and diabetes. In the UK today, the leading causes of death are dementia and Alzheimer's disease, closely followed by ischaemic heart disease (ONS, 2023). This shift in the causes of mortality led to further understanding of the links between lifestyle and disease and that the onus for prevention must be, in some capacity, down to the individual. Targeting high-risk patient groups through various screening programmes allowed the public health workforce to provide health education aimed at reducing mortality through preventable illness. For example, identifying those with high cholesterol and prescribing a statin where appropriate to reduce the risk of ischaemic heart disease. However, despite multiple public health campaigns and health education provided by the public health workforce, preventable disease and chronic conditions still consume a large proportion of health resources. This has led to a call, in recent years, for individual *and* shared responsibility in public health. Providing individuals with the knowledge, tools and resources they need for healthier behaviour will allow people to live well for longer and, in turn, reduce the burden on health services. This, however, can only be achieved if the wider determinants of health are fully understood and healthcare goals are aligned to reduce health inequalities.

Activity

Public health has developed into its own discipline, with health professionals compiling an annual calendar of campaigns, initiatives and events. Have a look at the campaigns listed below and consider incidents you either attended or that you might attend where you could draw on these campaigns to promote public health and assist in improving the health and wellbeing of everyone. Jot down your ideas.

- Action on Stroke Month
- Carers Week
- COPD Awareness Month
- Death Awareness Week
- Diabetes Week
- Dry January
- Epilepsy Awareness Purple Day
- International Day for the Elimination of Violence Against Women
- International Overdose Day
- Mental Health Awareness Week
- Movember: men's health awareness month
- National Obesity Awareness Week
- National Personal Safety Day
- National Stress Awareness Day
- No Smoking Day
- Sun Awareness Week
- World Asthma Day
- World Blood Donor Day
- World Health Day
- World Suicide Prevention Day

WIDER DETERMINENTS OF HEALTH AND HEALTH INEQUALITIES

Although public health initiatives have enabled significant progress in improving the health of the population, recently this progression has slowed. Whilst life expectancy has increased, the gap in life expectancy between the various socioeconomic groups has also increased and current data shows that individuals can spend approximately 20 per cent of their life in poor health (DHSC, 2021). The Office for National Statistics (2022) identified that in 2020, almost half of the UK population reported having at least one long-standing health problem. Approximately 50 per cent of hospital admissions and primary care consultations involve individuals who have two or more chronic health conditions (DHSC, 2021), meaning that paramedics are likely to be involved in the assessment and treatment of these patients in some capacity.

As a result of these figures, plans have been proposed to improve the outcomes of six major health conditions: cancer, cardiovascular disease, musculoskeletal disorders, mental health, dementia and chronic respiratory diseases. Together, these diseases account for over 60 per cent of early mortality and ill health in England (DHSC, 2021). These diseases share commonalities in that the risk factors for developing them, such as lifestyle factors, living conditions, employment, access to green spaces and education, are the same. The initial aim is to address the lifestyle choices that can lead to these adverse health outcomes through primary and proactive prevention to manage personalised risk factors. However, to be able to truly educate and enable individuals to be active participants in their own care, the wider determinants of health must be addressed.

The wider determinants of health are part of the complex interactions which contribute to an individual's health and wellbeing. This combination of individual or constitutional factors, such as age and genetics, specific lifestyle factors, community networks, and socioeconomic and environmental conditions, has a significant influence on long-term health, usually across many years. The variation in these factors can contribute to health and social inequalities, and these inequalities make it harder to achieve specific health goals as access to physical, social and personal resources to drive change are often limited. Addressing these factors specifically is argued to be more important than health care in isolation for developing a healthy population (Raleigh, 2023).

This leads to complexities for ambulance clinicians when trying to adopt a public health approach within their practice. Providing health education as a form of primary prevention may seem straightforward, but there may be significant obstacles out of individual control which prevent uptake of healthy behaviours. As Chadwick found in the 1800s, and which is still evident today, income and health are strongly connected. A low-income family, for example, may be more likely to purchase ultra-processed foods (UPF) due to their affordability, despite new research with shows that a high UPF diet has risk factors for cardiovascular disease, diabetes and early mortality (Chang et al., 2023). Whilst health promotion in this context is important so that individuals have the 'toolkits' available to help them make informed choices about their health, the socioeconomic status of an individual or family will limit the choices that can realistically be made.

The living environment of individuals can also greatly influence long-term health. Disadvantaged communities are often exposed to poor air quality and are more likely to be living close to highly polluted areas, such as busy roads and built-up urban environments. Whilst there has been considerable public health achievement with the reduction of smoking to reduce chronic respiratory conditions, the prevalence of both cardiac and respiratory issues for those living in areas with high levels of air pollution is on the rise (PHE, 2018d). Access to green spaces within urban environments has proven beneficial in health care as it encourages outdoor recreational activity and improves mental health. These green spaces are limited within areas of deprivation and the unequal distribution compared to areas of affluence is a likely contributor to risk factors such as exposure to air pollution and limited scope for exercise.

Many of these inequalities start early in life and have a significant influence on health over one's lifespan. Children born in deprived areas are at greater risk of a low birth weight, tooth decay and living with obesity (PHE, 2018a). In an assessment of children in the English school system aged 4–5 years, low-income areas were shown to have worse outcomes for 'school readiness', taking into account all aspects of social, behavioural and physical development. As a result of this, 'school readiness' is classed as a wider determinant of health due to its influence on long-term development, learning opportunities and educational qualifications. Education provides individuals with opportunities that can influence and contribute to positive health outcomes and access to health resources. Without the early and equal opportunity to thrive, the gap in health inequalities will continue to widen.

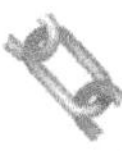

Chapter 9 and **Chapter 10** for relevant sociological theory, the complexities of social issues, and the social factors impacting individuals' decision-making about their own health and wellbeing.

THE IMPACT OF COVID-19 ON PUBLIC HEALTH

The aim in reducing health inequalities means that organisations involved with supporting individuals with their health and social care needs will attempt to move away from a reactive response and initiate proactive forms of care. However, the increased pressure on resources, cuts to funding, delays and backlogs caused by the COVID-19 pandemic create real challenges in reducing health inequalities and providing the support needed to address immediate issues. In fact, the COVID-19 pandemic played a pivotal role in unearthing health and societal issues which have been unaddressed and potentially misunderstood for many years. The pandemic was the greatest threat to public health in the twentieth century. In the UK, infection and mortality rates were highest amongst the elderly, ethnic minority communities and people living with disabilities. Evidence showed that people from ethnic minority groups were three times as likely to contact COVID-19 and five times more likely to suffer serious outcomes as a result (Lally, 2020). These data, combined with mortality figures and rates of infection, highlighted the need for preparedness regarding health security and future infectious diseases, and thus the UK Health Security Agency was set up. Health improvement and tackling the inequalities exposed by the pandemic became the responsibility of the Office for Health Improvement and Disparities.

Whilst the exacerbation of health inequalities resulting from the pandemic is evident, other public health issues are now being highlighted. A proportion of the population infected with COVID-19 have developed 'long covid': signs, symptoms and conditions which continue after the acute infection stage. These long-term effects can last from weeks to years and create chronic health problems. These chronic health problems lead to repeated contact with healthcare services, increasing demand and creating a new cohort of individuals living in poor health. Mental health outcomes have been documented globally in patients infected with COVID-19 as well as people generally as a result of lockdowns. There were higher reported levels of stress, anxiety and depression, especially amongst children and adolescents whose daily routines and education were disrupted beyond recognition.

The lasting effects of the pandemic are still being felt by healthcare services: the NHS waiting lists for secondary care and the consequences of delayed care, alongside these additional needs as a result of lockdown, means that the health and social care system is under severe pressure. An awareness of the wider determinants of health and health inequalities, the impact of the recent global pandemic and the subsequent effect of the delivery of health services is necessary for ambulance clinicians and paramedics to deliver a public health approach effectively. This means tailoring care, utilising suitable referral pathways and using clinical judgement to help make decisions in the best interests of their patients.

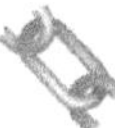 **Chapter 7** and **Chapter 8** for more on psychological theory and the effects of COVID-19.

THE PARAMEDIC'S ROLE IN PUBLIC HEALTH

The paramedic role has evolved not only in the UK but also globally. The increase in demand for the paramedic skill set, as well as the need to increase access to services and reduce the burden on emergency services, has led to developments which provide paramedics with the ability to address the wider determinants of health. Though it is an integral part of the role, there is no published framework or defined model of public health approach within the ambulance service or the wider paramedic profession. Therefore, the approach varies between clinicians and environments and could ultimately hinder the progress of public health activity.

In 2021, the Association of Ambulance Chief Executives published a paper on the development of a public health approach within the ambulance sector (AACE, 2021). The COVID-19 pandemic highlighted the prevalence of health inequalities in the UK and how people living in deprived areas were at greater risk of contracting coronavirus and potentially more serious outcomes as a result. The pandemic had a detrimental effect on the NHS as a whole, with longer waiting times, cancelled appointments and delays in routine care often impacting those already facing health inequalities. Paired with the economic recession, the lasting effects of the pandemic have widened the ever-growing disparities in health care. Recent government policy and the introduction of the Office for Health Improvement and Disparities has led to a focus on addressing inequalities through collaborative care and a public health approach. Therefore, incorporating a public health approach into practice is now the norm for all allied health professionals.

So, what would this look like in practice for paramedics and ambulance clinicians specifically? The paper by AACE (2021) discusses key approaches which underpin the public health approach. They are summarised below.

Population focus

Whilst front-line clinicians deal with the individual needs of patients they attend, the scope of the ambulance service allows health to be considered at a population level. This means improving the health and wellbeing of communities through targeted intervention and the way in which health and social care services are implemented. This can be actioned by utilising health-related data to identify populations or patient groups that ought to be considered a priority. Whilst such health data may not be relevant at an individual level, in practice, a population approach means that paramedics need to make a holistic assessment to identify those in greatest need and who require prioritised care. A patient who presents with a chronic health condition but is well supported by friends or family and related care services may not need additional advice or onward referral. A more isolated individual without a support network, however, may require additional advice and service input. This will involve ambulance clinicians considering possible safeguarding issues, identifying the most appropriate services and taking into account the time frame in which these services can provide help and support. Due to the demand on support services at the time of writing, it can take several weeks before contact is made with a patient in need. Unfortunately, this unprecedented demand results in accident and emergency (A&E) admissions due to health and social needs that cannot be met in the community. It is the responsibility of ambulance clinicians to identify where the greatest need lies, and consider how services can be implemented and over what time frame, all the while acting in the best interests of the patient.

Data-informed decisions

Improving population health requires an evidence-based approach, which can only evolve from the collation of data recorded during patient interactions. Ambulance data specifically can be utilised to improve the health and wellbeing of communities by establishing an overview of the needs of the population. Due to the nature of the service it provides, the ambulance sector holds a wide variety of historic and current data and patient activity which can be shared across systems to help provide the evidence to drive change in specific areas. Creating opportunities to collect this data helps to enable a public health approach across a wider system and therefore result in greater collective impact. Paramedics can collect data at incidents they attend by documenting a thorough patient history and completing the patient's clinical record. Due to the vast array of environments ambulance clinicians are exposed to, the wide range of data collected can be used to aid the development of research or implementation of evidence-based practice. This includes collecting information about a patient's social history, environment and housing issues, smoking status and diet, and previous contact with allied health professionals.

Other ways in which data has been used to inform clinical decisions and best practice in the ambulance service include the implementation of certain care bundles as a quality improvement initiative. Care bundles are tools used to provide evidence-based and reliable care, consisting of three to five elements or interventions that must be completed for full compliance to be achieved. Ambulance services across England adopted the STEMI (S-T segment elevation myocardial infarction) and stroke care bundles, and the data is measured and analysed as part of the ambulance system indicators. This allows standardised care to be delivered nationally and areas of poor outcome to be addressed. These care bundles and their measure of compliance were developed based on data collected by ambulance clinicians. This measure of compliance extends to other indicators which must be documented accurately, so information can be exchanged between services. For example, when attending a patient who has fallen, specific criteria must be documented in order to complete and close the patient's clinical record. This can include specific observations such as blood glucose level and blood pressure, whether the patient uses any walking aids, whether there was an intrinsic or extrinsic cause and the height from which the patient fell (e.g. from standing).

Focusing on prevention

The public health approach identifies three levels of prevention that can be implemented during patient care. As an example, attending 999 calls for falls in the elderly provide an opportunity to put the public health approach and prevention into practice. Primary prevention may include identifying slip or trip hazards within the home and mitigating these risks by putting preventative measures in place. Simple education or removal of objects from well-used thoroughfares throughout the patient's environment may reduce the risk of falls.

Secondary – or 'targeted' – prevention will not be relevant to all 'elderly fallers' but is more nuanced in that it attempts to facilitate behaviour change in those who display risk factors. A person who has type 2 diabetes, for example, which can be prevented by lifestyle changes, may suffer from peripheral neuropathy and as a result is more prone to falling. Providing education around diet and its impact on adequately controlling type 2 diabetes allows the opportunity for tailored support and onward referral to services that can provide continued care. There is also the opportunity to refer onwards for walking aid assessments or to have adaptations made to the home to reduce the risk of further falls.

Finally, tertiary prevention is focused on slowing the long-term impacts of a condition rather than prevention at the population level. This may be identifying when a patient's condition is deteriorating and referring on to the required health and social care sectors so that individual needs are met. From an ambulance service or primary care perspective, this may materialise as multiple attendances to a patient for similar episodes or increased contact with other health and social care services. Attendances of this nature usually provide an opportunity for ambulance clinicians to communicate with the patient's general practitioner, whether directly or via a GP summary sent electronically to the surgery where the patient is registered. This allows documentation of the patient's deterioration to be shared across services, and provides the opportunity for further holistic review of the patient and advance care planning to be initiated.

The wider determinants of health and reducing health inequalities

As already discussed, the wider determinants of health have an influence on an individual's health and wellbeing. These factors affect the ability or opportunity to access services and impact vulnerability and resilience directly. NHS ambulance trusts have the ability to connect with communities and identify the social determinants of health through interaction with their local populations. The 2021 paper by AACE goes on to discuss the size and scale of NHS ambulance trusts in the community and how, as an organisation, these trusts can reduce inequalities through the way in which they employ staff, purchase goods and address environmental issues. However, the relevance of this to ambulance clinicians is limited as their focus is on identifying and understanding the impact of health inequalities at an individual level. Paramedics should understand the relationship between patients of low economic status and the direct effect of a negative health event and lasting ramifications of this. This applies to ethnic minority groups and the disproportionate impact of COVID-19 on Black, Asian and ethnic minority communities.

Partnerships across systems

Public health remains the shared responsibility of a wide range of sectors which have the influence to improve population health. A successful public health approach unifies these sectors as part of a public health system to drive change and reduce inequalities. This unification or partnership between sectors allows for a wider reach and for specialisation to reduce overlap or replication of public health goals. This means that a public health goal can be targeted by various sectors working and supporting one another with similar objectives. In 2021, the government proposed a 10-year plan to tackle illegal drug use (GOV.UK, 2022). This drug strategy prioritises three important aspects: breaking drug supply chains, improving the treatment and recovery of drug users and changing societal attitudes towards drug use. This public health goal will necessitate collaboration across services to reach the desired outcome. Brighton and Hove City Council (2022), for example, are working in collaboration with local public services to help deliver the drug strategy laid out by the government due to the city's high percentage of drug trafficking offenders. These public services can often engage with and provide support to intravenous drug users to reduce the need for opiate-related ambulance calls or A&E attendances. The involvement of ambulance services in a public health goal such as this is unique, as front-line clinicians will be more exposed to drug-related incidents and in a position to collect data which can be shared across services. This can highlight where drug use may be more prevalent geographically or when adverse outcomes from drug-related incidents are on the rise. This can indicate that more dangerous or synthetically enhanced batches of drugs such as heroin are circulating, and this can be fed back to support services who can act accordingly. It is important in this example to understand how the wider determinants of health factor into a public health goal such as reducing drug use. Many factors can contribute to drug and alcohol use, including unemployment, deprivation, mental health issues, housing status, social networks and criminal activity.

The complexities of achieving a public health goal are further exacerbated by health inequalities. The key means of underpinning a public health approach within the ambulance sector can only be implemented successfully once the disparity of health inequalities is addressed. Paramedics, however, in whatever health or social care sector they work in, are in a position to make a difference at an individual level through the assessment and care they provide. Through an understanding of these key approaches and how they can be implemented, paramedics can play a key role in public health initiatives, tackling inequalities and improving the health and wellbeing of the population they serve.

Case study 12.1 provides a practical link between the public health theory discussed in this chapter and the potential for paramedics to apply it to patients in their care.

Case study 12.1

You receive an emergency call in the early hours of Saturday morning to a patient collapsed outside a popular nightclub in the city centre. On arrival, you find a patient medically well with no injuries, although they are vulnerable and intoxicated with no means of getting home.

Let us look at the burden of alcohol and think about what could be done from a public health perspective, considering initiatives and work already completed.

Facts

- Alcohol is the leading risk factor of ill health, early mortality and disability within the 15–49 age group and the fifth leading risk factor for ill health across all age groups.
- There has been a 4 per cent rise in licensed establishments, with 210,000 licensed premises in England and Wales alone.
- There are over one million alcohol-related hospital admissions each year with specific alcohol-related mortality at 54.3 years, a cost to the NHS of £3 billion (PHE, 2018b).
- The public health burden of alcohol can be seen in the associated health, social and economic harms; tangible, direct and indirect costs; and intangible costs, such as pain and suffering, and emotional distress.

Individual considerations and vulnerability factors

- The volume of alcohol consumed
- The frequency of drinking
- The quality of alcohol consumed
- Age
- Gender
- Familial factors
- Socioeconomic status

Current campaigns and initiatives

- Drink Responsibly
- Dry January
- Drink driving campaigns
- Drunk tanks

What could you do?

- Avoid an unnecessary hospital admission.
- Contact friends or family who have not been drinking to take responsibility for the individual and collect them.
- Transport the individual to a 'drunk tank' to sober up and be monitored safely.
- Provide information regarding health and wellbeing related to alcohol.
- Educate and spread awareness of the risks associated with excessive alcohol consumption.

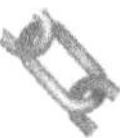

Chapter 1 for suggestions about communication strategies; **Chapter 4** for more about ethical and legal considerations; **Chapter 2** for suggestions on reflection.

CONCLUSION

Having an awareness of the development of public health and the wider determinants of health and health inequalities allows paramedics to underpin their practice with the knowledge and understanding of how societal health can be influenced. Though there is still no formal public health approach used by the ambulance service, the integration of paramedics into various healthcare roles allows for their thorough assessment skills and holistic nature of care to be implemented in different sectors, thus having a wider reach. Embedding these practices early allows opportunity for growth throughout their career and for continued professional development regarding their own public health approach.

Chapter key points:

- The development of the public health discipline was discussed.
- Education about public health is paramount to the practice of undergraduate paramedics.
- The development of a public health approach within the ambulance service was discussed.
- The importance of considering the wider determinants of health and health inequalities when discussing public health was emphasised.

REFERENCES AND SUGGESTED READING

Association of Ambulance Chief Executives (AACE) (2021) *Developing a public health approach within the ambulance sector*. Available at: https://aace.org.uk/news/phe-and-aace-publish-discussion-paper-developing-a-public-health-approach-within-the-ambulance-sector-2 (accessed 10 April 2024).

Brighton and Hove City Council (2022) *Brighton & Hove drugs and alcohol needs assessment*. Available at: https://www.brighton-hove.gov.uk/joint-strategic-needs-assessment-jsna/brighton-hove-drugs-and-alcohol-needs-assessment-2022#tab--5-pillar-2---delivering-a-world-class-treatment-and-recovery-service (accessed 10 April 2024).

British Medical Association (BMA) (2023) *The impact of the pandemic on population health and health inequalities.* Available at: https://www.bma.org.uk/advice-and-support/covid-19/what-the-bma-is-doing/the-impact-of-the-pandemic-on-population-health-and-health-inequalities (accessed 10 April 2024).

Centres for Disease Control and Prevention (CDC) (2023) *Long COVID or post-COVID conditions.* Available at: https://stacks.cdc.gov/view/cdc/133106 (accessed 10 April 2024).

Chang, K., Gunter, M.J., Rauber, F., Levy, R.B. et al. (2023) Ultra-processed food consumption, cancer risk and cancer mortality: a large-scale prospective analysis within the UK Biobank, *eClinicalMedicine,* 56: 101840. Available at: https://www.thelancet.com/journals/eclinm/article/PIIS2589-5370(23)00017-2/fulltext.

Department of Health and Social Care (DHSC) (2021) *Transforming the public health system: Reforming the public health system for the challenges of our times.* Available at: https://www.gov.uk/government/publications/transforming-the-public-health-system/transforming-the-public-health-system-reforming-the-public-health-system-for-the-challenges-of-our-times (accessed 10 April 2024).

GOV.UK (2022) *From harm to hope: A 10-year drugs plan to cut crime and save lives.* Available at: https://www.gov.uk/government/publications/from-harm-to-hope-a-10-year-drugs-plan-to-cut-crime-and-save-lives/from-harm-to-hope-a-10-year-drugs-plan-to-cut-crime-and-save-lives (accessed 10 April 2024).

Hamlin, C. (2010) *Public Health and Social Justice in the Age of Chadwick: Britain, 1800–1854* (Cambridge Studies in the History of Medicine). Cambridge: Cambridge University Press.

Health and Care Professions Council (HCPC) (2023) *Standards of Proficiency for Paramedics.* Available at: https://www.hcpc-uk.org/standards/standards-of-proficiency/paramedics/ (accessed 10 April 2024).

Holmes, J. (2022) *What is a population health approach?* London: The King's Fund. Available at: https://www.kingsfund.org.uk/publications/population-health-approach (Accessed 10th April 2024).

House of Commons Library (2022) *Office for Health Improvement and Disparities and health inequalities.* Available at: https://researchbriefings.files.parliament.uk/documents/CDP-2022-0015/CDP-2022-0015.pdf (accessed 10 April 2024).

Institute of Medicine (2003) *The future of the public's health in the 21st century,* Committee on Assuring the Health of the Public in the 21st Century. Washington, DC: National Academies Press.

Lally, S. (2020) *Impact of COVID-19 on different ethnic minority groups.* Available at: https://post.parliament.uk/impact-of-covid-19-on-different-ethnic-minority-groups/ (accessed 10 April 2024).

McCartney, G., Douglas, M., Taulbut, M., Katikireddi, S.V. et al. (2021) Tackling population health challenges as we build back from the pandemic, *British Medical Journal,* 375: e066232. Available at: https://doi.org/10.1136/bmj-2021-066232.

National Health Service (NHS) (2019) *NHS Long Term Plan.* Available at: https://www.longtermplan.nhs.uk/wp-content/uploads/2019/08/nhs-long-term-plan-version-1.2.pdf (accessed 10 April 2024).

Office for National Statistics (ONS) (2022) *UK health indicators 2019–2020*. Available at: https://www.ons.gov.uk/peoplepopulationandcommunity/healthand socialcare/healthandlifeexpectancies/bulletins/ukhealthindicators/2019 to2020 (accessed 10 April 2024).

Office for National Statistics (ONS) (2023) *Monthly mortality analysis, England and Wales July 2023*. Available at: https://www.ons.gov.uk/peoplepopulation andcommunity/birthsdeathsandmarriages/deaths/bulletins/monthlymortali-tyanalysisenglandandwales/july2023#:~:text=Dementia%20and%20Alzhei-mers%20disease%20had,in%20Wales%20(250%20deaths (accessed 10 April 2024).

Pettigrew, L.M., van Schalkwyk, M., Rechel, B. and Garlick, R. (2021) Where's the integration between public health and primary care in the response to covid-19?, *BMJ Opinion*. Available at: https://blogs.bmj.com/bmj/2021/02/18/wheres-the-integration-between-public-health-and-primary-care-in-the-response-to-covid-19/ (accessed 10 April 2024).

Public Health England (PHE) (2018a) Health of children in the early years, in *Health Profile for England: 2018*. Available at: https://www.gov.uk/government/publi-cations/health-profile-for-england-2018/chapter-4-health-of-children-in-the-early-years (accessed 10 April 2024).

Public Health England (PHE) (2018b) Inequalities in health, in *Health Profile for England: 2018*. Available at: https://www.gov.uk/government/publications/health-profile-for-england-2018/chapter-5-inequalities-in-health (accessed 10 April 2024).

Public Health England (PHE) (2018c) Wider determinants of health, in *Health Profile for England: 2018*. Available at: https://www.gov.uk/government/publica-tions/health-profile-for-england-2018/chapter-6-wider-determinants-of-health (accessed 10 April 2024).

Public Health England (PHE) (2018d) *Health matters: Air pollution*. Available at: https://www.gov.uk/government/publications/health-matters-air-pollution/ health-matters-air-pollution (accessed 10 April 2024).

Public Health England (PHE) (2019) *PHE strategy 2020–25*. Available at: https:// assets.publishing.service.gov.uk/media/5d7b72c8ed915d5257b5b66c/PHE_ Strategy_2020-25.pdf (accessed 10 April 2024).

Raleigh, V. (2023) *The health of people from ethnic minority groups in England*. Lon-don: The King's Fund. Available at: https://www.kingsfund.org.uk/publications/ health-people-ethnic-minority-groups-england (accessed 10 April 2024).

Rechel, B., Jakubowski, E., McKee, M. and Nolte, E. (2018) *Organization and financ-ing of public health services in Europe*. Copenhagen: WHO Regional Office for Europe. Available at: https://iris.who.int/handle/10665/326254.

Schofield, B. and McClean, S. (2022) Paramedics and health promotion, *Perspec-tives in Public Health*, 142 (3):135–36.

The Lancet Public Health (2022) Editorial: Covid-19 pandemic: what's next for pub-lic health?, *The Lancet Public Health*, 7 (5): e391. Available at: https://doi. org/10.1016/S2468-2667(22)00095-0.

UK Parliament (no date) *Poverty and the poor law*. Available at: https://www.parliament. uk/about/living-heritage/transformingsociety/livinglearning/19thcentury/overview/ poverty/ (accessed 10 April 2024).

World Health Organization (WHO) (2023) *Public health milestones throughout the years*. Available at: https://www.who.int/campaigns/75-years-of-improving-public-health/milestones#year-1945 (accessed 10 April 2024).
World Health Organization (WHO) (no date) *A brief history of vaccines*. Available at: https://www.who.int/news-room/spotlight/history-of-vaccination/a-brief-history-of-vaccination (accessed 10 April 2024).

USEFUL WEBSITES

Allied Health Professionals Federation: http://www.ahpf.org.uk
Department of Health and Social Care: https://www.gov.uk/government/organisations/department-of-health-and-social-care
Faculty of Public Health: http://www.fph.org.uk
HSC Public Health Agency: http://www.publichealth.hscni.net
Royal Society for Public Health: https://www.rsph.org.uk
Safe Lives: http://www.safelives.org.uk/about-us
World Health Organization: http://www.euro.who.int/en/health-topics/Health-systems/publichealth-services

13 Considering frailty in the pre-hospital setting

Georgina Gill

> **In this chapter:**
>
> - Introduction
> - Why is this relevant?
> - Sociology of ageing
> - Normal ageing
> - Frailty
> - Recognising frailty
> - Models of frailty
> - Frailty and ambulance workload
> - Conditions/complications associated with frailty
> - Urgent community response services
> - Carers
> - Decision-making and person-centred care
> - Shared decision-making
> - Conclusion
> - Chapter key points
> - References and suggested reading
> - Useful websites

INTRODUCTION

Globally, over the past 100 years, life expectancy has been rising and people are increasingly enjoying fulfilling lives well into their nineties. The average life expectancy for a child born in 1945 in the UK was 64.01 years, and in 2020, it was 81.14 years (Statista, 2024). As life expectancy rises, the demographics of the population become weighted to be older (Government Office for Science, 2016), and between 2020 and 2050, the population of over-85s is set to quadruple whilst the working population (20–64 years) is set to shrink by 20.1 per cent (International Longevity Centres, 2023). Older people are the largest user group for health and social care (BGS, 2023).

WHY IS THIS RELEVANT?

Frailty affects up to half of all people aged over 85 (Clegg et al., 2013). It is important to note that frailty is not a normal part of ageing and can be avoided (BGS, 2023). Not all older people are frail. All healthcare professionals working with older adults can recognise frailty and put interventions in place to reduce its progression and impact.

Higher levels of frailty are associated with increased mortality, increased rates of institutionalisation and geriatric syndromes such as falls, disability, mortality and excess healthcare costs (Romero-Ortuno et al., 2010). Moreover, frailty results in reduced independence, increased vulnerability, reduced quality of life and reduced psychological health for the people it impacts (Romero-Ortuno et al., 2010). Frailty also affects a person's family, creating demand for assistance and care (Romero-Ortuno et al., 2010).

This change in population increases pressure on health services to meet the ageing population's needs. This growth is further complicated by the increasing complexity of ageing, frailty and multimorbidity (NHS England, 2023), meaning people need more complex and time-consuming health care. People are living with more long-term conditions, requiring ongoing treatments and care to mitigate the impacts of ill health on daily life (Harper et al., 2020).

SOCIOLOGY OF AGEING

Ageing began to be considered as a sociological concept in the late nineteenth century, as the population began to live longer, creating a change in population demographics (Fletcher, 2021). As people began to live longer, there were concerns regarding the connection between ageing and poverty as many people reaching older age were considered paupers (Fletcher, 2021) even with the growth of state-delivered health care.

In western cultures, successful ageing is seen as the avoidance of disease and disability, maintaining an ability to function at high levels and being socially engaged (Preston et al., 2017a). Those who are unable to align with these norms can become disadvantaged within the societal structure. The main sociological theories related to ageing are presented in Table 13.1.

It is important to acknowledge the difference between frailty as a clinical syndrome and what frailty means to the lay person. Frailty may be seen by non-professionals – as well as some non-specialist clinicians – as a negative label, being associated with 'giving up'. Patients may resist the label of frailty, perceiving themselves as having two bodies: 'the body one is' (i.e. their sense of self, who they are, what makes them 'them') and the 'body

Table 13.1   Sociological theory related to ageing

Feminism	Men are the primary workers, and women have less social power when ageing, less time in work and less pension, but have a longer life expectancy, thus living longer in poorer conditions.
Marxism	Attitudes to old age are influenced by capitalism. Older people are not able to work in jobs and contribute less to the workplace economy, reducing their value within capitalist society.
Postmodernist perspectives	View ageing positively compared with other perspectives. As older people age they are able to remain independent, go on holiday, dress fashionably and have active social lives. They have high spending power to contribute to the economy.
Social construction	A person's experience of ageing is dependent on that person's social and cultural context. For example, eastern cultures value ageing and care for loved elderly family members, placing them on a pedestal within the family. In contrast, in the West, the elderly are cared for in residential homes and health settings as they become unable to contribute to the labour economy.

one has' (i.e. the physical self and its perception and place within society) (Preston et al., 2017a).

Becoming old in England is increasingly challenging. According to the Centre for Ageing Better (CAB), the proportion of older people living in rented accommodation is rising, and the number of pre-retirement aged adults in work is falling, leading to a generation of adults with reduced financial security in older age (CAB, 2022). From age 65, the poorest live twice as many years with disability and illness than the wealthiest (CAB, 2022).

Whilst people are increasingly living longer, they are not living healthier lives (CAB, 2022), and the number of disability-free life years is declining. Musculoskeletal disorders are the most common cause for years of poor health in adults over the age of 50 years (CAB, 2022). Additionally, the most deprived are twice as likely to be physically inactive than the wealthiest (CAB, 2022).

Engaging older people in social activity that is perceived to be supportive of both their social and psychological needs has been shown to be beneficial.

Engaging in several activities (e.g. volunteering; helping neighbours, friends and family members; taking part in political, community or religious organisations) improved their wellbeing, especially those who were considered to be the most vulnerable at the outset (Potocnik and Sonnentag, 2013).

The 2023 consensus statement on healthy ageing advocates the importance of reducing the disparity between the richest and poorest within society (Office for Health Improvement and Disparities, 2023). Research has shown that adults living in the most deprived areas – the lowest wealth quintiles – are 1.3 per cent more likely to be pre-frail or frail (Maharani et al., 2023). The work of Maharani et al. highlights a vast disparity in the incidence of frailty between those in the lowest wealth quintiles (20.9 per cent) and those in the wealthiest quintiles (3.7 per cent). The NHS Long Term Plan (NHS England, 2023) builds on the need to reduce these inequalities and address care for those living with frailty (NHS Assembly, 2023).

NORMAL AGEING

As ageing occurs, presentations of illness change and, in older adults, can be non-specific, resulting in difficulties in differentiation and diagnosis. Whilst ageing is something all of us experience, the rate at which it happens varies between individuals. Factors such as lifestyle, environment and genetics influence the rate at which we age. There are many physiological changes that occur with ageing that should be considered when caring for older adults.

Box 13.1 Physiological changes associated with normal ageing

- Cerebral atrophy
- Reduced cerebral blood flow
- Reduced thermoregulation
- Hearing impairment
- Vestibular changes
- Postural changes (kyphosis, scoliosis)
- Reduced fatty tissue
- Vision changes
- Joint degeneration (reduced mobility, reduced bursa size)
- Osteoporotic change
- Reduced muscle strength
- Slower new muscle synthesis
- Increased drug metabolism
- Build-up of atheroma within blood vessels

When caring for older adults, it is essential that paramedics are aware of the physiological changes of ageing and the impact upon diseases, treatment and decision-making.

In 1992, the geriatrician Bernard Isaacs described what he called the '5 geriatric giants':

- Incontinence
- Immobility
- Intellectual impairment
- Instability
- Iatrogenesis.

These 'geriatric giants' are presentations that are of significant burden to patients and present as secondary to more complex elements of ageing and illness combined.

When considering frailty, it is important to consider the wider and closely associated physiology that is normal ageing. Ageing is a physiological decline, and Bernard Strehler defined it as:

Universal: it happens to all members of a species.
Intrinsic: it does not depend on external factors to occur.
Progressive: it occurs progressively at a rate of about 1 per cent per year.
Deleterious: it is bad for the individual.

(Preston et al., 2017b)

Frailty does not affect everyone and it is possible for a person to age without becoming frail. Frailty occurs in around one in five older adults in England, and its prevalence is expected to increase to one in four by 2038 (Sinclair et al., 2022). This rise in prevalence will increase demand on the health and social care systems and is increasingly becoming recognised at policy level, with a shift to increase coordinated and community care to support older adults living with frailty (NHS Assembly, 2023).

FRAILTY

Frailty is a clinical syndrome in that a person gradually loses the ability to maintain homeostasis, reducing their physiological reserve and ability to respond physiologically to minor stressor events.

Developing a global consensus on defining frailty has been historically challenging (Rockwood et al., 2005). As can be seen by the definitions provided in Box 13.2, these vary based on the contextual use of the term, whether that be for recognising frailty, considering the physiological aspects of frailty or the implications of frailty. Whilst decline does occur across all physiological systems with normal ageing, the rate at which it occurs in a person with frailty is accelerated (Clegg et al., 2013).

Box 13.2 Definitions of frailty

Frailty is a distinctive health state related to the ageing process in which multiple body systems gradually lose their in-built reserves. (BGS, 2018b: 6)

Frailty is a state of increased vulnerability to poor resolution of homeo-stasis following a stress, which increases the risk of adverse outcomes including falls, delirium and disability. (Clegg et al., 2013: 1)

… clinically recognizable state of increased vulnerability resulting from ageing associated decline in reserve and function across multiple physi-ologic systems such that the ability to cope with everyday or acute stressors is compromised. (Xue, 2011: 1)

As highlighted by the definitions in Box 13.2, frailty is not a singular condition but rather a collection of multiple inter-occurring syndromes (Wyrko, 2015). This does not mean frailty is simply a collection of comorbidities, although an increased number of comorbidities can be an indicator for frailty. Frailty is not isolated to age, disability or having multiple long-term conditions; however, it is acknowledged that as frailty and age are bound together, there will be an age at which virtually all people would be frail (Rockwood et al., 2005).

Frailty is a spectrum, although a person's progression through the stages is not linear, and not every person experiences every stage; a person's frailty can both increase and decrease (BGS, 2018b). Generally, the time spent at each successive stage of the frailty journey reduces as a result of reduced physiological reserve.

For a person living with frailty, a minor stressor such as an infection, a change of environment or new medication can result in a disproportionate change in their health (Clegg et al., 2013). This may be reflected in a change from independent to dependent, a reduction in mobility, an increased likeli-hood of falling or delirium (Clegg et al., 2013). As someone recovers from a stressor events, they may regain functional ability, but with each episode, their baseline health declines, affecting their independence and functional ability and increasing their rate of decline.

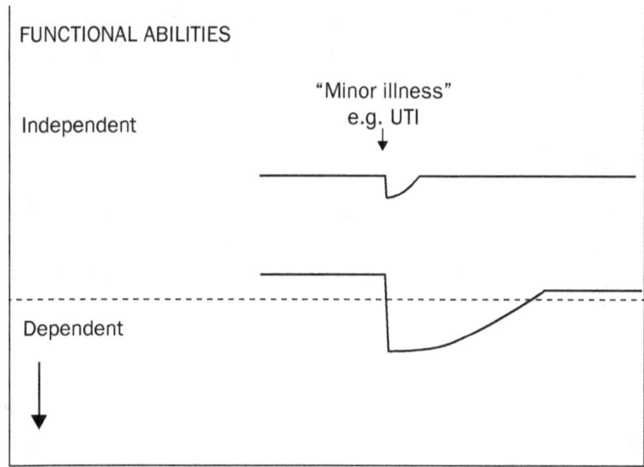

Figure 13.1 Difference in deterioration of a fit older person (top line) vs. that of a frail individual (bottom line) in response to a physiological stressor such as a urinary tract infection

Source: Clegg et al. (2013).

RECOGNISING FRAILTY

Recognising frailty can enable professionals to implement measures to slow or prevent further decline, enabling the person to be more independent for longer (BGS, 2023). This can improve quality of life and reduce poor health outcomes (BGS, 2018b) by reversing or postponing severe frailty (Green et al., 2018). Adults living with severe frailty are four times more likely to be admitted to hospital, be placed in a care home or to die than the non-frail (Harper et al., 2020). Older adults living with frailty are more likely to use community resources (Morley et al., 2013). The British Geriatric Society (BGS) advocates not labelling people as frail or not frail, but rather acknowledging they have frailty in order to identify where they are on the spectrum of disease (BGS, 2018b).

Ambulance clinicians are ideally placed to recognise patients who are pre-frail or living with frailty and are able to inform primary care services (Green et al., 2018). Gathering information and identifying frailty early in a patient's healthcare journey can enable appropriate treatment and referrals to be made. It can support ambulance clinicians to see changes in a patient, assisting with decision-making, especially in cases where patients are not conveyed to the hospital (Charlton et al., 2022). However, paramedics' current knowledge of frailty, relevant vocabulary and assessment structure are variable (Green et al., 2018). Staff knowledge, optimism and behaviours, as well as a failure to ascertain a patient's baseline abilities, have been identified as barriers to maximising independence during hospital admission (Dijk-Huisman et al., 2022).

MODELS OF FRAILTY

There is no ideal tool for measuring frailty but two models stand out: the Frailty Phenotype Model and Cumulative Deficit Model (BGS, 2018b). These should be considered as complementary to one another rather than as alternatives (Cesari et al., 2014).

The Frailty Phenotype Model involves a group of characteristics, which, if present, can predict frailty. These characteristics include unintentional weight loss, reduced muscle strength, self-reported exhaustion and low energy expenditure. If a person has three or more characteristics, they can be considered frail. The model, however, cannot be used to assess the efficacy of treatment interventions for a person who is living with frailty. The Cumulative Deficit Model, in contrast, assumes an accumulation of deficits associated with ageing that can combine to increase a person's frailty index, which increases the risk of an adverse outcome.

The main frailty scoring instruments used within UK clinical practice are the Electronic Frailty Index and Rockwood Clinical Frailty score, both of which are based on an accumulation of deficits model. Research has shown that frailty will fluctuate irrespective of the measurement tool (Hartley et al., 2023). Early recognition of whether someone's frailty is mild, moderate or severe is essential for improved patient-centred care and outcomes. Using standardised frailty assessment tools can support decision-making that is reflective of individual patient and carer needs (Reuben and Tinetti, 2012; Rockwood et al., 2005).

The Electronic Frailty Index (EFI) is a risk stratification tool. It is computer driven and creates a score that identifies people living with frailty, based on the accumulation of 36 deficits present in health records. Because it is not delivered by a clinician, it is reliant upon the accurate recording of routine data (Harper et al., 2020). It has been shown to have relatively high sensitivity, but low specificity in that it over-identifies frailty (NHS England, 2023). Once frailty has been identified using the EFI, it acts as a flag for primary care services to arrange a review by a clinician. During assessment by a clinician, targeted interventions can be considered.

The Clinical Frailty Scale (CFS), sometimes referred to as the 'Rockwood score', was developed by Kenneth Rockwood and his team (Rockwood et al., 2005). The CFS can be used to describe a person's frailty very quickly

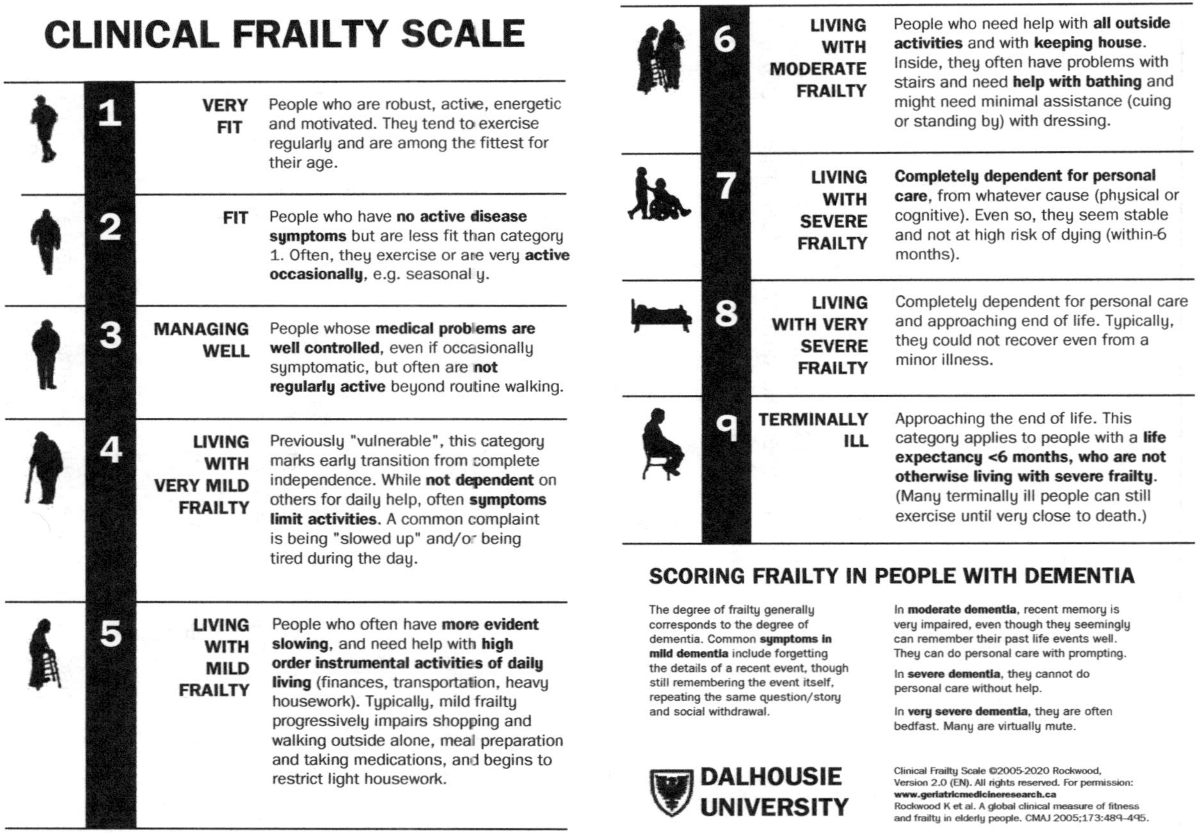

CLINICAL FRAILTY SCALE

1 VERY FIT — People who are robust, active, energetic and motivated. They tend to exercise regularly and are among the fittest for their age.

2 FIT — People who have **no active disease symptoms** but are less fit than category 1. Often, they exercise or are very **active occasionally**, e.g. seasonally.

3 MANAGING WELL — People whose **medical problems are well controlled**, even if occasionally symptomatic, but often are **not regularly active** beyond routine walking.

4 LIVING WITH VERY MILD FRAILTY — Previously "vulnerable", this category marks early transition from complete independence. While **not dependent** on others for daily help, often **symptoms limit activities**. A common complaint is being "slowed up" and/or being tired during the day.

5 LIVING WITH MILD FRAILTY — People who often have **more evident slowing**, and need help with **high order instrumental activities of daily living** (finances, transportation, heavy housework). Typically, mild frailty progressively impairs shopping and walking outside alone, meal preparation and taking medications, and begins to restrict light housework.

6 LIVING WITH MODERATE FRAILTY — People who need help with **all outside activities** and with **keeping house**. Inside, they often have problems with stairs and need **help with bathing** and might need minimal assistance (cuing or standing by) with dressing.

7 LIVING WITH SEVERE FRAILTY — **Completely dependent for personal care**, from whatever cause (physical or cognitive). Even so, they seem stable and not at high risk of dying (within ~6 months).

8 LIVING WITH VERY SEVERE FRAILTY — Completely dependent for personal care and approaching end of life. Typically, they could not recover even from a minor illness.

9 TERMINALLY ILL — Approaching the end of life. This category applies to people with a **life expectancy <6 months, who are not otherwise living with severe frailty.** (Many terminally ill people can still exercise until very close to death.)

SCORING FRAILTY IN PEOPLE WITH DEMENTIA

The degree of frailty generally corresponds to the degree of dementia. Common **symptoms in mild dementia** include forgetting the details of a recent event, though still remembering the event itself, repeating the same question/story and social withdrawal.

In **moderate dementia**, recent memory is very impaired, even though they seemingly can remember their past life events well. They can do personal care with prompting.

In **severe dementia**, they cannot do personal care without help.

In **very severe dementia**, they are often bedfast. Many are virtually mute.

DALHOUSIE UNIVERSITY

Figure 13.2 The Clinical Frailty Scale

Source: Rockwood et al. (2005).

using a standardised measure. It has been tested across a range of health-care departments, and is accurate and quick to deliver in busy environments (Fehlmann et al., 2023), with the mean time to complete the score in the emergency department as low as 41 seconds (Elliott et al., 2017). The scale has been shown to be a reliable predictor for both short- (Hwan-Lee et al., 2022) and long-term mortality (Rueegg et al., 2022).

The CFS can support clinicians to adopt a holistic approach to patient care and identify the goals of care for individual patients (Leeds Frailty Education, 2023). It can assist decision-making by aiding the identification of patients who may benefit from further assessment or an alternative care pathway (Green et al., 2018). The scale is not an isolated decision-making tool (Green et al., 2018). It requires clinicians to probe more deeply as part of their history-taking than they might do without the system in place (Leeds Frailty Education, 2023), such as asking what help and assistance a person has or needs at home and recording baseline activity. Initially, the CFS required concurrent comprehensive geriatric assessment (CGA), but since being validated across settings this is no longer required (Wallis et al., 2015).

As the CFS is designed to assess a patient's baseline activity; this will not be possible in the acute ambulance setting (Green et al., 2018). The score should be based on a person's condition two weeks previously (Rock-wood et al., 2005). Ambulance clinicians often attend in the patient's home environment, so additional environmental clues from the lived environment could lead to pre-hospital assessment of frailty being more accurate than in the emergency department (Fehlmann et al., 2023).

There is limited research to date of paramedic and pre-hospital emergency use of the CFS. Fehlmann et al. (2023) used clinical vignettes to assess paramedics' inter-rater reliability of frailty assessment using the scale. The authors reported excellent inter-rater reliability but moderate accuracy, although none of the 56 paramedics rated had used the scale in clinical practice previously. As use of the scale in clinical practice increases, ambulance clinicians may become more competent in its use.

FRAILTY AND AMBULANCE WORKLOAD

The undifferentiated nature of elderly patients' presentations, together with the complexity of their care, results in frequent referrals to other multidisciplinary services (Jadzinski et al., 2021). Research has suggested that up to 35 per cent of ambulance call outs are for adults aged over 75 (Buswell et al., 2016). The emergency ambulance call room is up to four times more likely to receive a call for an older adult living in a residential or nursing home than a community-dwelling older adult (Dwyer et al., 2018). They are also more likely to be considered of a slower response category than community-dwelling adults (Sinclair et al., 2023). Ambulance clinicians spend less time treating patients living in care homes per call than they do those who live in a community dwelling (Sinclair et al., 2023); however, research is at odds as to whether those living with frailty are more or less likely to be conveyed to hospital (Charlton et al., 2022; Sinclair et al., 2023).

Frailty in the older population necessitates ambulance personnel having to convey them to healthcare facilities. In the north east of England, almost 60 per cent of patients aged 50 or above are living with frailty (a CFS score of 5 or above, where 5 = 'mildly frail'), rising to over 88 per cent for those over 90 (Charlton et al., 2022). It is suggested that in south west England, 20 per cent of patients attended by the ambulance service in 2017 were living with frailty (CFS > 5) (Green et al., 2018).

Older people living in rural areas were less likely to be assessed as frail than those in urban areas (59.9 vs. 53.0 per cent) with the likelihood of being frail rising with deprivation (Charlton et al., 2022). This is in keeping with wider UK data from the English Longitudinal Study of Ageing (ELSA), where higher rates of frailty (CFS > 5) have been identified as more prevalent in the most deprived and urban areas (Sinclair et al., 2022).

CONDITIONS/COMPLICATIONS ASSOCIATED WITH FRAILTY

Returning to Isaacs' (1992) five geriatric giants, it is possible to match syndromes to commonly presenting complaints that ambulance clinicians see on a daily basis (see Figure 13.3).

These presentations are referred to as frailty syndromes (RCP, 2020). Understanding this can enable clinicians to undertake thorough assessments that not only address the acute presenting needs of the patient, but also consider their wider health and frailty.

Falls

Research has shown that the label of 'faller' and associated stigma may reduce healthcare-seeking behaviours (Hartley et al., 2023) when healthcare input could reduce future falls. The reasons for this non-contact are multifaceted. Falls are variable in their characteristics and clinicians should be aware of this. These characteristics can be divided into intrinsic and extrinsic factors (see Box 13.3).

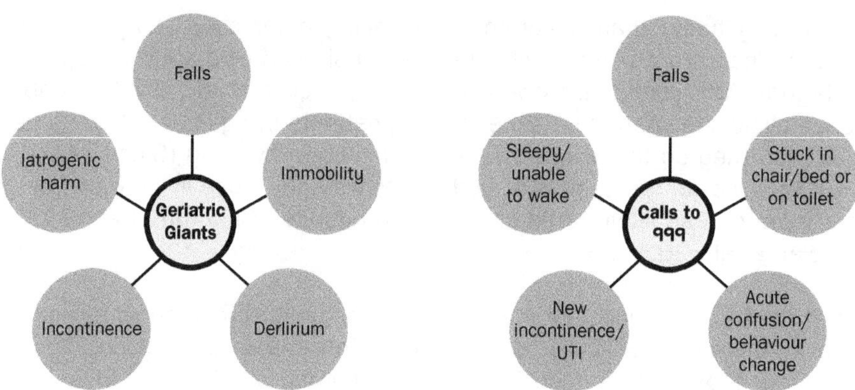

Figure 13.3 Matching Issac's 5 geriatric giants to front-line 999 presentations

Adapted from: Isaacs (1992).

Box I3.3 Intrinsic and extrinsic factors of falls

Intrinsic: factors resulting in falls from 'inside' the person include ongoing illness or injuries, vision or hearing loss, urinary urgency and balance problems.

Extrinsic: factors external to the person in the environment such as objects, trip and slip hazards and footwear.

For older adults reporting two or more falls in the previous year, the likelihood of reporting fewer falls at the one-year follow-up was higher for females, but lower per second to complete 'time to up and go' (11 per cent), lower for adults with orthostatic hypotension (28 per cent) and lower for adults taking antidepressants (35 per cent) (Hartley et al., 2023).

Ambulance clinicians have the opportunity to provide simple advice and health promotion on-scene to reduce the number of risk factors from first contact with a patient. Understanding risk factors associated with falls can enable clinicians to deliver person-centred advice. Falls prevention advice should consider physiological age-related changes, the multi-morbid conditions of the patient, and the history and nature of the reported falls. Potential advice includes that on:

- footwear;
- lighting;

- rugs and carpets;
- walking stick height, size and technique;
- postural hypotension;
- attending vision or hearing assessment;
- fluid intake and hydration;
- keeping walkways in the home clear of obstacles.

Whilst developed as a model to explain healthcare errors, the Swiss cheese model (Reason, 2000) is useful for considering the multifactorial nature of falls and the positive impact of falls prevention. Advice from ambulance clinicians attending patients at the time of a fall together with follow-up prevention can halt or reduce the number of falls. However, the possibility of falling cannot be ensured, and therefore some holes remain.

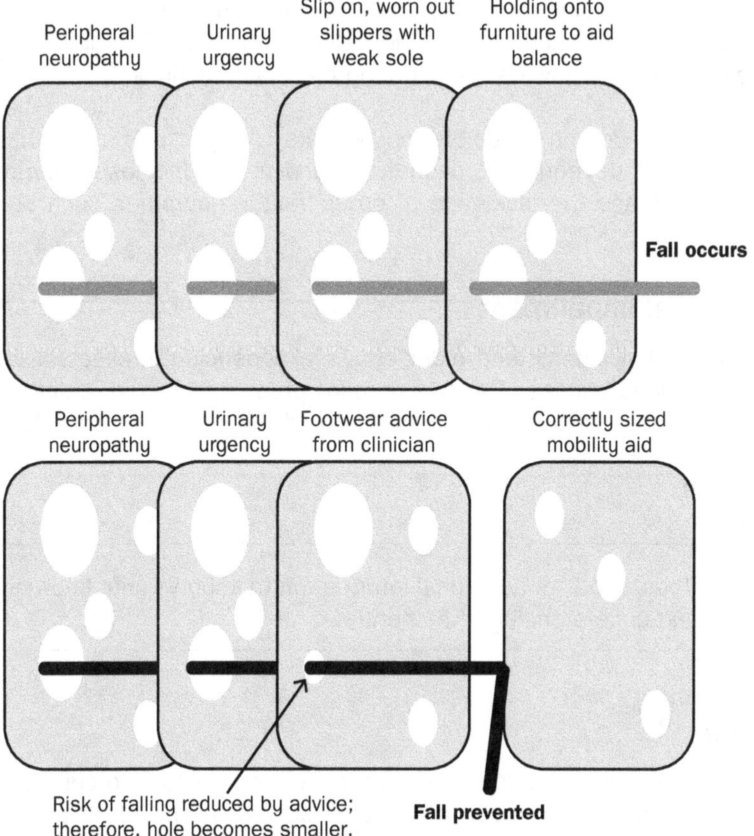

Figure 13.4 The impact of falls prevention on reducing the incidence of falling

Hypotension and the presence of orthostatic hypotension is associated with an increased risk of falling. Ambulance clinicians should have a good knowledge of national guidelines for older people (see Useful websites).

Referral to the appropriate follow-up service, such as the local specialist falls services or GP, should be made. Multiple concurrent interventions have been shown to be effective to reduce the numbers of falls (NHS Confederation, 2024). Home safety interventions are most effective when delivered by an occupational therapist (Gillespie et al., 2012).

Immobility

Often the assessment and onward advice for patients experiencing immobility is similar to that of people experiencing falls. Immobility may be acute on a call, such as when attending an elderly person stuck in a chair or on the toilet, and clinicians should consider whether this episode is a result of ongoing frailty and inactivity combined. Clinicians should manage the acute causes of immobility, whilst considering the frailty alongside.

Immobility has potentially deleterious effects on a person's strength, bone mass, level of dependence, confidence and mood. Increased immobility can also increase the incidence of other frailty syndromes such as falls and delirium.

Intellectual impairment

Ambulance clinicians attend older adults experiencing intellectual impairment of various causes. The two primary presentations are delirium and dementia. It is important that clinicians can differentiate between the two

Dementia

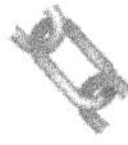

Chapter 15 for additional information to improve your knowledge and understanding of dementia.

Delirium

Delirium is a clinical syndrome with an acute and fluctuating course, characterised by a change in consciousness, cognitive function or perception (NICE, 2023b). Older adults and those living with dementia or severe illness or presenting with hip fracture have the highest risk of delirium; between 20 and 30 per cent experience delirium when admitted to a medical ward

Table 13.2   Signs of hyperactive and hypoactive delirium

Hyperactive	Hypoactive
Heightened arousal	Withdrawal
Changes in communication, mood or attitude	Sleepiness
Visual or auditory hallucinations	Quiet
Restlessness	Reduced activity, mobility or movement
Agitation	Slow responses
Aggression	Worsened concentration
	Reduced appetite

Source: NICE (2023b).

(NICE, 2023b). However, rates of recognition and reporting for delirium are low, so numbers may be higher.

Delirium can be categorised into three main presentations: hyperactive, hypoactive and mixed, which is where a person fluctuates between hyperactive and hypoactive presentations (see Table 13.2).

Left unrecognised and untreated, delirium can have serious consequences, such as increased length of stay, increased care needs, increased likelihood of admission to long-term care and increased risk of dementia and death (NICE, 2023b). Half of the patients with delirium on general and geriatric medicine wards will die within 6 months (BGS, 2020b).

Ambulance clinicians should be able to identify delirium and potential causes during an assessment. The PINCH ME acronym is useful for this. Remember, infections are frequently a cause for delirium but not the only cause, so you must complete a thorough assessment (see Table 13.3). Delirium is often multifactorial, and clinicians should make efforts to address all precipitating factors. Not all patients presenting with delirium require hospital admission; many can be managed in community settings.

Incontinence

Continence issues affect one in three people living in residential care settings and two in three in nursing homes (BGS, 2011). High rates of incontinence are associated with functional and cognitive decline, as well as reduced quality of life (Smith et al., 2019). Moreover, loss of bowel and bladder control is associated with discomfort, distress and pain (Smith et al., 2019). Patients who have indicated significant concerns related to a

---

Table 13.3 Applying PINCH ME to pre-hospital assessment

P	**P**ain: is the pain acute or chronic? Has the person had analgesia? Has the analgesia been reviewed or changed?
I	**I**nfection: is there a source of infection? Check chest, urine, abdomen, skin.
N	**N**utrition: what is the patient's appetite like? Has it changed?
C	**C**onstipation: has the patient moved their bowels in the last 24 hours? What was the stool like? – use a Bristol stool chart. If soft, could it be overflow round compaction?
H	**H**ydration: what has the patient's fluid intake been like in the past 48–72 hours? Are there any physical or environmental limitations reducing access to drinks? What has the patient's urine output been like? Are they passing enough urine, is there potential for retention?
M	**M**edication: consider side effects from medications such as opiates or anticholinergics. Have any medications been stopped recently, whether intentionally or unintentionally (BGS, 2020)
E	**E**nvironment: has the patient recently moved location/residence? Or, has their room been rearranged?

Adapted from: Dykes (2018).

---

loss of dignity at the end of their life are more likely to have difficulty with bowel functioning and heightened dependence (Smith et al., 2019).

Continence issues can result in acute admissions, particularly for adults living in nursing and residential settings (BGS, 2020a). Ambulance clinicians should have an understanding of the common causes and management options for frail older adults experiencing constipation, diarrhoea and urinary incontinence, as well as catheter complications.

Iatrogenic disability

Professionals working in pre-hospital settings are becoming increasingly aware of the potential negative impacts of hospitalisation on older persons. The process for decision-making related to adults living with frailty and frailty-related conditions is explored further later in the chapter.

The cumulative disabling effects of medical interventions on a person's function that results in an increase in dependence is termed 'iatrogenic disability'. This occurs as a result of a combination of pre-existing frailty, severe illness leading to admission and healthcare processes (Lafont et al., 2011).

Box 13.4 The impact of hospitalisation on the elderly

- Increased risk of falls.
- Longer length of stay concurrent with level of frailty at admission.
- Higher risk of secondary complications such as hospital-acquired pneumonia, new incontinence.
- High risk of readmission.
- Increased dependency in relation to activities of daily living.
- Increased likelihood of the need for some form of care once discharged.
- Trajectory is towards institutional care (residential or nursing home).
- Older adults in hospital settings often experience depersonalisation, losing the power to voice opinions related to their care.
- Many older adults would rather live with an element of risk in their own homes rather than have extended hospital stays with lower risk.
- This may be difficult for families and healthcare professionals providing care to accept and manage.

URGENT COMMUNITY RESPONSE SERVICES

Health systems are recognising the benefits of coordinated care at home for service users and the local healthcare system as a whole. One in seven people aged 85 or over permanently live in a care home, and those residing in care homes take up 1.46 million emergency bed days per year, of which 35–40 per cent are avoidable (NHS England, 2019). The NHS Assembly report (2023) pushed for increased universal care for those living with frailty, delivered by community services and hospital outreach teams. Across the UK, these services have a multitude of different names, but here we will refer to them as Urgent Community Response (UCR) services.

UCR services aim to complete assessment and begin short-term interventions within 48 hours, in efforts to avoid hospital admission due to crisis. This is usually for a person for whom hospital attendance within 24 hours is likely without onward intervention. Once a referral has been received, services aim to contact and begin assessment within a couple of hours. UCR services work in people's homes, whether that be a private residence, or care or nursing home.

Service delivery by UCR can be divided into three parts: clinical and nursing needs, care needs and therapy needs. The conditions UCR services could assist with include:

- falls (including those still on the floor and without apparent injury);
- decompensated frailty;
- reduced function or mobility;
- palliative/end-of-life care;
- provision of urgent equipment;
- confusion/delirium;
- urgent catheter care;
- carer breakdown.

Box 13.5 Typical interventions offered by UCR services

- Blood diagnostics: typical panels might include full blood count, urea and electrolytes, C-reactive protein testing, d-dimer.
- Urine diagnostics.
- Provision of equipment.
- Medicines optimisation.
- Administration of some medicines.
- Nurse assessment, including review of skin, continence, wound care, mobility, physical health.
- Catheter care.
- Access to hospital at home and virtual ward where intravenous antibiotics and outpatient input may be arranged.

Adapted from: NHS England (2022).

A common feature and strength of UCR services is multidisciplinary teams from a whole range of backgrounds to care for patients. A 2010 King's Fund report highlighted the value of integrated health and social care teams and multidisciplinary teams in admission-avoidance initiatives (Purdy, 2010). The goal is not only to prevent an acute admission but to prevent an acute crisis recurring in the future. UCR services are closely commissioned alongside other community services whilst remaining distinct services, enabling care to be passed onwards to long-term care services such as community nursing, podiatry or falls teams.

A challenge for ambulance clinicians is that UCR services are often locally funded by integrated care systems, meaning availability varies across an ambulance service's geographical area. Two-hour response times are a key pathway for ambulance services to help avoid conveying patients to hospital, and can also support some people who return home the same day without admission (NHS England, 2022).

Frailty-specific patient pathways are being developed nationally but remain variable in their delivery capabilities and hours of work. However, the set-up of these services is reliant on buy-in from all partners from the early design phases, along with an understanding of each service and clinician role, and the skill and knowledge to build trust (NHS Confederation, 2023).

CARERS

Across the UK, an estimated 1.4 million older people have unmet care needs, and the gap to meet these needs is often filled by friends and family (Age UK, 2019). An estimated 5.8 million people in the UK provide unpaid care to family members, friends and partners, and this unpaid care is estimated to save the UK economy up to £132 billion per year (Public Health England, 2021).

Many people do not self-identify as carers, especially those from a Black and Ethnic Minority (BME) background (The Carers Trust Wales, 2022). Carers may support a person in different ways, such as money management, transport to appointments and events, or assisting with personal care and mobility. Social expectations of families to care for loved ones often means that providing care is simply a part of life (The Carers Trust Wales, 2022). The Carers Trust reports that whilst this may not be a barrier to service access, it may reduce the chance of a person accessing services because they do not consider themselves and their role 'worthy' of support or feeling pressure to provide care. Misalignment between carers' concepts of care and organisational concepts of care – defined in terms of the time, tasks and space required – can create division between carers and organisations, leading to the care provided not meeting an individual's needs (The Carers Trust Wales, 2022).

When attending older people living with frailty, ambulance clinicians will often interact with their families and carers. These people know the patient best and it is important that clinicians include them in any discussions whilst keeping patients at the centre of care.

Ambulance clinicians have a responsibility to support carers and acknowledge the challenges and consequences of caring. Identifying challenges early can help support carers and reduce acute carer breakdown. Carers are often unaware of the support that is available, and some may assume due to circumstances such as working or finances that they are not eligible for assistance (The Carers Trust Wales, 2022). The 2021 White Paper, 'People at the Heart of Care', acknowledges that people often access care and support at times of crisis, and it can be difficult for people to understand what support is available to them and how to access it (DHSC, 2021: 5.4). Most areas of the UK have local carer support networks provided by local councils, as well as local careers charities. The Carers Trust is a useful organisation to help people find support services local to them.

DECISION-MAKING AND PERSON-CENTRED CARE

For a person living with frailty, care rarely follows a simple pathway (BGS, 2023). The multi-system complexity of frailty in combination with other health conditions means that a person may have input from multiple services at any one time. Ensuring services are aware of each other's roles and treatment priorities can help ensure care is cohesive and meets individual needs.

Considering a person's various health and care needs – symptoms, and physical and social function (Reuben and Tinetti, 2012) – alongside their priorities and goals for care, will help healthcare professionals to assess how well these goals are met, as well as what interventions, if any, are required. A challenge for ambulance clinicians is that assessment is needed at a time of acute need and patients may not be at their baseline activity, and clinicians often don't have access to patient records. Therefore, decisions are made based on the isolated findings and information gained at each attendance (O'Hara et al., 2014). This also means that ambulance clinicians need to be skilled in gathering accurate information from patients and their caregivers.

Making decisions related to the care of patients with frailty is far more complex and individualised than traditional protocol-driven presentations such as stroke or trauma (NIHR, 2016). It is important to consider frailty as well as the current presentation (Hwan Lee et al., 2022). A person's degree of frailty or age alone should never be the sole decision-making factor. Identifying frailty as part of decision-making may lead clinicians to consider both 'what can be done for the patient' and 'what should be done for the patient' (Harper et al., 2020). Best practice guidelines advise that identifying frailty and providing community support is best for patient outcomes (NHS Confederation, 2024), but the additional challenges of acute crisis presentations can add additional complexity to decision-making for ambulance clinicians.

Decisions related to the onward care of patients may be influenced by time of call and attendance. In recent years, ambulance services have struggled to meet target response times, leading to delays in care and some onward care services, such as primary care, may not be available outside of routine working hours (9–5 weekdays), which may influence conveyance decisions (Sinclair et al., 2023).

NHS England (2019) acknowledges that ambulance services are the heart of urgent and emergency care, and efforts are being made to reduce the number of conveyances to hospital. Ambulance services need to work closely with other services within the local health systems to design suitable pathways for onward patient care. Whilst some data has been collected reviewing a range of service interventions to support reducing conveyance of older adults, particularly those living with frailty, the variation in data collected and small area each programme serves (often a single county or Integrated Care Board) makes gathering a national picture of conveyance reduction difficult (Knowles et al., 2020). As top-down pressure increases from policy level, the gap in the evidence base for admission avoidance will widen.

SHARED DECISION-MAKING

Primary care and community services might undertake a comprehensive geriatric assessment of an older adult in some circumstances:

- the person presents to a GP with a frailty syndrome;
- the GP or clinician learns of an incident that suggests the person is frail (such as a fall requiring an ambulance response);
- the person is discharged from hospital following admission for a frailty syndrome with potential prolonged admission;
- a person moves to or is resident in a care or nursing home (BGS, 2019).

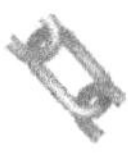 **Chapter 18** for more on decision-making.

Having goals of care that are relevant to a patient can enable them to be involved in healthcare decisions and express what is important to them (Reuben and Tinetti, 2012). An example of this may be a patient who chooses not to have further tests such as endoscopy for a suspected gastrointestinal bleed in the context of anaemia, instead. Choosing feeling

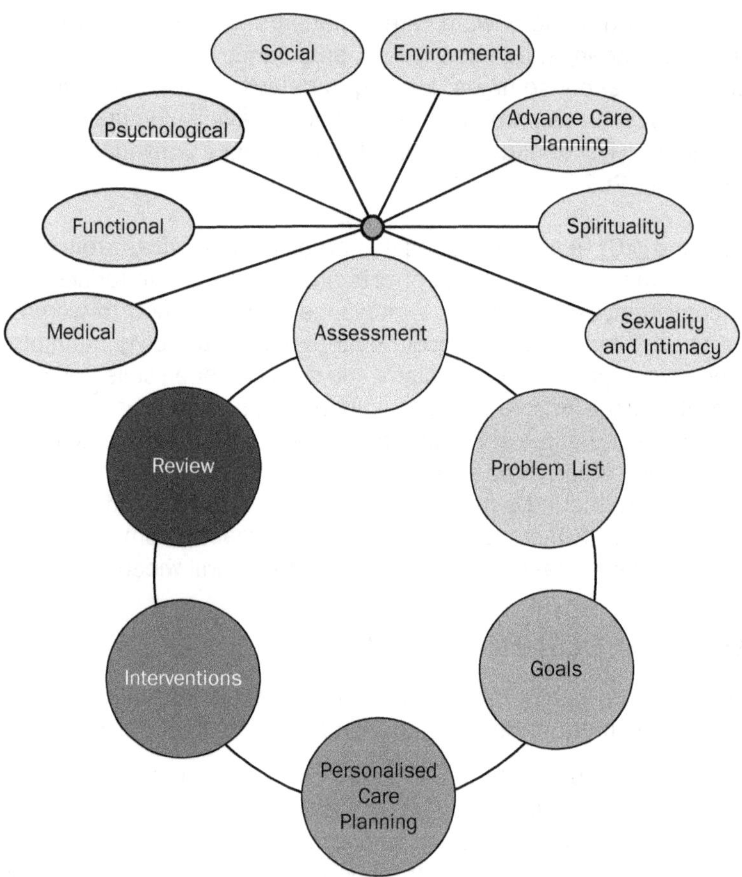

Figure 13.5 Comprehensive Geriatric Assessment Elements Framework

Source: Comprehensive Geriatric Assessment, CGA Toolkit Plus. https://www.cgakit.com/cga.

comfortable instead of diagnostic investigations. Knowing a person's health goals can enable healthcare professionals to work towards clear goals of care (Reuben and Tinetti, 2012), with the decision-making shared by a multidisciplinary team.

Considering a patient using this holistic approach can support decision-making by considering overall common treatment goals for multiple conditions (Reuben and Tinetti, 2012). This may lead to improvements in a person's social, functional and psychological health.

Whilst the Comprehensive Geriatric Assessment Elements Framework (see Figure 13.5) is designed to support clinicians to undertake a thorough and

Table 13.4 Applying the principles of the Comprehensive Geriatric Assessment Framework to the older person

Physical	What conditions do they live with? What acute illnesses or concerns are present? What are the physical assessment findings?
Socioeconomic/ environmental	What is their living environment like? Who is present at the time of assessment? What is the person's social support system like? What services support the person regularly?
Functional	What is their normal baseline activity (last two weeks)? For which tasks does the person need support to complete?
Mobility/balance	How do they mobilise? Can they do this today during assessment? Do they use a mobility aid? What is their balance like normally?
Psychological/ mental	What is their baseline cognition? What is their cognition like today? What is important to them about their care? Are they able to call for assistance should things change? Do they feel safe at home?
Medication review	Have they been taking their prescribed medicines? Have they started or stopped any new medications recently? Do they take any high-risk medications – anticoagulant or antiplatelet therapies? Opioids? Antipsychotics?

personalised in-depth assessment of an older person at a time without acute illness, the structure and elements of the model can be a useful way for clinicians attending patients living with frailty to structure assessment and gain an overall perspective of the person to support decision-making (see Table 13.4). Each and every patient will have different needs, priorities of care and lifestyle circumstances.

If a patient has pre-existing documentation, such as a comprehensive geriatric assessment (CGA), a Proactive Enhanced Advance Care Plan (PEACE) or a Recommended Summary Plan for Emergency Care and Treatment (ReSPECT), it can support and guide ambulance clinicians' decision-making

(Green et al., 2018). Such documentation can support clinicians to consider the risks and benefits of hospital attendance compared with other options available (Green et al., 2018).

End-of-life care for a person living with frailty should be inclusive of the needs and priorities of the individual, as well as of optimising their function and quality of life (Burns, 2020).

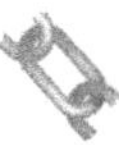 **Chapter 16** for more detail about Do Not Actively Resuscitate (DNAR).

CONCLUSION

The care of older adults living with frailty is complex and requires clinicians to undertake holistic assessments. People living with frailty should be considered as individuals, and clinicians should ensure that the care they provide remains person-centred and does not discriminate on the basis of a person's age, frailty or comorbidities. Care should consider the multifaceted nature of frailty and seek to provide further management and referral opportunities that address not only the acute presenting complaint, but also other aspects of a person's health which may enable them to have an improved quality of life and reduce the incidence of acute debilitating illness or injury.

Chapter key points

- Frailty is not simply a consequence of ageing or the presence of multiple health conditions.
- Frailty is a spectrum and people can both improve or decline along the spectrum of frailty.
- The Clinical Frailty Scale can assist in both recognising frailty and communicating a person's level of frailty to other professionals.
- Clinicians should be able to assess both acute presentations in adults living with frailty and recognise the presence of frailty syndromes.
- Clinicians should be able to make onward referrals to manage acute need, and also refer, where appropriate, to preventative services in order to promote positive long-term health outcomes.

REFERENCES AND SUGGESTED READING

Admi, H., Shadmi, E., Baruch, H. and Zisberg, A. (2015) From research to reality: minimizing the effects of hospitalization on older adults, *Rambam Maimonides Medical Journal*, 6 (2): e0017. Available at: https://www.ncbi.nlm.nih.gov/pmc/articles/PMC4422456/ (accessed 5 April 2024).

Age UK (2019) *Breaking point: The social care burden on women.* Available at: https://www.ageuk.org.uk/contentassets/c3dac0771e614672b363c5fe7e6f826e/breaking-point-age-uk.pdf (accessed 5 April 2024).

British Geriatric Society (BGS) (2011) *Quest for quality.* Available at: https://www.bgs.org.uk/sites/default/files/content/attachment/2019-08-27/quest_quality_care_homes.pdf (accessed 5 April 2024).

British Geriatric Society (BGS) (2018a) *Comprehensive geriatric assessment toolkit for primary care practitioners.* Available at: https://www.bgs.org.uk/sites/default/files/content/resources/files/2019-02-08/BGS%20Toolkit%20-%20FINAL%20FOR%20WEB_0.pdf (accessed 5 April 2024).

British Geriatric Society (BGS) (2018b) *Fit for frailty part 1.* Available at: https://www.bgs.org.uk/sites/default/files/content/resources/files/2018-05-23/fff_full.pdf (accessed 5 April 2024).

British Geriatric Society (BGS) (2019) *1. CGA in primary care settings: Introduction.* Available at: https://www.bgs.org.uk/cgatoolkit (accessed 5 April 2024).

British Geriatric Society (BGS) (2020a) *End of life care in frailty: Continence care.* Available at: https://www.bgs.org.uk/resources/resource-series/end-of-life-care-in-frailty (accessed 5 April 2024).

British Geriatric Society (BGS) (2020b) *End of life care in frailty: Delirium.* Available at: https://www.bgs.org.uk/resources/resource-series/end-of-life-care-in-frailty (accessed 5 April 2024).

British Geriatric Society (BGS) (2023) *Joining the dots: A blueprint for preventing and managing frailty in older people.* Available at: https://www.bgs.org.uk/Blueprint (accessed 5 April 2024).

Burns, E. (2020) *End of life care in frailty: Introduction and foreword.* London: British Geriatric Society. Available at: https://www.bgs.org.uk/resources/resource-series/end-of-life-care-in-frailty.

Buswell, M., Lumbard, P., Fleming, J., Ayres, D. et al. (2016) Using ambulance service PCRs to understand 999 call-outs to older people with dementia, *Journal of Paramedic Practice*, 8 (5): 246–51.

Centre for Ageing Better (CAB) (2022) *Health: The state of ageing 2022.* Available at: https://ageing-better.org.uk/health-state-ageing-2022 (accessed 5 April 2024).

Cesari, M., Gambassi, G., Abellan van Kan, G. and Vellas, B. (2014) The frailty phenotype and the frailty index: different instruments for different purposes, *Age and Ageing*, 43 (1): 10–12.

Charlton, K., Sinclair, D., Hanratty, B., Burrow, E. et al. (2022) Measuring frailty and its association with key outcomes in the ambulance setting: a cross sectional observational study, *BMC Geriatrics*, 22: 935. Available at: https://bmcgeriatr.biomedcentral.com/counter/pdf/10.1186/s12877-022-03633-z.pdf (accessed 5 April 2024).

Clegg, A., Young, J., Iliffe, S., Olde Rikkert, M. et al. (2013) Frailty in older people, *Lancet*, 3981 (9868): 752–62.

Comprehensive Geriatric Assessment, CGA Toolkit Plus. Available at: https://www.cgakit.com/cga (accessed 10 September 2024)

Dalhouse University (no date) *Clinical Frailty Scale*. Available at: https://pubmed.ncbi.nlm.nih.gov/26301980/ (accessed 5 April 2024).

Department of Health and Social Care (DHSC) (2021) *People at the heart of care*. Available at: https://assets.publishing.service.gov.uk/media/6234b0a6e90e0779a18d3f46/people-at-the-heart-of-care-asc-reform-accessible-with-correction-slip.pdf (accessed 5 April 2024).

Dijk-Huisman, H. van, Raeven-Eijkenboom, P.H., Magdelijns, F.J.H., Sieben, J.M. et al. (2022) Barriers and enablers to physical activity behaviour in older adults during hospital stay: a qualitative study guided by the theoretical domains framework, *BMC Geriatrics*, 22: 314. Available at: https://bmcgeriatr.biomedcentral.com/articles/10.1186/s12877-022-02887-x (accessed 5 April 2024).

Dwyer, R., Gabbe, B., Tran, T. D., Smith, K. et al. (2018) Patterns of emergency ambulance use, 2009–13: a comparison of older people living in residential aged care facilities and the community, *Age and Ageing*, 47 (4): 615–19.

Dykes, L. (2018) *Delirium: Top tips*. Available at: https://www.lindadykes.org/_files/ugd/bbd630_250fb9b676ed484aada7f89b6ce7d239.pdf (accessed 5 April 2024).

Elliott, A., Hull, L. and Conroy, S.P. (2017) Frailty identification in the emergency department: a systematic review focussing on feasibility, *Age and Ageing*, 46 (3): 509–13.

Falconi, G. and Daniel, T. (2018) *Delirium do's and dont's*. Available at: https://www.grepmed.com/images/3641/management-dos-guidelines-donts-geriatrics (accessed 5 April 2024).

Fehlmann, C.A., Stuby, L., Graf, C., Genoud, M. et al. (2023) Assessment of frailty by paramedics using the Clinical Frailty Scale: an interrater reliability and accuracy study, *BMC Emergency Medicine*, 23: 121. Available at: https://bmcemergmed.biomedcentral.com/articles/10.1186/s12873-023-00875-x (accessed 5 April 2024).

Fletcher, J.R. (2021) Age-associations in British politics: implications for the sociology of aging, *British Journal of Sociology*, 72 (3): 609–26.

Gillespie, L.D., Robertson, M.C., Gillespie, W.J., Sherrington, C. et al. (2012) Interventions for preventing falls in older people living in the community, *Cochrane Database of Systematic Reviews*, 9: CD007146. Available at: https://doi.org/10.1002/14651858.CD007146.pub3 (accessed 6 August 2024).

Government Office for Science (2016) *Future of an ageing population*. Available at: https://assets.publishing.service.gov.uk/media/5d273adce5274a5862768ff9/future-of-an-ageing-population.pdf (accessed 5 April 2024).

Green, J., Kirby, K. and Hope, S. (2018) Ambulance clinicians' perceptions, assessment and management of frailty: thematic analysis of focus groups, *British Paramedic Journal*, 3 (3): 23–33.

Harper, A., Wilkinson, I. and Preston, J. (2020) Geriatric medicine, frailty and multimorbidity, in A. Feather, D. Randall and M. Waterhouse (eds.) *Kumar and Clark's Clinical Medicine*, 10th edition, pp. 297–317. London: Elsevier.

Hartley, P., Forsyth, F., O'Halloran, A., Kenny, R.A. et al. (2023) Eight-year longitudinal falls trajectories and associations with modifiable risk factors: evidence from The Irish Longitudinal Study on Ageing (TILDA), *Age and Ageing*, 52 (3): afad037. Available from: https://doi.org/10.1093/ageing/afad037 (accessed 5 April 2024).

Hwan Lee, J., Seok Park, Y., Joung Kim, M., Jung Shin, H. et al. (2022) Clinical Frailty Scale as a predictor of short-term mortality: a systematic review and meta-analysis of studies on diagnostic test accuracy, *Academic Emergency Medicine*, 29 (11): 1347–56.

Isaacs, B. (1992) *The Challenge of Geriatric Medicine.* Oxford: Oxford University Press.

International Longevity Centres (2023) *One hundred not out: A route map for long lives.* Available at: https://ilcuk.org.uk/wp-content/uploads/2024/01/One-hundred-not-out-report-final.pdf (accessed 5 April 2024).

Jadzinski, P., Pocock, H., Lofthouse-Jones, C., King, P. et al. (2021) Improving recording and reporting of dementia and frailty via electronic patient record by ambulance staff in a single service (IDEAS), *British Paramedic Journal*, 6 (3): 31–40.

Knowles, E., Long, J. and Turner, J. (2020) *Reducing avoidable ambulance conveyance in England: Interventions and associated evidence.* Sheffield: University of Sheffield, School of Health and Related Research. Available at: https://aace.org.uk/wp-content/uploads/2020/08/ScHARR-report-SRAC-Final-020320-.pdf (accessed 5 April 2024).

Lafont, C., Gérard, S., Voisin, T., Pahor, M. et al. (2011) Reducing 'iatrogenic disability' in the hospitalized frail elderly, *Journal of Nutrition, Health and Aging*, 15 (8): 645–60.

Leeds Frailty Education (2023) 5 benefits of using the Clinical Frailty Scale, *YouTube*. Available at: https://www.youtube.com/watch?v=OFo79drrU5k (accessed 6 August 2024).

Maharani, A., Sinclair, D., Chandola, T., Bower, P. et al. (2023) Household wealth, neighbourhood deprivation and frailty amongst middle-aged and older adults in England: a longitudinal analysis over 15 years (2002–2017), *Age and Ageing*, 52 (3): afad034. Available from: https://www.ncbi.nlm.nih.gov/pmc/articles/PMC10061942/ (accessed 5 April 2024).

Morley, J.E., Vellas, B., Abellan van Kan, G., Anker, S.D. et al. (2013) Frailty consensus: a call to action, *Journal of the American Medical Directors Association*, 14 (6): 392–97.

National Institute for Health and Care Excellence (NICE) (2023a) *Hypertension.* Available at: https://cks.nice.org.uk/topics/hypertension/#:~:text=Age%20 under%2080%20years%20%E2%80%94%20clinic,based%20on%20standing%20 blood%20pressure (accessed 5 April 2024).

National Institute for Health and Care Excellence (NICE) (2023b) *Delirium: Prevention, diagnosis and management in hospital and long-term care*, Clinical guideline CG103. Available at: https://www.nice.org.uk/guidance/cg103/chapter/Context (accessed 5 April 2024).

National Institute for Health Research (NIHR) (2016) *Care at the scene: Research for ambulance services.* Available at: https://aace.org.uk/wp-content/uploads/2016/05/Care-at-the-scene-final-for-web.pdf (accessed 5 April 2024).

NHS Assembly (2023) *The NHS in England at 75: Priorities for the future*. Available at: https://www.longtermplan.nhs.uk/wp-content/uploads/2023/06/The-NHS-in-England-at-75-priorities-for-the-future.pdf (accessed 5 April 2024).

NHS Confederation (2023) *Providing urgent health care at home for older people living with frailty*. Available at: https://www.nhsconfed.org/case-studies/providing-urgent-health-care-home-older-people-living-frailty (accessed 6 August 2024).

NHS Confederation (2024) *Supporting people with frailty*. Available at: https://www.nhsconfed.org/publications/supporting-people-frailty (accessed 6 August 2024).

NHS England (2019) *The NHS Long Term Plan*. Available at: https://www.longtermplan.nhs.uk/wp-content/uploads/2019/08/nhs-long-term-plan-version-1.2.pdf (accessed 5 April 2024).

NHS England (2022) *Community health services two-hour urgent community response standard*. Available at: https://www.england.nhs.uk/wp-content/uploads/2021/07/B1406-community-health-services-two-hour-urgent-community-response-standard.pdf (accessed 5 April 2024).

NHS England (2023) *Electronic frailty index*. Available at: https://www.england.nhs.uk/ourwork/clinical-policy/older-people/frailty/efi/#why-is-clinical-judgement-important-can-clinicians-not-just-use-the-results-of-the-tool (accessed 5 April 2024).

Office for Health Improvement and Disparities (2023) *A consensus on healthy ageing*, Policy paper. Available at: https://www.gov.uk/government/publications/healthy-ageing-consensus-statement/a-consensus-on-healthy-ageing (accessed 6 August 2024).

O'Hara, R., Johnson, M., Hirst, E., Weyman, A. et al. (2014) A qualitative study of decision-making and safety in ambulance service transitions, *Health Services and Delivery Research*, 2 (56). Available at: https://www.ncbi.nlm.nih.gov/books/NBK269166/pdf/Bookshelf_NBK269166.pdf (accessed 5 April 2024).

Potocnik, K. and Sonnentag, S. (2013) A longitudinal study of well-being in older workers and retirees: the role of engaging in different types of activities, *Journal of Occupational and Organizational Psychology*, 86 (4): 497–521.

Preston, J., Wilkinson, I., Moffatt, T. and Lelkes, J. (2017a) Episode 3.06: Identity and ageing, *The Hearing Aid Podcasts* [online blog]. Available at: https://thehearingaidpodcasts.org.uk/wp-content/uploads/2017/05/Show-notes-Identity-and-Ageing.pdf (accessed 5 April 2024).

Preston, J., Wilkinson, I. and Ryan, S.J. (2017b) Episode 4.01: Theories of ageing, *The Hearing Aid Podcasts* [online blog]. Available at: https://thehearingaidpodcasts.org.uk/episode-4-01-theories-of-ageing/ (accessed 5 April 2024).

Public Health England (2021) *Caring as a social determinant of health*. Available at: https://assets.publishing.service.gov.uk/media/60547266d3bf7f2f14694965/Caring_as_a_social_determinant_report.pdf (accessed 5 April 2024).

Purdy, S. (2010) *Avoiding hospital admissions: What does the research evidence say?* Available at: https://assets.kingsfund.org.uk/f/256914/x/3aa73acab8/avoiding_hospital_admissions_2010.pdf (accessed 6 August 2024).

Reason, J. (2000) Human error: models and management, *British Medical Journal*, 320 (7237): 768–70.

Reuben, D. and Tinetti, M. (2012) Goal-orientated patient care: an alternative health outcomes paradigm, *New England Journal of Medicine*, 366 (9): 777–79.

Robertson, C.M., Gillespie, W.J., Sherrington, C., Gates, S. et al. (2012) Interventions for preventing falls in older people living in the community, *Cochrane Database of Systematic Reviews*, 2012 (9): CD007146. Available at: https://www.ncbi.nlm.nih.gov/pmc/articles/PMC8095069/ (accessed 5 April 2024).

Rockwood, K., Song, X., MacKnight, C., Bergman, H. et al. (2005) A global clinical measure of fitness and frailty in elderly people, *Canadian Medical Association Journal*, 173 (5): 489–95.

Romero-Ortuno, R., Walsh, C., Lawlor, B. and Kenny, R.A. (2010) A frailty instrument for primary care: findings from the Survey of Health, Ageing and Retirement in Europe (SHARE), *BMC Geriatrics*, 10: 57. Available at: https://www.ncbi.nlm.nih.gov/pmc/articles/PMC2939541 (accessed 5 April 2024).

Royal College of Physicians (RCP) (2017) *How to do lying and standing blood pressure*. Available at: https://www.rcplondon.ac.uk/projects/outputs/measurement-lying-and-standing-blood-pressure-brief-guide-clinical-staff (accessed 5 April 2024).

Royal College of Physicians (RCP) (2020) *Acute Care Toolkit 3: Acute care for older people living with frailty*. Available at: https://www.rcplondon.ac.uk/guidelines-policy/acute-care-toolkit-3-acute-care-older-people-living-frailty (accessed 5 April 2024).

Rueegg, M., Nissen, S. and Brabrand, M. (2022) The clinical frailty scale predicts 1-year mortality in emergency department patients aged 65 years and older, *Academic Emergency Medicine*, 29 (5): 572–80.

Sinclair, D.R., Maharani, A., Chandola, T., Bower, P. et al. (2022) Frailty among older adults and its distribution in England, *Journal of Frailty and Aging*, 11: 163–68.

Sinclair, D., Charlton, K., Stow, D., Burrow, E. et al. (2023) Care home residency and its association with ambulance service workload, *Journal of the American Medical Directors Association*, 24 (5): 657–60.

Smith, N., Hunter, K., Rajabali, S., Fainsinger, R. et al. (2019) Preferences for continence care experienced at end of life: a qualitative study, *Journal of Pain and Symptom Management*, 57 (6): 1099–1105.

Statista (2024) *Life expectancy (from birth) in the United Kingdom from 1765 to 2020*. Available at: https://www.statista.com/statistics/1040159/life-expectancy-united-kingdom-all-time/ (accessed 6 August 2024).

The Carers Trust Wales (2022) *Experiences of unpaid carers from Black and Minority Ethnic Communities Report*. Available at: https://carers.org/downloads/carers-trust-report-final.pdf (accessed 5 April 2024).

Wallis, S.J., Wall, J., Bram, R.W.S. and Romero-Ortuno, R. (2015) Association of the clinical frailty scale with hospital outcomes, *QJM: Monthly Journal of the Association of Physicians*, 108 (12): 943–49.

Wyrko, Z. (2015) Frailty at the front door, *Clinical Medicine*, 15 (4): 377–81.

Xue, Q.-L. (2011) The frailty syndrome: definition and natural history, *Clinics in Geriatric Medicine*, 27: 1–15.

USEFUL WEBSITES

British Geriatric Society discussing uncertainty in the context of acute deterioration: https://www.bgs.org.uk/resources/end-of-life-care-in-frailty-urgent-care-needs# anchor-nav-discussing-uncertainty-in-the-context-of-acute-deterioration

Clinical Frailty Scale: https://www.acutefrailtynetwork.org.uk/Clinical-Frailty-Scale/ Clinical-Frailty-Scale-App

5 Reasons to use the Clinical Frailty Score: https://www.youtube.com/watch? v=OFo79drrU5k

NICE guidelines for older people: https://www.nice.org.uk/guidance/population-groups/older-people

The Carers Trust: https://carers.org

14

Safeguarding adults

Gwenan Jones-Parry

In this chapter:

- Introduction
- Why is this relevant?
- UK legislation and guidance
- Who is at risk?
- Harm, abuse and neglect
- Types of abuse
- Reporting safeguarding concerns
- Professional concerns
- Case studies
- Conclusion
- Chapter key points
- References and suggested reading

INTRODUCTION

This chapter relates to safeguarding people over 18 years of age. An adult should be able to live safely, free from harm (Butler, 2022). This area of work can provide a challenging dichotomy for healthcare professionals, as adults with capacity will sometimes make unwise decisions. Adults with capacity may choose to remain in a situation where there is risk of abuse and neglect, contrary to the advice and support offered by attending healthcare professionals. Paramedics must not judge, and need to understand some adults risk-assess on a daily basis. Adult safeguarding is a balance between respecting individuals' right to live as they wish and protecting those adults who are unable to protect themselves, and meet the 'adult at risk' definition.

Regardless of what kind of environment paramedics find themselves working in, safeguarding adults training must be a fundamental element of all induction and ongoing education. Historically, there has been greater emphasis on safeguarding children. Several UK Acts of Parliament and sets of guidance have been published in recent years that address the past imbalance between safeguarding children and safeguarding adults.

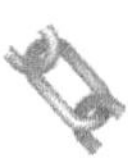 **Chapter 11** for more on safeguarding children.

This chapter will provide the essential knowledge to enable paramedics to practise, with a suitable level of awareness regarding the theory of safeguarding adults. Healthcare professionals of all grades and roles must consider safeguarding essential knowledge to their work, and it should be considered with every service user interaction.

WHY IS THIS RELEVANT?

Adult safeguarding concerns may be highlighted at any time by paramedics both in a professional capacity and via personal non-work exposure to neglect and abuse. In professional forums, safeguarding concerns may be identified at any point; call handling, attendance at 999/urgent calls, during transportation, primary care consultations and remote clinical work. Safeguarding concerns may also be identified through single or integrated governance processes such as high impact service users, complaints, audits or reviews.

Paramedics are in a very privileged and unique position to identify safeguarding adult concerns due to the nature of working in out-of-hospital emergency care settings. Paramedics are often the first professionals to interact with an adult at risk and can identify/report initial concerns (JRCALC Plus, 2024). Emergency calls to the ambulance service dictate that paramedics are often the only professionals to gain entry to certain premises or speak to victims of abuse/neglect. This was especially true during the COVID-19 pandemic when many services stopped home visits or face-to-face consultations, but ambulance services did not. There were also additional safeguarding challenges during the pandemic as many people were further isolated, putting them at greater risk. The College of Paramedics (CoP) asked at the time that paramedics be vigilant for signs of abuse/neglect (CoP, 2020).

The Joint Royal Colleges Ambulance Liaison Committee (JRCALC Plus, 2024) guidelines have a safeguarding adults section which clearly summarises the expectation for paramedics to stop abuse/neglect, respect adults' wishes where possible, report concerns appropriately and document fully concerns/actions (JRCALC Plus, 2024). There is no expectation for paramedics to investigate safeguarding concerns; the expectation is to recognise and report appropriately and in a timely manner.

Any suspicion of adult abuse and neglect must be addressed by sharing information with the police and other services, such as social care. If a paramedic is unsure of how to respond to circumstances, an initial discussion with a more specialist colleague in their own organisation would be appropriate. Occasionally, the threshold for safeguarding concerns may not be met but there may be an expectation that concerns are reported via a different route, for example via serious incident reporting mechanisms. The Health and Care Professions Council's (HCPC) *Standards of Proficiency for Paramedics* includes specific standards in relation to safeguarding. Standard 6.3 evidences safeguarding as a paramedic's responsibility: 'recognise and respond in a timely manner to situations where it is necessary to share information to safeguarding service users, carers and/or the wider public' (HCPC, 2023).

To think that human beings are able to abuse and neglect one another is both distressing and disturbing for healthcare professionals, and historically has not be considered at the beginning of a paramedic's career. The Dreyfus model proposes that to acquire a new skill, individuals should progress through its various stages (Mangiante and Peno, 2021), and the same is true of newly qualified paramedics.

Safeguarding concerns may be immediately upsetting or emotionally corrosive over time and it is important that professionals seek help should this be necessary. Involvement in incidents causing such distress must be acknowledged by individuals/organisations, prompting them to seek/provide welfare and support. Each organisation will have its own welfare arrangements and personnel should embrace these. Service users can only be provided with the highest level of care by a healthy workforce (Meadley et al., 2020).

UK LEGISLATION AND GUIDANCE

Safeguarding adults is governed by many Acts of Parliament and national guidelines. The following is not an exhaustive list but captures the main elements of UK legislation currently influencing adult safeguarding practice.

- Adult Support and Protection (Scotland) Act 2007 (Legislation.gov. uk, 2007)
- Care Act 2014 (Legislation.gov.uk, 2014a)

- Counter-Terrorism and Security Act 2015 (Legislation.gov.uk, 2015a)
- Domestic Abuse Act 2021 (Legislation.gov.uk, 2021a)
- Domestic Abuse and Civil Proceedings Act (Northern Ireland) 2021 (Legislation.gov.uk, 2021b)
- Domestic Abuse (Scotland) Act 2018 (Legislation.gov.uk, 2018b)
- Equality Act 2010 (Legislation.gov.uk, 2010)
- Female Genital Mutilation Act 2003 (Legislation.gov.uk, 2003a)
- Female Genital Mutilation (Protection and Guidance) (Scotland) Act 2020 (Legislation.gov.uk, 2020)
- Human Rights Act 1998 (Legislation.gov.uk, 1998)
- Mental Capacity Act 2005 (Legislation.gov.uk, 2005)
- Modern Slavery Act 2015 (Legislation.gov.uk, 2015b)
- Sexual Offences Act 2003 (Legislation.gov.uk, 2003b)
- Serious Crime Act 2015 (Legislation.gov.uk, 2015f)
- Social Services and Well-being (Wales) Act 2014 (Legislation.gov.uk, 2014b)
- Violence Against Women, Domestic Abuse and Sexual Violence (Wales) Act 2015 (Legislation.gov.uk, 2015e)

Although there are UK-wide Acts, each country within the UK has specific legislation. Paramedics should ensure they comprehend the legislation where they practice and are apprised of their employer's safeguarding policies and reporting mechanisms.

Wales was the first of the UK nations to publish legislation on domestic abuse with the Violence Against Women, Domestic Abuse and Sexual Violence (Wales) Act 2015. There has since been the publication of the Domestic Abuse (Scotland) Act 2018, Domestic Abuse and Civil Proceedings Act (Northern Ireland) 2021 and the Domestic Abuse Act 2021 for England. Each piece of legislation has different definitions and remits. It is important paramedics understand the Acts that are relevant to their jurisdiction.

Of note, there is a new criminal offence in England and Wales called '*non-fatal strangulation or suffocation*'. It was created as part of the Domestic Abuse Act 2021, which amends the Serious Crime Act 2015 (Home Office, 2023a). The offence clarifies there is no 'attempted strangulation' if an individual applies pressure to the throat and impedes oxygen reaching the brain: they have strangled the victim (even if not fatally) (Home Office, 2023a).

WHO IS AT RISK?

It is imperative paramedics understand that everyone, at some point in their lives, may be at risk of harm, abuse, neglect and/or exploitation (JRCALC

Plus, 2024). An adult can be victimised due to circumstances or following a specific event: loss of a job, bereavement and/or poor health. Different to safeguarding children, adults must meet the definition of an 'adult at risk'. The Social Services and Well-being (Wales) Act (2014) defines an 'adult at risk' as an adult who

> *(a) Is experiencing or is at risk of abuse or neglect,*
> *(b) Has needs for care and support (whether or not the authority is meeting any of those needs), and*
> *(c) As a result of those needs is unable to protect himself or herself against the abuse or neglect or the risk of it.*

The Adult Support and Protection (Scotland) Act (2007), Care Act (England) (2014) and Northern Ireland's Adult Safeguarding: Prevention and protection in partnership policy (Department of Health, Social Services and Public Safety, 2015) contain similar definitions. The crux is there must be an aspect of an adult's life which makes them unable to protect themselves. Consideration must be given to implementation of these principles during all service user contact (face-to-face or hear and treat). All three of the above descriptors must be met prior to concerns being reported to local authority adult safeguarding teams. When paramedics are unsure, they must seek advice.

When considering whether an individual meets the criteria, the following should be considered:

- physical frailty/chronic illness;
- older person with care needs;
- physical/sensory disability;
- mental health/dementia/lacking capacity;
- alcohol/substance misuse;
- autistic spectrum disorder.

'Adults at risk' were previously known as vulnerable adults (see Table 14.1 for further updated safeguarding terminology). In this chapter, I use the word 'victim', and paramedics need to understand that all individuals who have suffered abuse are survivors.

Safeguarding discussions should only be conducted if safe to do so. Paramedics must not place themselves or the adult at risk of harm by discussing safeguarding concerns in the presence of the perpetrator. There will also be times when the 'adult at risk' is unconscious and unable to provide information. If paramedics have safeguarding concerns and are unable to discuss, a 'best interest' decision can be made, and a safeguarding report submitted without consent (Office of the Public Guardian, 2009).

Table 14.1 Safeguarding terminology

Previous term/wording	Updated term/wording
Vulnerabilities	Needs for care and support
Adult protection	Adult at risk
POVA – protection of vulnerable adult	Adult at risk safeguarding report
Safeguarding referral	Safeguarding report
Safeguarding issues	Safeguarding concerns

A key consideration is whether the individual has capacity and provides consent for a safeguarding report. Paramedics will need to practise in line with the principles of capacity legislation relevant to them: the Mental Capacity Act (2015) in Wales and England; the Mental Capacity Act (Northern Ireland) 2016 and the Adults with Incapacity (Scotland) Act (2000). It is recommended practice to have consent from an adult with capacity, but the Data Protection Act (2018) does permit the submission of safeguarding reports for 'adults at risk' without consent. Box 14.1 lists the key principles from the Care Act (2014) that are to be considered for those involved in adult safeguarding. The paramedic role is clearly highlighted.

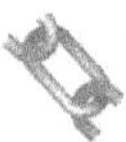 **Chapter 4** for more on mental capacity and consent.

Paramedics often find themselves in very challenging safeguarding situations, in possession of limited medical histories and social backgrounds. Decisions must not be made in isolation; internal support and external agency guidance should be considered. Often challenging, discussions and decisions to report (or not report) safeguarding concerns should be documented with the relevant rationale (JRCALC Plus, 2024). Understandably, certain times of the day can present unique challenges. Many complex safeguarding events occur during the night, but there are always other professionals available. On-call social service professionals can receive immediate safeguarding concerns.

Box 14.1 The six principles for adult safeguarding

1 Accountability: *Accountability and transparency in delivering safeguarding.* For paramedics, there is a need to adhere to current clinical guidelines and ensure that actions are commensurate with professional registration.

2 Empowerment: *People being supported and encouraged to make their own decisions and provide informed consent.* Paramedics must implement the practice of making safeguarding personal and placing the individual at the centre of their care.

3 Partnership: *Local solutions through services working with their communities.* Paramedics must share their concerns with local authorities. May relate to a service user or carer, or escalation of concerns about a service user, professional or colleague.

4 Prevention: *It is preferable to take action before harm occurs.* Paramedics possess information regarding individuals other agencies may not be aware of.

5 Proportionality: *The least intrusive response appropriate to the risk presented.* It is essential paramedics adhere to guidance regarding dignity and respect. When faced with a challenging adult safeguarding concern, consider all options, including the individual's wishes.

6 Protection: *Support and representation for those in greatest need.* Paramedics must act swiftly to protect adults at risk when abuse/neglect is identified. May require police attendance.

Source: Care Act 2014 (Legislation.gov.uk, 2014a).

Adult victims can be any age, but in consideration of the service users paramedics often treat, they should always be suspicious of elder abuse (Shepperd, 2021). In June 2022, the World Health Organization published a factsheet stating that elder abuse is a global public health problem; one in six people over the age of 60 had experienced some form of abuse within the previous year (WHO, 2022). Elder abuse can be a single or repeated act (or lack of appropriate action) which causes distress/harm to an older adult within a trusting relationship. It often involves the loss of dignity and respect (WHO, 2022). Age UK (2023) states that individuals over 85 years are most likely to be the subject of a safeguarding enquiry.

Reflection: points to consider

You do not need proof that an adult is being abused or neglected; you need reasonable grounds to suspect and evidence that the adult meets the 'adult at risk' definition. If an adult lacks capacity, report your concerns as you can make a 'best interest' decision. When in doubt regarding whether an adult has capacity, or whether an individual meets the 'adult at risk' definition, seek advice.

HARM, ABUSE AND NEGLECT

The impairment of intellectual, social, physical or behavioural development causes harm (Social Care Wales, 2019). The *Oxford English Dictionary* defines 'abuse' as a chronic corrupt practice/custom or improper usage (OED, 2023). Neglect is when an individual deliberately withholds (or fails to provide) adequate care to another (NI Direct Government Services, 2023).

To cause harm, all a perpetrator/abuser requires is the opportunity (Starns, 2019). Perpetrators can be known to the individual (carer, friend, colleague, family member) or a stranger, have any background and be of any, religion, race, gender or age. Every adult has the right to live free from harm (JRCALC Plus, 2024).

Incidents of abuse/neglect may be one-off or repeated over a period of time. The abuse may affect one person or a group of people. Paramedics must remain vigilant and raise concerns, no matter the environment/situation, when witnessing harm to 'adults at risk'. Even a snippet of information could be enough to trigger an enquiry. It is essential paramedics are familiar with local inter-agency processes and feel confident reporting concerns when required. It is useful to consider safeguarding as a jigsaw puzzle the local authority is trying to complete. Information paramedics hold could be critical in providing the missing piece to the puzzle, thus enabling the local authority to act.

TYPES OF ABUSE

High quality education is one of the most important elements to safeguarding adults; knowledge and awareness will improve recognition and reporting. An understanding of the different categories and their indicators is crucial if paramedics are to report concerns appropriately. There is a wide range of types of abuse, which can be committed in isolation or in combination. Not recognising the type of abuse should not prohibit the paramedic from reporting concerns. The receiving local authority can investigate and decide definitively the type of abuse involved. In this section, possible indicators of each type of abuse are provided; although not exhaustive, these lists should help to raise paramedics' awareness.

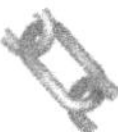

Chapter 11 to compare the similarities and differences between child and adult safeguarding indicators.

Physical abuse

This type of abuse considers anything physical that is done to an individual that may cause actual or potential harm: punching, kicking, slapping, biting, scratching or beating with an object (see Box 14.2). The use of inappropriate or excessive restraint, the intentional incorrect administration of medication, and fabricated/induced illness are also classified as physical abuse.

Box 14.2 Indicators of physical abuse

- History of unexplained falls/injuries
- Not being allowed to go where you'd like, when you'd like
- Illegal use of restraint
- Rough handling
- Intentional improper medication administration
- Fractures
- Burns/marks in unexpected places
- Not wanting to be touched, recoiling from professionals
- 'Finger pattern' marks
- Untreated medical problems/injuries

Adapted from: NHS Choices (2021), NI Direct Government Services (2023), Southern Health & Social Care Trust (2024).

Sexual abuse

Sexual abuse can be perpetrated against anyone, no matter their age or gender (Home Office, 2020), can take many forms and has significant psychological and physical impacts. It includes sexual harassment, rape, being forced or pressured to take part in sexual acts, being forced to watch sexual acts or pornography, sexual photography or inappropriate looking/touching (NHS Choices, 2021) (see Box 14.3). If anyone (including partner or ex-partner) has sex with an adult without their consent, it is rape (CPS, 2022b). Paramedics must be patient, supportive, understanding and provide opportunities for victims to disclose. Remind victims it is not their fault and it is a crime, no matter who the perpetrator is or where the offence occurred (NHS England, 2021).

Conveyance to the emergency department may not always be the most appropriate care pathway for a victim of sexual abuse, and close working with the police is necessary. Paramedics must make themselves familiar with the local procedures for dealing with cases of sexual abuse, including processes for accessing the local Sexual Assault Referral Centre (SARC) or similar in the local area.

Box 14.3 Indicators of sexual abuse

- Altered sleep patterns
- Sexually transmitted diseases
- Unexpected or unexplained behaviour changes
- Soreness/discomfort in the genital area
- Torn, stained or bloody underwear
- Preoccupation with anything sexual
- Withdrawal, spending the majority of the time alone
- Sudden onset of soiling, wetting or confusion

Adapted from: Southern Health & Social Care Trust (2024), Tameside Metropolitan Borough Council (2022).

Emotional/psychological abuse

Emotional/psychological abuse is the persistent emotional maltreatment of an individual and can significantly damage health and wellbeing (Social Care Wales, 2019). It is often difficult to detect as behavioural changes may develop over time (AMIS, 2020). The Domestic Abuse and Civil Proceedings Act (Northern Ireland) 2021 states that psychological harm includes causing fear, alarm or distress. Perpetrators of emotional abuse are often affectionate, which confuses the victim and provides hope the situation may improve (AMIS, 2020). Such abuse may only become apparent upon disclosure by the victim or based on the perpetrator's behaviour. See Box 14.4 for the indicators of emotional/psychological abuse abuse.

Box 14.4 Indicators of emotional/psychological abuse

Victim

- Not able to focus
- Very eager to please
- Compulsive behaviours
- Being withdrawn, isolated from family and friends

Adapted from: NI Direct Government Services (2023).

Perpetrator behaviours

- Enforces isolation, often with threats of abandonment
- Deprives all wider support by ensuring lack of contact with others (isolation)
- Intimidation and threats
- Persistently embarrasses or humiliates the victim (in person or via social media)
- Controlling or coercive behaviour aimed at disempowering and undermining
- Threatens physical violence

Adapted from: Home Office (2020, 2023a).

Neglect and acts of omission

Neglect is the impairment of an individual's wellbeing (e.g. health), based on a failure to meet their basic needs: social, psychological, emotional, care or physical needs (Social Care Wales, 2019). It is sometimes a real challenge for professionals to make the distinction between neglect and poor standards of care. Concerns should be discussed (seek advice and support) and reported; a multi-agency safeguarding meeting (strategy meeting/case conference) will be held if considered necessary. See Box 14.5 for the main indicators of neglect.

Box 14.5 Indicators of neglect

- Poor physical condition/personal hygiene
- Pressure sores
- Poor environment
- Malnutrition/unexplained weight loss
- Accumulation of untaken medication
- Inappropriate or inadequate clothing
- Untreated injuries/medical problems
- Delay seeking medical assistance

Adapted from: SCIE (2020).

Self-neglect

Self-neglect is the neglect of one's own personal health and surroundings, unwillingness to manage one's affairs and failure to seek help or access services (SCIE, 2018). It often leads to harm as the individual is unable to care for themselves. Paramedics have witnessed self-neglect for years, but historically, if the adult had capacity, no action would be taken without their consent. Current legislation recognises this as part of safeguarding responsibilities – when the way an 'adult at risk' lives has an adverse effect on their health and wellbeing, paramedics can report their concerns without the adult's consent. See Box 14.6 for the main indicators of self-neglect.

Consider whether the person is a hoarder; fire and rescue services (FRS) nationally have cluttering tools to assess risk in properties. Paramedics may consider contacting their local FRS to share information if consent is forthcoming, and the local authority environmental health team as they possess legislative powers to assist/act.

Self-neglect also includes a failure to self-care through poor personal hygiene, which would likely be evident during a face-to-face assessment. It is a complex situation for paramedics when visiting personal residences and decision-making can be difficult, so seek advice if you are at all uncertain how to act.

Box 14.6 Indicators of self-neglect

- Poor personal hygiene
- Property in disrepair, cluttered garden
- Poor security, lack of locks on doors/windows
- Hoarding affecting access/egress
- Evidence of fire risks
- Signs of vermin/infestation
- Unsafe or out-of-date utility fittings
- Lack of heating, plumbing, electricity
- Non-compliance with health and care services

Adapted from: SCIE (2020).

Financial abuse

There are many methods that perpetrators of financial or material abuse use to access money and/or possessions. These may range from simple opportunistic thefts/fraud to large multi-million pound internet-based scams (Social Care Wales, 2019). Paramedics may attend victims of assault or robbery where further disclosure of ongoing financial abuse is shared by the adult at risk. These allegations must be taken seriously, as the perpetrator may be a close family member or another professional or carer in close contact with the victim. Your concerns must be raised immediately, highlighting whether the alleged perpetrator is a person in a position of trust (further information can be obtained by reading the 'professional concerns' section on p. 308). Financial abuse may involve property, inheritance, wills and lasting power of attorney arrangements. See Box 14.7 for more details.

Box 14.7 Indicators of financial abuse

- Poor living conditions as unable to invest in maintenance and repairs
- Poor self-care through a lack of money to buy new clothes and toiletries
- Mounting bills as unable to pay utilities
- Cold or poorly heated property
- Unable to locate debit/credit cards or money
- Unusual activity or unapproved withdrawals from bank account
- Changes to financial documents such as wills
- Frequent telephone calls from unknown persons
- Lack of food and drink in the home leading to weight loss

Adapted from: SCIE (2020), Southern Health &
Social Care Trust (2024).

Domestic abuse

Domestic abuse is pervasive and can be found in all cultures, communities and social groupings. It includes a range of abusive behaviours, and there is often a pattern of abusive behaviour over a long period – all with the aim of maintaining power and control over the victim. It includes aspects of the other types of abuse discussed here. The Domestic Abuse Act 2021 defines domestic abuse as any incident between two persons aged over 16 years, where the abuser and abused are partners, ex-partners, relatives or parents who had at one time had a parental relationship to the same child.

A survey for England and Wales by the Office for National Statistics estimated that 2.1 million individuals over 16 years old experienced domestic abuse in the year ending March 2023 (ONS, 2023). Of those, it is estimated that 1.4 million were female and 751,000 were male (historically male victims are less likely to report abuse). The highest numbers of victims were in the 16–19 year age range – both males and females. A person who was ill or at home looking after family was more likely to be a victim than if they were employed (ONS, 2023).

The perpetration of domestic abuse can have an effect on all members of the family, and paramedics must always consider the impact on the household. A holistic, whole-family approach should be adopted to ensure all concerns are included as part of any dynamic risk assessments and ongoing care plans. This will include carers, relatives and anyone else living at the residence. Children living, visiting or being cared for part-time in a domestic abuse household are being emotionally abused and this must be reported. Paramedics do not need to see children to report their concerns; an awareness of children within the family dynamic is sufficient to report child safeguarding concerns.

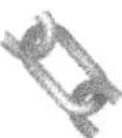 **Chapter 11** to read more on the effect of domestic abuse on children.

The Duluth Wheel is a resource used to understand the different tactics perpetrators of domestic abuse adopt (Domestic Abuse Intervention Programs, 2017). It has been around for decades and adapted for different genders, sexual orientations and religions to highlight that perpetrators will target an individual's most personal traits. What is consistent between all the wheels is that 'power and control' are at the centre. Everything a perpetrator does is to maintain power/control and anything that affects this is considered by them a threat. A gender-neutral Duluth Wheel has the following key elements:

- coercion and threats;
- intimidation;
- isolation;
- minimising, denying, blaming;
- using children;
- using privilege;
- financial abuse;
- emotional abuse.

Specialised Duluth wheels provide further detail regarding specific situations. For example, a female perpetrator may tell her male victim that he cannot be abused because he's a man; a perpetrator in a same-sex relationship may threaten to 'out' their partner; religious perpetrators may use their faith/religion as a weapon – gaining obedience by threatening repercussions in the afterlife or specifying it is a Deity's will they provide appropriate discipline.

In relation to non-fatal strangulation, abusers utilise strangulation to demonstrate power/control and inflict terror. It is a sign of escalating behaviour and there is high risk of domestic homicide as a result. Strangulation is the second most common means of death of women as a result of domestic violence in England and Wales (Home Office, 2023a).

Modern slavery

Modern slavery is an illegal trade in which humans are treated like commodities being bought and sold. It is an umbrella term that includes human trafficking, forced labour, servitude and slavery (GOV.UK, 2017). Human trafficking is defined as being transported from one place to another for the purpose of being exploited. The distance between destinations is irrelevant, as it might be from one country to another or from one house to another in the same town. Exploitation can involve forced labour or services, slavery, servitude, removal of organs, prostitution and sexual exploitation (CPS, 2022a). In 2022, 16,938 potential victims of modern slavery were referred to the Home Office, the highest number since the national referral mechanism was introduced in 2009 (Home Office, 2023c).

Labour exploitation can involve poor working conditions, unacceptably low pay, reductions in wages and being kept against one's will. Victims of domestic servitude, who usually work in private residences, are humiliated, treated poorly and made to work long hours for low (or no) pay in unbearable conditions. Sexual exploitation is when there is sexual abuse, or an individual is coerced into sex. Having been warned of the severe consequences and with their documents (e.g. passports) taken from them, victims find it hard to highlight their predicament. Modern slavery can be found everywhere in the UK: in the agricultural and fishing sectors, nail salons, car washes, building sites and the sex industry (GOV.UK, 2017).

Paramedics must be cognisant of modern slavery and be able to recognise indicators, report concerns and refer victims to support services (see Box 14.8). Any concerns regarding victims of modern slavery must be reported in accordance with safeguarding reporting mechanisms and consideration should be given to informing the police. The Modern Slavery Act 2015 (England and Wales), Human Trafficking and Exploitation (Scotland) Act 2015 and the Human Trafficking and Exploitation (Criminal Justice and Support for Victims) Act (Northern Ireland) 2015 provide information on offences, prevention orders, enforcements and victim protection (if they have committed crimes under duress).

Box 14.8 Indicators of modern slavery

- Fear of police/authorities
- Fear of trafficker and belief that their lives or family members' lives are at risk
- Limited freedom of movement
- Someone else possesses their passport/ID
- Seem to be in debt to someone
- Total reliance on another for translation
- Cramped/squalid living conditions

Adapted from: GOV.UK (2017), Home Office (2023b).

Organisational abuse

Organisational abuse, or institutional abuse, is the neglect or maltreatment of an 'adult at risk' by a regime of individuals. This could be in any organisational/institutional setting within the health and social care sector (NI Direct Government Services, 2023). Paramedics are familiar with working in out-of-hospital environments and are ideally placed to witness and report suspicions of abuse/neglect in organisations. These may be nursing, care or residential homes of disparate provision, with varying standards of care offered to service users and residents. This issue may also be prevalent in a hospital or other clinical settings. The events may be singular in nature or a series of incidents of ongoing poor care/ill treatment. It can happen when systems/routines result in poor care, where there is acceptance of poor practice, where human rights and dignity are violated or where there is a cultural acceptance of denying/restricting an individual's choice or independence (NI Direct Government Services, 2023) (see Box 14.9).

If you have safeguarding concerns that a person in a position of trust could be a perpetrator, you have a legislative responsibility to report your concerns (even if the victim does not provide consent) as there are wider safeguarding concerns – for example, the perpetrator could be abusing other service users who are 'adults at risk' and paramedics must advocate for them.

Box 14.9 Indicators of organisational abuse

- Repeated poor clinical practice
- Lack of procedures/policies
- Paucity of staff training

- Unsafe staffing levels
- Incorrect placements of residents
- No care plan in place
- No personal belongings for service user
- Professionals acting in a way that could be harmful
  Adapted from: NI Direct Government Services (2023).

Discriminatory abuse

Discriminatory abuse includes any forms of bullying, harassment, derogatory remarks or similar due to any of the current nine protected characteristics within the Equality Act 2010: age; disability; gender reassignment; marriage and civil partnership; pregnancy and maternity; race; religion or belief; sex; and sexual orientation (GOV.UK, 2013). This type of abuse may overlap with hate incidents and hate crimes which are reportable to the local police as appropriate.

Radicalisation

There are responsibilities to safeguard individuals who may be vulnerable or susceptible to radicalisation and extremism. The objective of the 2023 UK counter-terrorism strategy (CONTEST) is to reduce the risk of terrorism and ensure UK citizens can go about their lives safely. The CONTEST framework – Prevent, Pursue, Protect and Prepare – aims to ensure multi-agency cooperation to counter terrorism (HM Government, 2023). Paramedics need to complete Prevent training and be familiar with their Prevent reporting process. Ask your practice educator about this on your next shift.

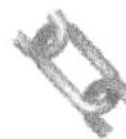 **Chapter 11** for information on child radicalisation.

REPORTING SAFEGUARDING CONCERNS

Organisations have reporting mechanisms in place for when their employees have adult safeguarding concerns. It is a paramedic's responsibility to ensure they are aware of these mechanisms, as reporting safeguarding concerns in a timely manner is part of a paramedic's professional registration and *Standards of Proficiency for Paramedics* (HCPC, 2023).

When completing safeguarding reports, they should be factual and evidence based. These are professional documents which may be used as part of legal proceedings. Their content should comply with the Data Protection Act 2018, including that the information reported is adequate, relevant and necessary. Schedule 8 of the Act details the circumstances in which it is acceptable to share information without consent for 'safeguarding children and individuals at risk'. It is imperative when reporting concerns regarding adults to show they meet the 'adult at risk' definition.

Police should be contacted if a paramedic suspects a crime has been committed. When there are immediate safeguarding concerns – for example, concern that an adult at risk has been abused by their carer who is making medical decisions on their part – direct contact should be made with the local authority emergency duty team. A local authority emergency duty social worker is always on call. There is a duty to document safeguarding concerns: if a paramedic has a discussion with social workers, a safeguarding report must be completed.

PROFESSIONAL CONCERNS

Paramedics have a statutory obligation to report safeguarding concerns they have regarding colleagues (employed or voluntary). There is a responsibility to put the safety and wellbeing of service users first. The HCPC are clear that employers should encourage a culture that positively supports practitioners to report their concerns (HCPC, 2016). The reporting method will vary depending on who the safeguarding concern involves. A concern relating to a healthcare professional can be raised with their employer and if they are on the HCPC register, it can also be reported to the HCPC. Organisations should have internal policies which provide further bespoke guidance. There are several regulatory bodies within the UK, so any concerns regarding the management or practices of a health or social care service can be reported to the relevant responsible body. Paramedics need to be vigilant, as some UK healthcare professionals have been prosecuted for abuse.

CASE STUDIES

Read the following case studies and reflect on some of the main points covered in this chapter.

Case study 14.1

999 call to Nora, an 82-year-old female who has activated her care alarm following a fall at home. When you arrive, the carers meet you at the door and you discover that Nora lives alone with a twice-daily

care visit to support her with personal hygiene. You are told by her carers that Nora's mobility is declining gradually, and that she uses a walking aid and rarely leaves the house. During your assessment, you notice Nora's arms are covered with marks and contusions. The carers leave and you ask Nora about her arms. After some discussion, Nora mentions that the carers haven't been letting her wash and they just change her clothes when they visit. When she tried asking them to let her wash, on two separate occasions, the carers were physically rough with her, leaving the marks on her arms. They told her to be quiet and to stop complaining. When you explain to Nora you need to report this information, she says she does not want you to, as the carers are the only people she sees regularly and she does not want them to stop visiting.

1   What categories of abuse are evident here?
2   What actions, if any, would you take?
3   Would you document your discussion? If so, where?
4   Would your safeguarding actions be different if Nora lacked capacity?
5   Would you have asked Nora about her arms if the carers had not left?

Having read case study 14.1 and thought about questions 1–5, look at the reflection box below. Were your thoughts about potential action at all similar?

Reflection: points to consider

1   Physical – carers being rough and leaving marks on her body. Neglect – carers are being paid to provide a level of care, which they are not providing by not washing Nora. Possibly organisational – could be the result of specific individuals or an organisational culture/training issue.
2   Complete a safeguarding report, specifying that Nora did not consent. The report is required as the carers are individuals in a position of trust and could be providing care to an unknown number of clients. You need to safeguard Nora and other clients.

3   Yes – complete an adult safeguarding report and note on your clinical documentation that you have safeguarding concerns and that a safeguarding report has been submitted (follow your local and employer guidance).

4   No – an adult safeguarding report is always required in such circumstances.

5   No – as possible perpetrators, you might have put both yourself and Nora at risk in the presence of the carers. You could report your concerns based on what you witnessed (without the information Nora disclosed). You must include in the report that there was no opportunity to have a discussion with Nora as the carers were present during your assessment.

Case study 14.2

999 call to 38-year-old Morgan, who has been assaulted by her partner. The perpetrator is no longer at the address and your clinical assessment determines there is no need to convey Morgan to hospital. You discover this is not the first time Morgan's partner has been physically abusive and he is verbally abusive to everyone in the household. You ask who else lives at the property and you learn there are two children who are at school and Morgan's elderly, bed-bound Dad is upstairs. You check on Dad who is unharmed and advise Morgan the assault should be reported to the police. Morgan says she does not want you telling anyone about the assault.

1   What categories of abuse are evident here?
2   What actions, if any, would you take in relation to Morgan?
3   What actions, if any, would you take in relation to anyone else?
4   Would your safeguarding actions be different if Morgan lacked capacity?
5   Who you could ask for advice?

Reflection: points to consider

1   Physical – Morgan states she was assaulted. Domestic – the assault was by an intimate partner. Emotional – children and adult at risk living in a domestic abuse household.
2   Discuss the situation and ask Morgan whether she feels safe to remain in the property. Suggest seeking support from domestic abuse specialists; refer to the service directly if Morgan consents. Recommend reporting the assault to the police.
3   Yes – complete an adult safeguarding report for Morgan's elderly, bed-bound Dad as he is unable to remove himself from the property/protect himself. Also complete a child safeguarding report for the children as they are victims of domestic abuse (witnessing the abuse of others).
4   Yes – if Morgan lacked capacity, an adult safeguarding report would be submitted for Morgan and the police contacted from the scene as Morgan would meet the definition of an 'adult at risk', unable to protect herself, and you would make a 'best interest' decision.
5   You can contact a senior clinician or the safeguarding team within your organisation. A local authority emergency duty social worker is also available if you feel there is an immediate risk. Remember, if you discuss safeguarding concerns with the local authority, you must submit a written safeguarding report. As Morgan has been assaulted, suggest she report the assault to the police.

CONCLUSION

Safeguarding adults is everyone's responsibility and paramedics should report concerns using the appropriate reporting mechanisms. Information that paramedics have is invaluable for safeguarding investigations and it is essential that safeguarding adults training is firmly embedded within paramedic training and continuous professional development.

Chapter key points:

- Adult safeguarding is everyone's responsibility.
- Paramedics are in a unique position within the community to identify adult safeguarding concerns.

- Paramedics must be aware of current adult safeguarding legislation (specific to the country in which they work).
- Safeguarding adult cases may be complex and due consideration must be given to the 'adult at risk' definition, consent and mental capacity (in accordance with the Data Protection Act 2018).
- Paramedics are professionally obligated to report adult safeguarding concerns in a timely manner.
- Organisations employing paramedics need to ensure their adult safeguarding training, policies and support are of high quality, effective and accessible.

REFERENCES AND SUGGESTED READING

AMIS (2020) *Emotional abuse*, Abused Men In Scotland. Available at: https://abusedmeninscotland.org/knowledge/types-of-abuse/emotional/ (accessed 5 April 2024).

Age UK (2023) *Safeguarding older people from abuse and neglect*. Available at: https://www.ageuk.org.uk/globalassets/age-uk/documents/factsheets/fs78_safeguarding_older_people_from_abuse_fcs.pdf (accessed 5 April 2024).

Butler, D. (2022) Safeguarding: recognising, reporting and recording adult abuse, *Journal of Community Nursing*, 36 (1): 60–65.

College of Paramedics (CoP) (2020) *Safeguarding during COVID-19*. Available at: https://collegeofparamedics.co.uk/COP/News/Covid-19/Safeguarding_During_Covid19.aspx (accessed 5 April 2024).

Crown Prosecution Service (CPS) (2022a) *Modern slavery and human trafficking: Offences and defences, including the section 45 defence*. Available at: https://www.cps.gov.uk/legal-guidance/modern-slavery-and-human-trafficking-offences-and-defences-including-section-45 (accessed 5 April 2024).

Crown Prosecution Service (CPS) (2022b) *Sexual offences*. Available at: https://www.cps.gov.uk/crime-info/sexual-offences (accessed 5 April 2024).

Department of Health, Social Services and Public Safety (2015) *Adult safeguarding: Prevention and protection in partnership policy*. Available at: https://www.health-ni.gov.uk/publications/adult-safeguarding-prevention-and-protection-partnership-key-documents (accessed 5 April 2024).

Domestic Abuse Intervention Programs (2017) *Understanding the power and control wheel*. Available at: https://www.theduluthmodel.org/wheels/understanding-power-control-wheel/ (accessed 5 April 2024).

GOV.UK (2013) *Equality Act 2010: Guidance*. Available at: https://www.gov.uk/guidance/equality-act-2010-guidance (accessed 5 April 2024).

GOV.UK (2017) *Modern slavery awareness and victim identification guidance.* Available at: https://assets.publishing.service.gov.uk/media/5a82b7a3ed9 15d74e3403349/6.3920_HO_Modern_Slavery_Awareness_Booklet_web.pdf (accessed 5 April 2024).

Health and Care Professions Council (HCPC) (2016) *Standards of Conduct, Performance and Ethics.* Available at: https://www.hcpc-uk.org/standards/standards-of-conduct-performance-and-ethics/ (accessed 5 April 2024).

Health and Care Professions Council (HCPC) (2023) *Standards of Proficiency for Paramedics.* Available at: https://www.hcpc-uk.org/standards/standards-of-proficiency/paramedics/ (accessed 5 April 2024).

HM Government (2023) *CONTEST: The United Kingdom's strategy for countering terrorism 2023.* Available at: https://www.gov.uk/government/publications/counter-terrorism-strategy-contest-2023 (accessed 5 April 2024).

Home Office (2020) *Domestic abuse: Recognise the signs.* Available at: https://www.gov.uk/government/publications/domestic-abuse-recognise-the-signs/domestic-abuse-recognise-the-signs#how-to-recognise-domestic-abuse-in-a-relationship (accessed 5 April 2024).

Home Office (2023a) *Controlling or coercive behaviour: Statutory guidance framework.* Available at: https://www.gov.uk/government/publications/controlling-or-coercive-behaviour-statutory-guidance-framework (accessed 5 April 2024).

Home Office (2023b) *Modern slavery.* Available at: https://www.gov.uk/government/collections/modern-slavery (accessed 5 April 2024).

Home Office (2023c) *Modern slavery: National referral mechanism and duty to notify statistics UK, end of Year Summary 2022.* Available at: https://www.gov.uk/government/statistics/modern-slavery-national-referral-mechanism-and-duty-to-notify-statistics-uk-end-of-year-summary-2022/modern-slavery-national-referral-mechanism-and-duty-to-notify-statistics-uk-end-of-year-summary-2022#:~:text=In%202022%2C%20the%20NRM%20received,the%20NRM%20began%20in%202009. (accessed 5 April 2024).

Joint Royal Colleges Ambulance Liaison Committee Plus (JRCALC Plus) (2024) *Joint Royal Colleges Ambulance Liaison Committee Plus.* Available at: https://jrcalcplusweb.co.uk/ (accessed 5 April 2024).

Legislation.gov.uk (1998) *Human Rights Act 1998.* Available at: https://www.legislation.gov.uk/ukpga/1998/42/contents (accessed 5 April 2024).

Legislation.gov.uk (2000) *Adults with Incapacity (Scotland) Act 2000.* Available at: https://www.legislation.gov.uk/asp/2000/4/contents (accessed 5 April 2024).

Legislation.gov.uk (2003a) *Female Genital Mutilation Act 2003.* Available at: https://www.legislation.gov.uk/ukpga/2003/31/contents (accessed 5 April 2024).

Legislation.gov.uk (2003b) *Sexual Offences Act 2003.* Available at: https://www.legislation.gov.uk/ukpga/2003/42/contents (accessed 5 April 2024).

Legislation.gov.uk (2005) *Mental Capacity Act 2005.* Available at: https://www.legislation.gov.uk/ukpga/2005/9/contents (accessed 5 April 2024).

Legislation.gov.uk (2007) *Adult Support and Protection (Scotland) Act 2007.* Available at: https://www.legislation.gov.uk/asp/2007/10/contents (accessed 5 April 2024).

Legislation.gov.uk (2010) *Equality Act 2010.* Available at: https://www.legislation.gov.uk/ukpga/2010/15/contents (accessed 5 April 2024).

Legislation.gov.uk (2014a) *Care Act 2014*. Available at: https://www.legislation.gov.uk/ukpga/2014/23/contents (accessed 5 April 2024).

Legislation.gov.uk (2014b) *Social Services and Well-being (Wales) Act 2014*. Available at: https://www.legislation.gov.uk/anaw/2014/4/contents (accessed 5 April 2024).

Legislation.gov.uk (2015a) *Counter-Terrorism and Security Act 2015*. Available at: https://www.legislation.gov.uk/ukpga/2015/6/contents (accessed 5 April 2024).

Legislation.gov.uk (2015b) *Modern Slavery Act 2015*. Available at: https://www.legislation.gov.uk/ukpga/2015/30/contents/enacted (accessed 5 April 2024).

Legislation.gov.uk (2015c) *Human Trafficking and Exploitation (Criminal Justice and Support for Victims) Act (Northern Ireland) 2015*. Available at: https://www.legislation.gov.uk/nia/2015/2/contents (accessed 5 April 2024).

Legislation.gov.uk (2015d) *Human Trafficking and Exploitation (Scotland) Act 2015*. Available at: https://www.legislation.gov.uk/asp/2015/12/contents (accessed 5 April 2024).

Legislation.gov.uk (2015e) *Violence Against Women, Domestic Abuse and Sexual Violence (Wales) Act 2015*. Available at: https://www.legislation.gov.uk/anaw/2015/3/contents (accessed 5 April 2024).

Legislation.gov.uk (2015f) *Serious Crime Act 2015*. Available at: https://www.legislation.gov.uk/ukpga/2015/9/contents (accessed 5 April 2024).

Legislation.gov.uk (2016) *Mental Capacity Act (Northern Ireland) 2016*. Available at: https://www.legislation.gov.uk/nia/2016/18/contents/enacted (accessed 5 April 2024).

Legislation.gov.uk (2018a) *Data Protection Act 2018*. Available at: https://www.legislation.gov.uk/ukpga/2018/12/schedule/8/crossheading/safeguarding-of-children-and-of-individuals-at-risk (accessed 5 April 2024).

Legislation.gov.uk (2018b) *Domestic Abuse (Scotland) Act 2018*. Available at: https://www.legislation.gov.uk/asp/2018/5/contents/enacted (accessed 5 April 2024).

Legislation.gov.uk (2020) *Female Genital Mutilation (Protection and Guidance) (Scotland) Act 2020*. Available at: Available at: https://www.legislation.gov.uk/asp/2020/9/contents (accessed 5 April 2024).

Legislation.gov.uk (2021a) *Domestic Abuse Act 2021*. Available at: https://www.legislation.gov.uk/ukpga/2021/17/contents/enacted (accessed 5 April 2024).

Legislation.gov.uk (2021b) *Domestic Abuse and Civil Proceedings Act (Northern Ireland) 2021*. Available at: https://www.legislation.gov.uk/nia/2021/2/enacted (accessed 5 April 2024).

Mangiante, E.M.S. and Peno, K. (eds.) (2021) *Teaching and Learning for Adult Skill Acquisition: Applying the Dreyfus and Dreyfus Model in different Fields*. Charlotte, NC: Information Age Publishing.

Meadley, B., Caldwell, J., Parraton, L., Bonham, M. et al. (2020) The health and well-being of paramedics: a professional priority, *Occupational Medicine*, 70 (3): 149–51.

NHS Choices (2021) *Abuse and neglect of vulnerable adults*. Available at: https://www.nhs.uk/conditions/social-care-and-support-guide/help-from-social-services-and-charities/abuse-and-neglect-vulnerable-adults/#:~:text=physical%20signs%20%E2%80%93%20such%20as%20bruises,or%20alone%20with%20particular%20people (accessed 5 April 2024).

NHS England (2021) *Help after rape and sexual assault*. Available at: https://www.nhs.uk/live-well/sexual-health/help-after-rape-and-sexual-assault/ (accessed 5 April 2024).

NI Direct Government Services (2023) *Recognising adult abuse, exploitation and neglect*. Available at: https://www.nidirect.gov.uk/articles/recognising-adult-abuse-exploitation-and-neglect#:~:text=Institutional%20abuse%20is%20the%20mistreatment,Health%20and%20Social%20Care%20sector. (accessed 5 April 2024).

Office for National Statistics (ONS) (2023) *Domestic abuse prevalence and trends, England and Wales: Year ending March 2023*. Available at: https://www.ons.gov.uk/peoplepopulationandcommunity/crimeandjustice/articles/domesticabuseprevalenceandtrendsenglandandwales/yearendingmarch2023#main-points (accessed 5 April 2024).

Office of the Public Guardian (2009) *Making decisions: A guide for people who work in health and social care*. Available at: https://assets.publishing.service.gov.uk/government/uploads/system/uploads/attachment_data/file/348440/OPG603-Health-care-workers-MCA-decisions.pdf (accessed 5 April 2024).

Oxford English Dictionary (OED) (2023) Available at: https://www.oed.com/ (accessed 5 April 2024).

Shepperd, L. (2021) *Domestic abuse of older people*, House of Lords Library. Available at: https://lordslibrary.parliament.uk/domestic-abuse-of-older-people/ (accessed 5 April 2024).

Social Care Institute for Excellence (SCIE) (2018) *Self-neglect at a glance*. Available at: https://www.scie.org.uk/self-neglect/at-a-glance (accessed 5 April 2024).

Social Care Institute for Excellence (SCIE) (2020) *Safeguarding adults: Types and indicators of abuse*. Available at: https://www.scie.org.uk/safeguarding/adults/introduction/types-and-indicators-of-abuse#neglect (accessed 5 April 2024).

Social Care Wales (2019) *Wales Safeguarding Procedures*, Safeguarding Wales. Available at: https://safeguarding.wales/en/ (accessed 5 April 2024).

Southern Health & Social Care Trust (2024) *Signs and indicators of adult abuse*. Available at: https://southerntrust.hscni.net/involving-you/community-development-and-user-involvement/community-sector-training/adult-safeguarding-information-and-resources/adult-safeguarding/signs-and-indicators-of-adult-abuse/ (accessed 5 April 2024).

Starns, B. (2019) *Safeguarding Adults Together Under the CARE Act 2014: A Multi-agency Practice Guide*. St Albans: Critical Publishing.

Tameside Adults Safeguarding Partnership Board (2022) *What is abuse and neglects?* Available at: https://www.tameside.gov.uk/TamesideMBC/media/adultservices/(3)-what-is-abuse-and-neglect.pdf (accessed 10 August 2024).

World Health Organization (WHO) (2022) *Abuse of older people*. Available at: https://www.who.int/news-room/fact-sheets/detail/abuse-of-older-people (accessed 5 April 2024).

15

Caring for people with dementia

John Krohne and Vicky Gooch

In this chapter:

INTRODUCTION

Dementia is a progressive, irreversible clinical syndrome (NICE, 2022a) characterised by neurocognitive impairment in the cognitive domains of memory, executive functioning, attention, language, social cognition, judgement, psychomotor speed and visuo-perceptual or visuo-spatial functioning (WHO, 2023). Paramedics play a vital role in the emergency health care of people living with dementia (Jones et al., 2023), with over 20 per cent of paramedic call-outs to those aged over 75 likely to be related to dementia (Buswell et al., 2016).

A diagnosis of dementia can take many months (SCIE, 2020) and is made following a series of comprehensive assessments, which include taking the history from the patient/family/carer (cognitive, behavioural and psychologi-cal symptoms, and the impact that the symptoms have on their daily life), conducting a physical examination and undertaking appropriate blood and urine tests to exclude reversible causes of cognitive decline (NICE, 2018). In addition, cognitive assessment (with a validated tool) should be performed in all people with suspected dementia (NICE, 2022a). If a diagnosis is in doubt, magnetic resonance imaging (MRI) scans, computed tomography (CT) scans and examination of cerebrospinal fluids may be performed (NICE, 2018).

To provide the best individualised, holistic care, it is important for paramed-ics to understand the different symptoms associated with the main types of dementia, rather than assuming all patients with dementia will present in the same way. Although there are many different types of dementia, the most commonly seen in paramedic practice will be Alzheimer's dementia (60 per cent), vascular dementia (15 per cent), dementia with Lewy bodies (10 per cent) and frontotemporal dementia (2 per cent), with up to 10 per cent of dementia cases having a mixed pathology (Alzheimer's Research UK, 2023).

 **Reflection: points to consider**

Before interacting with a person with dementia, it would be useful to know the specific dementia diagnosis and the likely symptoms. How might you do this?

Which parts of your brain did you use to get to work today? For example, remembering to go to work, deciding what to have for breakfast, the coordi-nation and emotional control needed to drive to work. Now consider if you lost the ability to do one of those things. This does not mean you would not be able to get to work, but you would need to develop alternative strategies and support mechanisms to ensure you arrived at your destination. This is the same when living with dementia, particularly those types with slower onset such as Alzheimer's and frontotemporal dementia. The individual can spend several (and in some cases, many) years still able to function inde-pendently with support, so it is important for paramedics to include the person living with dementia in the decision-making process as much as possible. Using this person-centred approach enables you to look beyond the label of dementia, focusing on the humanity of the person rather than just the disease (Kitwood, 1997). Literature on dementia refer to 'person', 'patient' and 'service user', which are used interchangeably in this chapter.

Reflection: points to consider

Do you tend to refer to your patients/service users by their diagnosis? Consider how this may make a person feel. Could you use a more person-centred approach?

WHY IS THIS RELEVANT?

Attending an older person in the pre-hospital environment can pose many challenges, which are further complicated when the patient is cognitively impaired by dementia (Harvey, 2014). Dementia can be a significant barrier to clinical assessment in the emergency care setting (Voss et al., 2020) and may result in people with dementia being more likely to be taken to hospital because paramedics cannot assess them properly (Buswell et al., 2016).

In a highly pressurised, busy pre-hospital environment, it is important to remember that taking a few extra moments to consider the person living with dementia will improve that patient's experience. The actions you take at the start of the interaction can make a big impact on how the situation will play out, both positively and negatively. Think of the ripples spreading out in a pond when you drop a stone into it; taking a few moments at the start of your interaction to review the approaches you need to take will improve patient care in the long run, stopping some of these 'ripples' from forming and impacting negatively on the overall outcome. This chapter will provide you with the underpinning theory on dementia, including assessment and communication strategies, which will make a significant difference when attending patients who have dementia. Case study 15.1 at the end of the chapter will help you to assess what you have learnt.

Reflection: points to consider

- 944,000 people in the UK have a diagnosis of dementia (Alzheimer's Research UK, 2023), of which 70,800 are under the age of 65 (Alzheimer's Society, 2024a).
- One in three people aged over 65 will develop dementia before they die (NHS England, 2014).
- Between 60 and 80 per cent of people with dementia experience a fall (Alzheimer's Society, 2016).

ALZHEIMER'S DEMENTIA

Alzheimer's dementia is characterised by progressive memory and neuronal loss culminating in cognitive impairment (Hsiao et al., 2018) and is the dementia most commonly seen by paramedics in practice. Those with Alzheimer's dementia live up to eight years on average after diagnosis but can live as long as 20 years (Alzheimer's Association, 2024). Symptoms vary considerably, from those which may present earlier in the disease progression to those presenting later (see Table 15.1).

Table 15.1 Potential symptoms of Alzheimer's dementia

Earlier symptoms	Later symptoms
Forgetting recent events/misplacing items	Unable to recognise family members
Forgetting places, object names and faces	Hallucinating and suffering delusions
Repetition of speech	Problems with speech and language
Mood swings and increased anxiety	Aggressive and demanding behaviour
Restlessness	Disturbed sleep
Problems with concentration	Physical issues – incontinence, difficulty eating and swallowing, weight loss or significant weight gain

VASCULAR DEMENTIA

Vascular dementia is the second most prevalent dementia you will encounter in paramedic practice. It is a progressive disease caused by impaired blood flow to the brain. Potential symptoms are listed in Box 15.1.

Box 15.1 Potential symptoms of vascular dementia

- Impaired memory
- Reduction in cognitive abilities
- Paralysis on one side of the body
- Balance issues
- Swallowing issues
- Pain and extreme tiredness
- Incontinence
- Vision issues
- Speech and language problems

DEMENTIA WITH LEWY BODIES

Dementia with Lewy bodies is less prevalent than Alzheimer's dementia and vascular dementia but unlike these dementias, memory impairment is not usually a symptom in the early stages (Box 15.2).

Box I5.2 Main symptoms of dementia with Lewy bodies

- Parkinsonism-type symptoms (including slowing of movement, tremor, stiffness)
- Visual hallucinations
- Fluctuating levels of alertness
- Reduced ability to smell
- Sleep disturbance

FRONTOTEMPORAL DEMENTIA

Although only accounting for 2 per cent of dementia diagnoses (Alzheimer's Research UK, 2023), frontotemporal dementia (FTD) is the second most common neurodegenerative dementia in people under the age of 65 (Pressman and Miller, 2014). Frontotemporal dementia is classified into three clinical variants: (1) behavioural variant FTD; (2) non-fluent variant primary progressive aphasia; and (3) semantic-variant primary progressive aphasia (Bang et al., 2015). Behavioural variant FTD is the most common type of FTD (Alzheimer's Society, 2024b) (Box 15.3).

Box I5.3 Main symptoms of behavioural variant FTD

- Disinhibition
- Impulsive behaviour
- Inability to grasp consequence of actions
- Apathy
- Loss of empathy
- Loss of planning, organising and decision-making abilities

The patient is unlikely to be aware of the symptoms of behavioural variant FTD listed in Box 15.3. For the other two types of FTD – non-fluent variant primary progressive aphasia and semantic-variant primary progressive aphasia – the main symptoms are linked to speech and language issues.

Reflection: points to consider

Some older adults have more memory or thinking problems than other adults their age. This condition is called mild cognitive impairment (MCI) (National Institute on Aging, 2021). MCI affects memory and other abilities, but not as severely as dementia. The cognitive changes associated with MCI are usually not serious enough to interfere with a person's daily life and independence (Alzheimer Society of Canada, 2024). MCI symptoms can improve for some people, although those with a diagnosis of MCI have a higher risk of developing dementia in later life (Roberts et al., 2014).

VISUO-PERCEPTUAL AND VISUO-SPATIAL DIFFICULTIES

Paramedics interacting with patients living with dementia need to be aware of the impact of potential vision and perception changes (Box 15.4). These changes will vary dependent on the type of dementia diagnosis.

Box 15.4 Visual, perceptual and spatial difficulties that may impact on the paramedic's interaction and care of the person living with dementia

- Depth perception – e.g. unable to judge distance when transferring from chair to stretcher.
- Peripheral vision acuity/narrowing of the visual field – e.g. inability to see the paramedic who approaches from the side of the patient.
- Misperceptions – e.g. shiny flooring mistaken for water or dark carpet mistaken for a hole in the ground.
- Hallucinations – although people living with dementia do experience hallucinations, it tends not to be common. Often the person's visual and perceptual deficits are interpreted as hallucinations, when the person is actually just mistaking what they have seen.

Reflection: points to consider

Hold your hands up to your eyes like a pair of binoculars. How does this restrict your peripheral vision? As a paramedic, how would you need to approach a person with impaired peripheral vision? Peripheral vision issues are common in people living with dementia, but they will not be obvious to you.

If you were asked to walk across a big hole in the road, would you do it? So why is it 'difficult' or 'unhelpful' behaviour when a patient with perceptual deficit refuses to cross a dark carpet if they think it is a hole?

COMMUNICATION

Communication and developing a rapport are two of the main challenges for paramedics delivering person-centred care for people with dementia (Choonara and Williams, 2021). Do not assume the person with dementia is incapable of making decisions based on their diagnosis alone (Smebye et al., 2012). They should have the opportunity to be involved in decisions about their care whenever possible. To enable this, good communication between paramedics and the patient/family/carer is vital.

The carer/family member can often compensate for the impaired person's inability to stay focused on one topic (Teten et al., 2015) but it is important to ensure that the individual patient is included in conversations.

Personal information records in dementia care are increasing in prevalence – for example, the Alzheimer's Society (2023) has produced the support tool 'This is me'. Paramedics should review this document and any care plans, where available, to best provide person-centred care. Topics such as family background, likes and dislikes, routines and personality may be included; having an awareness of such information can aid communication and enable a more positive experience for the patient.

Paramedics are responsible for facilitating decision-making and ensuring the participation of the person with dementia wherever possible. This can be done by using adapted communication strategies (Table 15.2).

Table 15.2 Common dementia communication issues and possible solutions

Problem	Possible solution
Building relationships	Smiling Open body language Calm tone of voice Orientating the person by informing them where they are, who they are with and what is going on Using names rather than 'he/she/they' Referring to the dementia personal information record/people who know the patient well Taking an interest in objects in the patient's personal environment to establish rapport, e.g. pictures, ornaments and pets
Understanding language	Avoid using complex language Use gestures/demonstrations Use pictures when possible
Physical assessment	Explain each step of the procedure, e.g. 'I am going to place a blood pressure cuff around your arm, it will feel tight for a few seconds' Avoid making the person feel rushed
Maintaining conversation threads	Offering verbal prompts about topic of conversation One point at a time
Visual and perceptual deficits	Interact one-on-one Slow down your movements
Making decisions	Use closed rather than open questions Involve family members
Environment	Reduce distractions, e.g. background noise, consider moving to a quieter room Remember an unfamiliar environment may be unsettling

Reflection: points to consider

The singular most important thing in communicating with people who are cognitively impaired is **PATIENCE!!!**

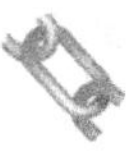

Chapter 1 for more about various communication strategies.

UNMET NEEDS

As well as visuo-perceptual and visuo-spatial difficulties, the presentation and behaviour of a person with dementia may be impacted by an unmet need. Everyone uses behaviour as an attempt to fulfill a need, communicate a need or as an outcome of frustration (Cohen-Mansfield et al., 2009), but when the person with dementia tries to meet this need, their behaviour may be interpreted as disruptive or difficult. For example, when you feel unwell, your own behaviour can change. You could be less tolerant of others, you might seek relief or reassurance (e.g. medication/contacting a health professional) as well as eating less and sleeping more. You are likely to be able to meet your 'needs' to improve the way you feel physically and emotionally, but the person with dementia may not be able to do this, so their needs remain unmet. This could lead to distress and behaviour changes.

Unmet needs can be due to physical discomfort from illness (e.g. fatigue, pain), functional needs (e.g. body position) or physiological needs that impair comfort (Jung Lee et al., 2020). In addition, unmet needs can also be due to psychosocial needs such as mental discomfort, the need for social contacts, uncomfortable environmental conditions or an inadequate level of stimulation (Cohen-Mansfield et al., 2015).

Reflection: points to consider

Consider what it would feel like if two strangers came into your own room at home? How might you feel? How might you react? If they approached you and started grabbing your arm or taking your clothes off, how might this escalate your behaviour?

All your reactions in the reflection box above could be considered 'normal behaviour' if this happened to a person who does not have dementia. Why might the person with dementia be reacting in a certain way? It is likely that their behaviour is normal based on their interpretation of the situation, even if it does not seem that way to those observing the behaviour.

Strangers, ambulance journeys and medical procedures can provoke fear and disorientation in people with dementia (Choonara and Williams, 2021), so it is important for the paramedic to consider what unmet need the person with dementia is trying to communicate through their behaviour. What might be the alternative meaning of this behaviour (Mental Health Foundation, 2016)? A sympathetic, caring approach by the paramedic is important in the identification of this discomfort (Jung Lee et al., 2020).

People living with dementia have individual needs which are specific to them and vary from person to person. This will be dependent on the type of dementia a person has, where they are on their dementia journey, and their individual character and personality. It is important to try to establish that person's 'baseline'. For example, a person with dementia is normally orientated to place, but today is not, so could this be due to an unmet need? Perhaps they have an infection? Similarly, if the person with dementia is usually calm and able to answer closed questions but now, following a fall, is agitated and repetitive, could they be in pain? Talking with them and their family/carers will help you establish what is 'normal' for them (their baseline) and thus identify any potential unmet need.

VALUES AND ETHICS

Paramedics' values and attitudes will have a significant impact on their practice (Choonara and Williams, 2021). A paramedic harbouring negative emotions about people with dementia, based on the paramedic's previous experiences of dementia, can affect how they act towards someone with the condition (Krohne, 2022). 'Mentalising' is a process in which the paramedic becomes more in touch with what they themselves are thinking and feeling. This allows the paramedic to take note of how the environment, time pressures and the behaviour of the person with dementia may be affecting the paramedic's own interactions and adapt their approach accordingly (Bray and Janner, 2014).

Kitwood (1997) referred to the concept of 'malignant social psychology' in dementia. This highlights 17 behaviours and traits in the delivery of care by health professionals which can intensify a patient's sense of loss of independence and feelings of being devalued (Read et al., 2017). Table 15.3 addresses these behaviours/traits with reference to the Health and Care Professions Council's *Standards of Conduct, Performance and Ethics* (HCPC, 2024).

Table 15.3 Malignant social psychology behaviours/traits and the potential impact on paramedic practice

Behaviour/trait	Description	Links to the HCPC's *Standards of Conduct, Performance and Ethics*
Accusation	Blaming a person for their lack of ability/ understanding	Standard 1.1: Treat service users as individuals, respecting their privacy and dignity
Infantilisation	Communicating with a person as a parent would a young child	
Labelling	Treating the person as a diagnosis rather than as an individual with an illness	
Disempowerment	Not recognising a person's abilities	Standard 1.2: You must work in partnership with service users and carers, involving them, where appropriate, in decisions about the care, treatment or other services to be provided
Ignoring	Treating the person as if they were not there	
Imposition	Forcing a person to go against their preferred choice	Standard 1.4: You must make sure that you have valid consent, which is voluntary and informed, from service users who have capacity to make the decision or other appropriate authority before you provide care, treatment or other services
Stigmatisation	Treating a person as if they were a diseased object/ outcast	Standard 1.5: You must treat people fairly and be aware of the potential impact that your personal values, biases and beliefs may have on the care, treatment or other services that you provide to service users and carers and in your interactions with colleagues

Disruption	A sudden intrusion that disturbs the individual	Standard 2.1: You must be polite and considerate
Objectification	Treating a person as if they were an object rather than a person	Standard 2.2: You must listen to service users and carers and take account of their needs and wishes
Invalidation	Not recognising how a person might be feeling about a situation	
Outpacing	Presenting information at a rate too fast for the person to understand	
Banishment	Physically or psychologically excluding a person from a situation	Standard 6.2: You must not do anything, or allow someone else to do anything, which could put the health or safety of a service user, carer or colleague at unacceptable risk
Treachery	Use of deception to manipulate, distract or control the person	Standard 9: Be honest and trustworthy
Disparagement	Verbal or psychological messages that tell a person they are incompetent or worthless	Standard 9.1: You must make sure that your conduct justifies the public's trust and confidence in you and your profession
Intimidation	Inducing fear through threats or intimidation	
Mockery	Making fun of the person, or teasing or humiliating them	
Withholding	Refusing to give attention/treatment	

Adapted from: Kitwood (1997), HCPC (2024).

COMMON MEDICATIONS IN DEMENTIA

Table 15.4 Common medications used in dementia

	Acetylcholinesterase (AChE) inhibitors	NMDA (*N*-methyl-D-aspartate) receptor antagonist	Antipsychotics
Examples	Donepezil Rivastigmine Galantamine	Memantine	Risperidone (maximum 6 weeks) Haloperidol* (maximum 6 weeks) Lorazepam**
Intention of action	May reduce symptoms/help people to function better for a while		Helps reduce symptoms of severe agitation and distress
Alzheimer's dementia	Yes (mild to moderate severity)	Yes – if AChE inhibitors are ineffective or there is intolerance to the same OR suffering severe Alzheimer's dementia	Yes, but increases risk of stroke***
Vascular dementia	Not effective	Not effective	Yes, but increases risk of stroke***
Lewy bodies dementia	Yes (mild to moderate severity) – donepezil or rivastigmine initially	Yes – if AChE inhibitors are ineffective or there is intolerance to the same	No – increased risk of severe adverse reactions
Fronto-temporal dementia	Not effective	Not effective	Only used in rare cases to relieve severe symptoms****

*Haloperidol is licensed for treatment in Alzheimer's and vascular dementias but only used in emergencies as a last resort due to severe side effects.
**Lorazepam is a benzodiazepine (not an antipsychotic) but occasionally used in the short term to reduce agitation/distress instead of an antipsychotic.
*** A doctor may choose to prescribe an off-label antipsychotic drug (e.g. quetiapine) when it offers a better balance of benefits and risks for an individual patient.
**** Antidepressants called selective serotonin reuptake inhibitors (SSRIs) may help control the loss of inhibitions, overeating and compulsive behaviours seen in some people with FTD.
Sources: NICE (2018, 2022b), NHS (2020), Alzheimer's Society (2021), Alzheimer's Research UK (2022).

DEMENTIA AND PAIN

In the community, over 50 per cent of patients with dementia experience daily pain and this can be as high as 80 per cent for people with dementia in nursing homes (Achterberg et al., 2020). There is evidence of under-detection of pain in patients with dementia due to the challenge of accurately assessing their pain (Lichtner et al., 2014). In addition, people with dementia are typically pre-scribed fewer analgesics than people without dementia, indicating a potential difference in how pain is identified and treated in these populations (Tan et al., 2014). With this knowledge, paramedics need to give careful consideration to assessing pain and administering analgesia to patients with dementia.

Self-report of pain should be attempted in all people with dementia because it is the most readily available means of assessing the subjective experience of pain (Hadjistavropoulos et al., 2014). It is recommend that paramedics use the Verbal Numeric Rating Scale (VNRS) to guide decisions relating to pain manage-ment and analgesia administration (JRCALC/AACE, 2022). Using the VNRS, patients are asked to self-report and score their pain on a scale of 0–10. Para-medics should attempt to facilitate this for patients with cognitive impairment when possible. Although this approach is encouraged as part of patient-centred care, the process of assessing pain in cognitively impaired patients is a difficult and complex process, with the inability to successfully communicate pain in severe dementia a major barrier to effective assessment and treatment (Had-jistavropoulos et al., 2014). The most popular pain assessment tool designed specifically for cognitively impaired patients in paramedic practice is the Abbey Pain Scale. It considers both acute and chronic pain and can be completed in a

Table 15.5 Commonly used pain assessment tools in paramedic practice and their application for cognitively impaired patients

Pain assessment tool	Description	Application for cognitively impaired patients
Verbal Numeric Rating Scale (VNRS)	Self-report score of pain from 0–10	Difficult for patients with moderate-to-severe cognitive impairment
Verbal Rating Scale (VRS)	Self-report ranking of pain – mild, moderate or severe	No discrete pain score Potentially, patients who are unable to perform VNRS may have the cognitive ability to perform VRS

Wong-Baker FACES	Visual aid – patients identify which face best describes their pain	Can be used with non-verbal patients Difficult for patients as their cognitive impairment increases Originally designed for children
FLACC scale	Considers face, legs, arms, cry and consolability. Scored 0–2 for each, giving a score out of 10	Difficulties arise if the clinician assessing does not know the patient
The Abbey Pain Scale	Observation for six areas: physiological changes, physical changes, vocalisation, facial expressions, body language and behaviours	Designed specifically for cognitively impaired patients Relatively quick to complete Considers acute and chronic pain Considers physiological changes
PAINAD	Consists of five behaviours which need to be observed: breathing, negative vocalisation, facial expression, body language and consolability	Recommended for use in advanced dementia Simple to use Does not consider physiological changes

timely manner. PAINAD is recommended for use in advanced dementia. Table 15.5 presents commonly used pain assessment tools in paramedic practice.

The JRCALC/AACE (2022) state that patients who are cognitively impaired may not be able to score their pain and that behavioural cues should be considered and assessed in these patients (Box 15.5). Paramedics need to be more aware of physical cues and changes in behaviour in order to assess pain, as well as considering the injury or potential acute medical pain that is being suspected. Having a greater appreciation of these communication challenges will allow paramedics to give more thought and consideration to assessing pain and administering analgesia for potentially painful injuries or conditions.

> ## Box 15.5 Recommended steps in pain assessment and management for cognitively impaired patients
>
> - Physical assessment – indication of injury.
> - Patient's behaviour – agitation, facial expressions, body language, etc.
> - Information from others – information from dementia personal information record/people who know patient well.
> - Consider the use of a pain assessment tool.
> - Consider an analgesic trial to see how the patient's behaviour changes.
>
> Adapted from: Lord (2009).

DELIRIUM

Delirium is an acute, fluctuating encephalopathic syndrome of inattention, impaired level of consciousness and disturbed cognition (NICE, 2021). Delirium is an abrupt onset of reduced orientation to the environment usually lasting from hours to days, in contrast to dementia, which is a gradual neurodegenerative process (Gogia and Fang, 2023). Delirium is a common and serious problem among acutely unwell people (EDA/ADA, 2014). It is likely that previous episodes of delirium increase the risk of a diagnosis of dementia (Vardy et al., 2014).

Delirium can lead to poorer outcomes if untreated, yet it is often missed. It can be difficult to distinguish between delirium and dementia, and some people may have both conditions. Paramedics may be called to patients with dementia who have vague or non-specific conditions, such as increased confusion or drowsiness. It is important that you consider a possible cause for this change in behaviour rather than attributing it solely to the dementia. Assuming the person's 'new' symptoms are a result of their dementia and ignoring other possible conditions could be an example of diagnostic overshadowing (Voss et al., 2017). If clinical uncertainty exists about the diagnosis, the person should be managed initially for delirium (NICE, 2023).

Depending on the type of delirium, the person may display hyperactive or hypoactive symptoms (or a mix of both) (Table 15.6). There is likely to be significant impairment to the person's ability to stay focused and symptoms can fluctuate rapidly during the day. Unlike dementia, hallucinations are common in delirium. With treatment, the person is likely to recover from delirium.

<table>
<tr><td colspan="2">Table 15.6 Potentially modifiable risk factors in delirium</td></tr>
<tr><td>Risk factor</td><td>Comment</td></tr>
<tr><td>Physical factors</td><td>

- Infection
- Vascular compromise – e.g. stroke, myocardial infarction
- Urinary catheterisation
- Constipation
- Pain
- Dehydration
- Malnutrition

</td></tr>
<tr><td>Environmental factors</td><td>

- Sleep deprivation
- Physical restraint/immobilisation
- Emotional distress
- Unfamiliar/change in environment

</td></tr>
</table>

Source: Adapted from: Anand and MacLullich (2017).

Case study 15.1

Betty is an 88-year-old who identifies as female and has a diagnosis of Alzheimer's dementia. Her cognitive function has declined over the last five years, and she is now non-verbal. She lives at home with her husband Harry and cat Toby. It is 03:30 and you have been called to attend Betty at home after Harry was woken by Betty screaming as she has fallen in the kitchen. On arrival, you find Betty on the floor of the kitchen, unable to get up and in a state of agitation, clearly in some distress and discomfort.

Reflection: points to consider

Based on the points discussed in this chapter, what strategies could you employ to ensure that Betty is assessed and treated appropriately? Some suggested strategies are outlined below.

Communication/unmet need

Due to Betty being non-verbal, you may need to adapt your own communication. When interacting with Betty, ensure that you smile, refer to 'Betty' and 'Harry' by name and make friends with Toby the cat who is sitting nearby. You know Harry is an important person in Betty's life, so consider involving him in the assessment. Use simple language: verbally explain, step by step, your actions and demonstrate the procedures you would like to carry out. An example could be putting the oxygen saturation probe on Harry's finger before attempting to put it on Betty's finger. You should consider slowing down your movements and doing one thing at a time, for example, taking the oxygen saturations reading before attempting to record blood pressure. Consider how Betty's unmet needs might be contributing to her distress, agitation and discomfort. For example, when did Betty last use the toilet? How long has she been lying in same position on the floor? Is she scared by the presence of strangers in her kitchen in the middle of the night?

Pain assessment

Using Lord's (2009) suggested steps in pain assessment for cognitively impaired patients, you make a physical assessment of the injury. A fracture to Betty's hip is suspected as she has shortening and rotation to her left leg. Consider Betty's behaviour – she is agitated, upset and tearful. Harry may be able to advise if this is normal behaviour for Betty, but it is also important for you to try and involve Betty in the pain assessment if possible. How might you do this? Using a non-verbal pain assessment tool could be advantageous to help support your decision to consider an analgesic trial.

Values and ethics

Where possible, involve Betty in decisions surrounding her care, using her husband Harry to support her when required. This would ensure you treat Betty as an individual, respecting her dignity.

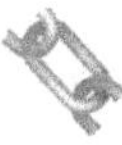

Chapter 4 for more about ethical and legal considerations; **Chapter 9** and **Chapter 10** for sociological perspectives; and **Chapter 14** for detail on safeguarding adults.

CONCLUSION

It is important to use a person-centred approach, considering the person rather than just the dementia diagnosis. Paramedics need to take a few extra moments at the beginning of their interaction and during assessment to review their approach. This chapter has demonstrated how an increased understanding of dementia-related issues will have significant positive impact on the experiences of both the person with dementia and the attending paramedics.

Chapter key points:

- The four main types of dementia are Alzheimer's dementia, vascular dementia, dementia with Lewy bodies and frontotemporal dementia.
- The main symptoms are disturbances of multiple higher cortical functions and visual and perceptual deficits.
- It is important to adapt your communication strategies when interacting with a patient with dementia.
- Unmet needs can have a significant impact on the presentation of the person with dementia.
- Assessing behavioural traits and physical cues is a crucial part of pain assessment for patients with dementia.
- Delirium should be considered if an acute behavioural change is reported.
- Paramedics need to be aware of their own behaviour and its potential impact on the patient.

REFERENCES AND SUGGESTED READING

Achterberg, W., Lautenbacher, S., Husebo, B. et al. (2020) Pain in dementia, *Pain reports*, 5 (1): e803. Available at: https://doi.org/10.1097/PR9.0000000000000803.

Alzheimer Society of Canada (ASC) (2024) *Mild cognitive impairment*. Available at: https://alzheimer.ca/en/about-dementia/other-types-dementia/conditions-related-dementia/mild-cognitive-impairment (accessed 6 April 2024).

Alzheimer's Association (2024) *What is Alzheimer's disease?* Available at: http://www.alz.org/alzheimers_disease_what_is_alzheimers.asp (accessed 6 April 2024).

Alzheimer's Research UK (2022) *Types of dementia*. Available at: https://www.alzheimersresearchuk.org/dementia-information/types-of-dementia/ (accessed 6 April 2024).

Alzheimer's Research UK (2023) *Statistics about dementia*. Available at: https://dementiastatistics.org/about-dementia/ (accessed 6 April 2024).

Alzheimer's Society (2016) *Exercise therapy in early dementia*. Available at: https://www.alzheimers.org.uk/research/care-and-cure-research-magazine/exercise-therapy-early-dementia (accessed 6 April 2024).

Alzheimer's Society (2021) *Antipsychotics and other drug approaches in dementia care*. Available at: https://www.alzheimers.org.uk/about-dementia/treatments/drugs/antipsychotic-drugs (accessed 6 April 2024).

Alzheimer's Society (2023) *This is me*. Available at: https://www.alzheimers.org.uk/sites/default/files/2020-03/this_is_me_1553.pdf (accessed 6 April 2024).

Alzheimer's Society (2024a) *Young-onset dementia*. Available at: https://www.alzheimers.org.uk/about-dementia/types-dementia/young-onset-dementia#:~:text=Whenper cent20aper cent20personper cent20developsper cent20dementia,theper cent20earlyper cent20stagesper cent20ofper cent20dementia (accessed 6 April 2024).

Alzheimer's Society (2024b) *Frontotemporal dementia*. Available at: https://www.alzheimers.org.uk/info/20007/types_of_dementia/11/frontotemporal_dementia (accessed 6 April 2024).

Anand, A. and MacLullich, A.M.J. (2017) Delirium in hospitalized older adults, *Medicine in Older Adults*, 45 (1): 47–50.

Bang, J., Spina, S. and Miller, B.L. (2015) Frontotemporal dementia, *Lancet*, 386 (10004): 1672–82.

Bray, J. and Janner, M. (2014) *Brief Encounters: Easier Relationships with Emotionally Vulnerable Patients*. London: CreateSpace Independent Publishing.

Buswell, M., Lumbard, P., Fleming, J. et al. (2016) Using ambulance service PCRs to understand 999 call-outs to older people with dementia, *Journal of Paramedic Practice*, 8 (5): 246–51.

Choonara, E. and Williams, J. (2021) What factors affect paramedics' involvement of people with dementia in decisions about their care? A qualitative study, *British Paramedic Journal*, 5 (4): 1–8.

Cohen-Mansfield, J., Dakheel-Ali, M. and Marx, M.S. (2009) Engagement in persons with dementia: the concept and its measurement, *American Journal of Geriatric Psychiatry*, 17 (4): 299–307.

Cohen-Mansfield, J., Dakheel-Ali, M., Marx, M.S. et al. (2015) Which unmet needs contribute to behavior problems in persons with advanced dementia?, *Psychiatry Research*, 228 (1): 59–64.

European Delirium Association and American Delirium Association (EDA/ADA) (2014) The DSM-5 criteria, level of arousal and delirium diagnosis: inclusiveness is safer, *BMC Medicine*, 12: 141. Available at: https://doi.org/10.1186/s12916-014-0141-2.

Gogia, B. and Fang, X. (2023) Differentiating delirium versus dementia in the elderly, *StatPearls*. Available at: https://www.ncbi.nlm.nih.gov/books/NBK570594/ (accessed 6 April 2024).

Hadjistavropoulos, T., Herr, K., Prkachin, K.M. et al. (2014) Pain assessment in elderly adults with dementia, *Lancet Neurology*, 13 (12): 1216–27.

Harvey, C. (2014) Is there scope for an observational pain scoring tool in paramedic practice?, *Journal of Paramedic Practice*, 6 (2): 84–88.

Health and Care Professions Council (HCPC) (2024) *Standards of Conduct, Performance and Ethics*. Available at: https://www.hcpc-uk.org/standards/standards-of-conduct-performance-and-ethics/.

Hsiao, Y.H., Chang C.H. and Gean, P.W. (2018) Impact of social relationships on Alzheimer's memory impairment: mechanistic studies, *Journal of Biomedical Science*, 25: 3. Available at: https://doi.org/10.1186/s12929-018-0404-x.

Joint Royal Colleges Ambulance Liaison Committee and Association of Ambulance Chief Executives (JRCALC/AACE) (2022) *JRCALC Clinical Guidelines*. Bridgwater: Class Professional Publishing.

Jones, D., Capstick, A., Faisal, M. et al. (2023) The impact of dementia education on student paramedics' preparedness to care, knowledge, confidence and attitudes towards dementia: an analytic survey, *British Paramedic Journal*, 8 (1): 9–17.

Jung Lee, S., Sun Park, M., Young-Rim, C. et al. (2020) Concept development of identification of discomfort for nursing home patients with advanced dementia, *International Journal of Nursing Knowledge*, 32 (4): 274–85.

Kitwood, T.M. (1997) *Dementia Reconsidered: The Person Comes First*. Buckingham: Open University Press.

Krohne, J. (2022) Reframing nurses' time to enhance interpersonal interactions in dementia care, *Nursing Older People*. Available at: https://doi.org/10.7748/nop.2022.e1402.

Lichtner, V., Dowding, D., Esterhuizen, P. et al. (2014) Pain assessment for people with dementia: a systematic review of systematic reviews of pain assessment tools, *BMC Geriatrics,* 14: 138. Available at: https://doi.org/10.1186/1471-2318-14-138.

Lord, B. (2009) Paramedic assessment of pain in the cognitively impaired adult patient, *BMC Emergency Medicine*, 9: 20. Available at: https://doi.org/10.1186/1471-227X-9-20.

Mental Health Foundation (MHF) (2016) *Dementia Truth Inquiry: Review of evidence.* Available at: https://www.mentalhealth.org.uk/explore-mental-health/publications/what-truth-inquiry-about-truth-and-lying-dementia-care (accessed 6 April 2024).

National Health Service (NHS) (2020) *Treatment: Frontotemporal dementia.* Available at: https://www.nhs.uk/conditions/frontotemporal-dementia/treatment/ (accessed 6 April 2024).

National Institute for Health and Clinical Excellence (NICE) (2018) *Dementia: Assessment, management and support for people living with dementia and their carers.* Available at: https://www.nice.org.uk/guidance/ng97/chapter/Recommendations#diagnosis (accessed 6 April 2024).

National Institute for Health and Clinical Excellence (NICE) (2021) *Delirium.* Available at: https://cks.nice.org.uk/topics/delirium/ (accessed 6 April 2024).

National Institute for Health and Clinical Excellence (NICE) (2022a) *Dementia.* Available at: https://cks.nice.org.uk/topics/dementia/#!backgroundsub:1 (accessed 6 April 2024).

National Institute for Health and Clinical Excellence (NICE) (2022b) *Dementia: Antipsychotics.* Available at: https://cks.nice.org.uk/topics/dementia/prescribing-information/antipsychotics/ (accessed 6 April 2024).

National Institute for Health and Clinical Excellence (NICE) (2023) *Delirium: Prevention, diagnosis and management.* Available at: https://www.nice.org.uk/guidance/cg103/chapter/Recommendations#assessment-and-diagnosis (accessed 6 April 2024).

National Institute on Aging (NIA) (2021) *What is mild cognitive impairment?* Available at: https://www.nia.nih.gov/health/what-mild-cognitive-impairment (accessed 6 April 2024).

NHS England (2014) *Five year forward view.* Available at: http://www.england.nhs.uk/wp-content/uploads/2014/10/5yfv-web.pdf (accessed 6 April 2024).

Pressman, P.S. and Miller, B.L. (2014) Diagnosis and management of behavioural variant fronto-temporal dementia, *Biological Psychiatry*, 75 (7): 574–81.

Read, S.T., Toye, C. and Wynaden, D. (2017) Experiences and expectations of living with dementia: a qualitative study, *Collegian*, 24 (5): 427–32.

Roberts, R.O., Knopman, D.S., Mielke, M.M. et al. (2014) Higher risk of progression to dementia in mild cognitive impairment cases who revert to normal, *Neurology*, 82 (4): 317–25.

Smebye, K., Kirkevold, M. and Engedal, K. (2012) How do persons with dementia participate in decision making related to health and daily care? A multi-case study, *BMC Health Services Research*, 12: 241. Available at: https://doi.org/10.1186/1472-6963-12-241.

Social Care Institute for Excellence (SCIE) (2020) *Getting a dementia diagnosis.* Available at: https://www.scie.org.uk/dementia/symptoms/diagnosis/getting-a-diagnosis.asp (accessed 6 April 2024).

Tan, E.C.K., Visvanathan, R., Hilmer, S.N. et al. (2014) Analgesic use, pain and day-time sedation in people with and without dementia in aged care facilities: a cross-sectional, multisite, epidemiological study protocol, *BMJ Open*, 4: e005757. Available at: https://doi.org/10.1136/bmjopen-2014-005757.

Teten, A.F., Dagenais, P.A. and Friehe, M.J. (2015) Auditory and visual cues for topic maintenance with persons who exhibit dementia of Alzheimer's type, *International Journal of Alzheimer's Disease*, 2015: 126064. Available at: https://doi.org/10.1155/2015/126064.

Vardy, E., Holt, R., Gerhard, A. et al. (2014) History of a suspected delirium is more common in dementia with Lewy bodies than Alzheimer's disease: a retrospective study, *International Journal of Geriatric Psychiatry*, 29 (2): 178–81.

Voss, S., Black, S., Brandling, J. et al. (2017) Home or hospital for people with dementia and one or more other multimorbidities: what is the potential to reduce avoidable emergency admissions? The HOMEWARD Project Protocol, *BMJ Open*, 7: e016651. Available at: https://doi.org/10.1136/bmjopen-2017-016651.

Voss, S., Brandling, J., Pollard, K. et al. (2020) A qualitative study on conveyance decision-making during emergency call outs to people with dementia: the HOMEWARD project, *BMC Emergency Medicine*, 20: 6. Available at: https://doi.org/10.1186/s12873-020-0306-6.

World Health Organization (WHO) (2023) Dementia, in *International Classification of Diseases (ICD-11)*, 11th revision. Available at: https://icd.who.int/browse11/l-m/en#/http://id.who.int/icd/entity/546689346 (accessed 6 April 2024).

16 Palliative and end-of-life care

Ptolemy Neoptolemos, Alison Robinson and Ann French

> **In this chapter:**
>
> - Introduction
> - Why is this relevant?
> - History of palliative care
> - Policy and guidance
> - Gold Standards Framework
> - Advance care planning
> - Mental Capacity Act 2005
> - Do not attempt cardiopulmonary resuscitation
> - Preferred priorities of care
> - Breaking bad/significant news
> - Conclusion
> - Chapter key points
> - References and suggested reading

INTRODUCTION

Since the early 2000s, a number of policies and frameworks have been developed which provide structure and guidance for everyone involved in the care of patients at the end of their lives. This chapter will introduce you to the history of palliative care and the key policies which have emerged to underpin end-of-life care for patients and their families. As paramedics you will, all too often, attend patients who are in the end stages of life with or without clear directives in place. This chapter will encourage you to think about your role and your contribution in meeting the challenge of providing optimum end-of-life care for individuals.

WHY IS THIS RELEVANT?

As people approach the end of their life, their health needs generally increase, requiring more frequent access to healthcare providers. There is projected to be a 26 per cent increase in the number of annual deaths in England between 2016 (490,791) and 2040 (616,479) (Public Health England, 2018). Etkind et al. (2017) predicted that by 2040, 42.4 per cent of people (161,842 more people per year, total 537,240) will have palliative care needs. However, during 2020, the impact of the COVID-19 pandemic resulted in an increase in the demand for palliative care, reaching levels of need similar to that which had previously only been expected to be reached in 2040 (Higginson et al., 2021).

Current trends in England indicate that people are living longer and the number of people living with frailty associated with ageing, long-term conditions and multimorbidity is projected to increase by 37 per cent. The majority (80 per cent) of that projected increase in major illness will be among those aged 70 years and older (Watt et al., 2023).

People dying in their 'usual place of residence' (i.e. at home or in care homes) had risen from 35 per cent in 2004 to 50 per cent in 2022. During the pandemic, the number of deaths at home was above the average of the previous five years (ONS, 2022). More people dying in their place of residence can be attributed to the increasing awareness of the importance of end-of-life care and the implementation of policies to ensure patients have more involvement in their treatment plans and more choice over where they are cared for at this phase of their life. The pattern of more people dying at home remains higher (28.7 per cent) than before the pandemic (24.4 per cent). Hospital remains the most common place of death (43.4 per cent of all deaths), with nearly half of people dying in the community, either at home (28.7 per cent) or in a care home (20.5 per cent). Only 4.7 per cent of people die in a hospice or other locations, such as public places or someone else's home (2.6 per cent) (Office for Health Improvement and Disparities, 2023). The 'A Place for Everyone' policy project (Marie Curie, 2021) not only highlights the importance of everyone having the right to express a choice on where they receive their end-of-life care and where they die, but also explores the diverse groups for whom choice in place of death is limited.

As a paramedic or healthcare professional, you will be actively involved in the care of patients at the end of their life and this can be challenging and emotionally demanding, but also rewarding and immensely satisfying when everything goes well. You need to be able to communicate effectively with family and carers, understand the legal obligations and know when to withhold unwanted interventions. Knowledge and understanding of the policies and frameworks underpinning end-of-life care and how they should be applied will support your decision-making and provide you with the tools to ensure the care you provide meets the needs and preferences of the individual.

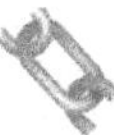 **Chapter 1** for more on communication skills; **Chapter 4** for legal and ethical issues; **Chapter 13** for more on frailty.

Definition of palliative and end-of-life care (PEoLC)

Palliative care is defined by the World Health Organization (WHO, 2020) as an approach that improves the quality of life of patients (adults and children) and their families who are facing problems associated with life-limiting illness, usually progressive. It prevents and relieves suffering through the early identification, correct assessment and treatment of pain and other problems, whether physical, psychosocial or spiritual.

Palliative care does the following (WHO, 2023):

- provides relief from pain and other distressing symptoms;
- affirms life and regards dying as a normal process;
- intends neither to hasten nor postpone death;
- integrates the psychological and spiritual aspects of patient care;
- offers a support system to help patients live as actively as possible until death;
- offers a support system to help the family cope during a patient's illness and their own bereavement;
- uses a team approach to address the needs of patients and their families, including bereavement counselling, if indicated;
- will enhance quality of life, and may also positively influence the course of illness;
- is applicable early in the course of illness, in conjunction with other therapies that are intended to prolong life, such as chemotherapy or radiation therapy, and includes those investigations needed to better understand and manage distressing clinical complications.

In England, the term 'end-of-life care' refers to the final year of life (NHS England, 2023).

Reflection: points to consider

Before reading on, do you know of any important policies, frameworks or guidelines, nationally or locally, related to palliative and end-of-life care?

HISTORY OF PALLIATIVE CARE

Caring for people at the end of life has always been an integral part of health care, from nursing nuns who cared for the dying many years ago to the development of the hospice movement. Dame Cicely Saunders, founder of the modern hospice movement, has been credited with the development of palliative care. As a nurse, social worker and latterly a physician, she explored not only the best way to care for the holistic needs of a patient but also what the patient was experiencing. Through her work at St Joseph's Hospice in Hackney, the concept of total pain evolved (Clark et al., 2005). She aspired not only to provide excellent clinical care but emphasised the importance of education and research. Dame Cicely founded St Christopher's Hospice in Sydenham, South London, in 1967 following eight years of fundraising and planning (Saunders, 2005). This independent organisation, which focused on the care of people when they were dying, became a source of inspiration around the world and the modern hospice movement was born. The concept of 'palliative care' was devised by the Canadian surgeon Balfour Mount, who visited St Christopher's in 1973 and then explored how the idea of hospice care could be combined with hospital medicine. In 1987, the Royal Colleges of Physicians and of General Practitioners recognised palliative care as a specialty, which is considered a turning point in palliative care.

One of the major criticisms of palliative care over the years has been the focus on patients with cancer. The House of Commons Health Committee (2004) suggested that the greatest inequality was the lack of provision of palliative care services for patients with a non-cancer diagnosis. In the same year, Dame Cicely suggested to the WHO that 'the next stage is surely the introduction of palliative care into mainstream medicine'. Since then, there have been many major policies and drivers that have advocated for the provision of palliative care for all, regardless of where the patient is being cared for or what their diagnosis is.

In 2008, the first national strategy for end-of-life care in England brought together the health and social care systems to redress three main areas of concern: that people didn't die in their place of choice; that we needed to prepare for larger numbers of dying people; and that not everybody received high-quality care. This prompted much change and investment in palliative and end-of-life care services, particularly through the work of national charities and governmental priorities for the NHS and social care.

However, the focus on end-of-life care has not always been positive. In 2012, a series of articles was published in the media that raised concerns over the use of the Liverpool Care Pathway (LCP), recommended as good practice by the End of Life Care Strategy (DH, 2008). The LCP was originally developed by the Royal Liverpool University Hospital and the Marie Curie Hospice in Liverpool to guide the care of patients within the last few days of life. The aim of the LCP was to ensure that wherever a person died, the care they received in the last days of life was uniformly good. The main concerns raised in the media related to the inappropriate use of the pathway and the withdrawal or withholding of medication, nutrition and hydration. This led to an independent inquiry into the use of the pathway by Baroness Julia Neuberger (DH, 2013a).

The recommendation of the inquiry was that the Liverpool Care Pathway should be phased out and instead there should be more emphasis on the individual care of the patient and their family. The inquiry highlighted the need for open and honest communication between healthcare professionals, patients and families, and the need to ensure both patients and their families are involved in discussions relating to care. Indeed, the review made 44 recommendations, including calls for more guidance on how to diagnose dying, along with guidance for healthcare professionals on decision-making at this stage of life.

In the years since the review of the LCP, there have been a number of key documents to help guide healthcare professionals to provide end-of-life care. However, the controversy about the pathway has shown that end-of-life care cannot be reduced to merely following a number of guidelines. All healthcare professionals need to be able to respond to a person and their family with compassion, using a variety of skills and, above all, treating them as unique individuals.

POLICY AND GUIDANCE

The End of Life Care Strategy (DH, 2008) was the first in the UK and covers adults in England. The strategy recognised the excellent innovative work of the hospice movement and the experience of the National End of Life Care Programme (2007).

The overall aim of the End of Life Care Strategy was to provide a 10-year vision for the provision of end-of-life care, ensuring access to high quality care for all people approaching the end of their life, irrespective of their age, gender, ethnicity, religious belief, disability, sexual orientation, socioeconomic status and diagnosis. It encompasses all adults with advanced, progressive illness and care delivered in all settings, including the home environment. Since the launch of the strategy in 2008, public awareness of end-of-life care has increased, partly owing to the work of Hospice UK (2015) and the need to plan for the end of life is now seen as a priority. Since 2008, other policies and guidance have shaped the provision of care for the dying, such as the NICE Quality Standard QS13 (2021); however, the emphasis now is on local decision-making and delivery. The National Palliative and End of Life Care Partnership (2021) built on the work of the End of Life Care Strategy with its publication of *Ambitions for Palliative and End of Life Care*. This framework encourages organisations to develop more effective ways of working and promotes the effective and creative use of resources (see Box 16.1). The framework recognises that the successful provision of good end-of-life care lies in working in partnership and collaboratively. Examples of this include shared record-keeping, 24/7 access to services and effective leadership.

Box 16.1 The six ambitions for palliative and end-of-life care

- Everyone is seen as an individual and should be treated as such.
- Each person gets fair access to care.
- Comfort and wellbeing of the individual should be maximised.
- Care is coordinated.
- All staff are prepared to care.
- Each community is prepared to help.

Source: National Palliative and End of Life Care Partnership (2021).

To realise these ambitions, building blocks must be in place such as having honest conversations, clear expectations, an integrated approach to care and the opportunity for people to take control of their own care. The focus of this framework is to create an impetus for better care at the end of life.

The NHS Long Term Plan (NHS England, 2019) equally commits to improving personalised palliative and end-of-life care for people of all ages and to address health inequity.

Reflection: points to consider

The objectives above set many challenges for all healthcare providers and organisations. What would you envisage these to be for you in your role as a paramedic?

GOLD STANDARDS FRAMEWORK

The Gold Standards Framework (GSF, 2019) is a systematic approach to formalising best practice so that quality end-of-life care becomes standard for every patient. It is concerned with helping people to live well until the end of life and includes care in the final years of life for people with any end-stage illness in any setting.

According to the GSF, the majority of people will spend 90 per cent of the final year of their life at home, yet over half of the population do not die where they choose. It has been previously stated that there is a significant gap between preferred and actual place of death, with too many people dying in hospital and too few in their own home, care home or hospice. A key goal of the GSF is to enable more people to die in their preferred place, reducing unnecessary hospital admissions and the numbers who inappropriately die on acute hospital wards. Over 95 per cent of GP practices in the UK have a palliative care support register (GSF, 2019). This ensures that patients who have palliative care needs are identified and information related to their illness, preferred priorities of care and choices are known to all the members of the primary healthcare team and out-of-hours services. Box 16.2 highlights the five goals of the GSF.

Box 16.2 The five goals of the Gold Standards Framework

1. Ensuring patients are well symptom controlled.
2. Enabling patients to live and die well in their preferred place of care.
3. Encouraging security and support via better advance care planning, involving the patient and their family.
4. Empowering carers through increased communication, listening and addressing issues proactively.
5. Educating staff and developing increased competence and confidence.

As a paramedic, you are a key advocate for patients and carers, reducing the need for admission by mobilising other services, advising how to access services and calming difficult situations. Patients at the end of their life frequently need care from multiple services and transfer between locations, such as home and hospital for treatment, investigations or respite care. This in itself will increase the amount of contact that you as ambulance personnel will have with them. They need access to care and support 24/7 to avoid being admitted to hospital as an emergency rather than being cared for in their home or normal place of residence. The End of Life Care Strategy (DH, 2008) identified that as a society, we do not talk openly about death and dying. It is suggested that relatively few adults, including older adults, have discussed their preferences for care with a close family member or friend. This makes it difficult or impossible for ambulance personnel and other healthcare professionals to ensure patients' wishes are met. The introduction of advanced care planning has provided structure and advice to ensure individuals are in a position to make their wishes known.

ADVANCE CARE PLANNING

The NHS defines advance care planning (ACP) as follows:

> *ACP is a voluntary process of person-centred discussion between an individual and their care providers about their preferences and priorities for their future care, while they have the mental capacity for meaningful conversation about these. The process, which is likely to involve a number of conversations over time, must have due consideration and respect for the person's wishes and emotions at all times. As a result, the person should experience a greater sense of involvement and the opportunity to reflect and share what matters most to them. (NHS England, 2022: 6)*

These discussions might include the preferences for their treatment, such as how and where they would like to be cared for. Some local areas have addressed issues regarding planning for the end of life. An example of this is Deciding Right (Northern Cancer Alliance, 2022), working across the entire integrated care system in the North East and North Cumbria to ensure the same approach is taken to advance care planning and 'do not attempt cardiopulmonary resuscitation' by using the same recognisable documentation across the area.

An advance care plan can take three forms:

1. **Advance statement:** this is a verbal or written statement of a person's wishes and preferences, beliefs and values. It must be stated by someone who has capacity for those care decisions,

and only becomes active when that person loses capacity for those decisions. It is not legally binding but all carers are required to take it into account if the person loses capacity and a care decision has to be made according to the best interests process on the Mental Capacity Act 2005 (Legislation.gov.uk, 2005). An example of this is a preferred priorities of care document.

2. **Advance decision to refuse treatment (ADRT):** this is a verbal or written refusal of treatment. It must be stated by someone who has capacity for those care decisions, and it only becomes active when that person loses capacity for those decisions. An ADRT must be prepared if life-sustaining treatment is refused, and must state that the treatment is being refused 'even if my life is at risk'. An ADRT is legally binding if it is valid and applicable to the situation. The National End of Life Care Programme (2013) lists several key elements relating to the making of an ADRT:

    - An advance decision should be made voluntarily.
    - The individual needs to be over 18 years of age.
    - The individual must have capacity to make an ADRT.
    - The advance decision should specify the treatment which is to be refused and the circumstances in which refusal applies.
    - The decision must be valid.
    - The decision must be in writing, signed and witnessed for it to apply.
    - An advance decision can only be used to refuse treatment and not to demand treatment or request any procedure that is against the law such as euthanasia.
    - A copy should be retained in the relevant patient records.

3. **Lasting power of attorney (LPA):** when an individual has capacity, they can legally nominate a person to make decisions on their behalf should they lose capacity for those decisions in the future. A Property and Affairs LPA cannot make healthcare decisions. These can only be made by a Personal Welfare LPA, and such an LPA can only make life-sustaining treatment decisions if this is authorised in the original LPA order. An LPA is bound by the same Mental Capacity Act process of best interests.

MENTAL CAPACITY ACT 2005

The Mental Capacity Act 2005 was implemented in 2007 and all health and social care professionals have a duty to abide by the code of practice within it. The Act gives individuals the right to make an advance decision to refuse treatment (ADRT).

The Mental Capacity Act has five main principles:

- A person must be assumed to have capacity unless it is established that they lack capacity.
- A person is not to be treated as unable to make a decision unless all practicable steps to help them to do so have been taken without success.
- A person is not to be treated as unable to make a decision merely because they make an unwise decision.
- An act done or decision made, under this Act for or on behalf of a person who lacks capacity must be done, or made, in their best interests.
- Before the act is done, or the decision made, regard must be had to whether the purpose for which it is needed can be as effectively achieved in a way that is less restrictive of the person's rights and freedom of action.

(Legislation.gov.uk, 2005: 5)

Brady (2014) expresses the importance of the patient's voice and the recording of their wishes, what they wish to receive, and the setting or location where they wish to be cared for. He suggests that there needs to be a clear understanding of the Mental Capacity Act as it is an integral part of end-of-life care.

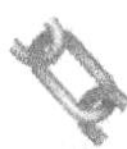

Chapters 4, 8 and **14** for more details on the Mental Capacity Act.

Reflection: points to consider

As a paramedic, think about how the management of some of your patients might change if they have an advance care plan. Have you considered this yourself?

DO NOT ATTEMPT CARDIOPULMONARY RESUSCITATION

A decision regarding 'do not attempt cardiopulmonary resuscitation' (DNACPR) needs to be considered as part of wider discussions about end-of-life care and must be facilitated by a professional who possess up-to-date knowledge, skill and confidence in order to support individuals in making such a decision (CQC, 2021). DNACPR decisions are an important element of care and a clear example of when advance decisions documenting the patient's wishes must be known in relation to future care and treatment. This will result in informed decisions being made in what can be stressful and emergency situations following calls from distressed relatives, carers or the general public. Moffat et al. (2019) interviewed paramedics about DNACPR and concluded that whilst there has been a significant increase in the number of DNACPR forms, most paramedics report inappropriate CPR attempts and find it difficult to make clinical judgements for those at the end of life. Coleman et al. (2020) identified that, crucially, DNACPR decisions are different to ADRTs, and Keeley and Generous (2017) state that communication with the individual and their family at the end of life can relieve anxiety and can ensure that final wishes for the end of life can be honoured.

The British Medical Association (RCUK, 2016) offers guidance on decision-making for a person who is nearing the end of life due to a terminal illness, when death is imminent and cardiopulmonary resuscitation (CPR) would not be successful, and there is no formal decision made and recorded. In such circumstances, any healthcare professional who makes a carefully considered decision not to start CPR should be supported by their senior colleagues, employers and professional bodies (RCUK, 2016). This will no doubt involve sensitive and distressing discussion. Education for paramedics on patient-centred end-of-life care (EoLC) is essential to help increase confidence in DNACPR, which is only applicable to CPR.

The Resuscitation Council UK (RCUK, 2023) has recommended the roll out of the Recommended Summary Plan for Emergency Care and Treatment (ReSPECT) process across the UK, with many health and social care communities already adopting this process. The ReSPECT process aims to create personalised recommendations and plans for an individual's future treatment and care if and when they are unable to express choice towards the end of their lives. These recommendations will be created through honest conversations between clinicians, individuals and their families so that everyone is aware not only of the individual's wishes but also what treatment and care is realistic. The plan should remain in the possession of the elderly person, so that it is readily available to anyone that needs to make an immediate decision in an emergency, such as paramedics. This approach of using standardised processes and documentation will allow for appropriate and timely support to be put in place in a consistent manner, easily recognisable to all involved, allowing for an individual's wishes to be accounted for at the end of life.

The RCUK (2016) suggests that the ultimate responsibility for initiating or withholding CPR falls to the most senior clinician in charge, and given the frequency of this type of call, this will often be a paramedic.

There are a variety of factors to take into account at the scene of a resuscitation, including family wishes and emotions, which can result in ethical conflicts between guidelines and the care requested, particularly where there is a lack of formal documentation (Milling et al., 2022). Consequently, invasive treatments and resuscitation procedures can be initiated in situations when death is expected or imminent.

The final decision regarding the application or not of the CPR decision in an emergency rests with the healthcare professionals responsible for managing the patient's immediate situation. These healthcare professionals may, on attending a cardiac arrest, make a clinical assessment resulting in a different decision from the one on the CPR decision form. As with any clinical decisions, healthcare professionals must be able to justify their decision; in particular, clinicians should be cautious of overriding a DNACPR decision where the CPR decision form records that the patient has expressed a clear wish not to receive attempted CPR (RCUK, 2016: 26).

In addition, patients who have valid DNACPR orders may undergo unwanted resuscitation if their documents are questioned or unknown by family members, friends and healthcare providers. To ensure paramedics and healthcare providers are aware of the needs and wishes of individuals, information systems must facilitate the sharing of information. The Electronic Palliative Care Coordination System (EPaCCS) is an example of practice initiatives to provide a joined-up solution to information-sharing in order to meet the needs of those requiring end-of-life care, allowing a range of clinicians to access and record individuals' preferences and needs about their end-of-life care (Humber and North Yorkshire Health and Care Partnership, 2023).

Clinical guidelines issued by the Association of Ambulance Chief Executives advise paramedics that in the case of cardiopulmonary arrest, they should always initiate CPR unless the patient has a condition unequivocally associated with death, specifically decapitation, massive cranial and cerebral destruction, hemicorporectomy or similar massive injury, rigor mortis, hypostasis, decomposition/putrefaction or incineration. The Ambulance Service guidelines also state that resuscitation can be discontinued where there is a formal DNACPR 'order', a ReSPECT form that indicates resuscitation should not be attempted or a valid advance decision that states the wish of the patient not to undergo attempted resuscitation, or where a patient is in the final stages of a terminal illness where death is imminent and unavoidable and CPR would not be successful, but for whom no formal DNACPR decision has been made. You are urged to read the full Ambulance Service guidelines for more detailed information on ambulance clinicians' response if cardiorespiratory arrest is required.

To ensure that paramedics do not start CPR against the recorded wishes of the patient, it is important that ambulance services have robust systems in place to record ADRTs and decisions about CPR, and to communicate these immediately to the paramedics who respond to an emergency call to a patient for whom such a document exists. With increasing use of electronic records, such documents may be stored centrally. As paramedics have to satisfy themselves that the document exists and is valid in the circumstances encountered, an agreed method of emergency communication of any such decision, and of the basis for it, is necessary and should be subject to clinical governance (RCUK, 2016: 29). Where documentation does not exist, the advice offered by the JRCALC guidelines (JRCALC/AACE, 2022) suggests that CPR may be discontinued or withheld, if 'a person is known to be in the final stages of an advanced, irreversible condition in which CPR would be both inappropriate and unsuccessful'.

Another initiative is the 'Message in a Bottle' scheme. This scheme encourages healthcare professionals to leave information which is vital for paramedics in a labelled container in the fridge. A sticker is placed on the back of the patient's front door alerting them to the fact that they are part of the scheme.

PREFERRED PRIORITIES OF CARE

The Universal Principles for Advance Care Planning (ACP) (NHS England, 2022) record a variety of aspects to be considered in planning for person-centred end-of-life care. This document highlights several pertinent tools to support and record discussions about treatment preferences, including Treatment Escalation Plans (TEPs), Anticipatory Clinical Management Plans, ReSPECT and Deciding Right. Such tools are not legally binding, unless a specific decision is recorded in a valid ADRT; however, they do allow patients and carers to discuss their main priorities at the end phase of life and promote honest and open communication. Topics covered include an understanding of current health preferences and priorities for future care, including preferred location of care.

Many patients express a wish to die at home (RCUK, 2016), one result of which is that ambulance staff and paramedics will come into contact with patients who are nearing the end of their life, either as a result of planned transfers or where a sudden crisis occurs (JRCALC/AACE, 2022). These contacts may be due to a sudden change in their health or as the result of something completely unrelated to their main illness. Current JRCALC guidelines (JRCALC/AACE, 2022) offer robust advice regarding the management of this type of patient alongside clear guidance for dealing with any exacerbation of the underlying condition. Paramedics may find themselves attending a patient in the dying phase due to a sudden deterioration of the condition or unexpected complications that family members might not yet be prepared for. Although it is crucial that the paramedic respects all concerned, they must attempt to establish the patient's wishes, while acknowledging the possibility of differing views between family members and carers. Some key points are noted in Box 16.3. The competent patient's right to make an autonomous decision to stay at home and to receive palliative care must be supported by the practitioner, liaising with the GP to arrange that the patient receives the right care at the right time.

The National Ambulance Service Medical Directors (NASMeD, 2014), when considering the future clinical priorities for ambulance services in England, acknowledged the involvement of the ambulance service in end of life care, and many ambulance services now have strategies and dedicates services in place to support those needing end of life care. Paramedics are frequently at the scene or shortly after the point of death and have to make decisions on whether resuscitation is required or would be futile, often based on limited knowledge of the patient's wishes. The Joint Royal Colleges Ambulance Liaison Committee notes that as a result of an ageing population, there will be increased demand for high-quality end-of-life care, which will be reflected in the workload of ambulance personnel (JRCALC/AACE, 2022).

Box 16.3 Key points to consider in end-of-life care

- Pain relief is a right of the patient and the duty of all clinicians when attending a patient at the end of their life.
- Escalating or acute pain is a medical emergency.
- It is easier to prevent pain than to relieve it.
- Morphine should be the first option for breakthrough pain where opioids are already prescribed and pain is severe.
- The presence or absence of a DNACPR should not direct treatment options. If a patient is diagnosed as dying, a clinician is not obliged to commence CPR at the point of death, even in the absence of a DNACPR form.
- A patient's own Just in Case (JIC) medication can be administered by a trained clinician.
- JIC medication carried by a clinician can be administered via patient-specific direction or via verbal order, depending on the Trust.
- Local guidelines and policies regarding end -of-life care should be referred to.

Source: JRCALC/AACE (2022).

As already stated, paramedics can find themselves attending a patient who is near the end of their life. Any conversation with the patient or family members who are in attendance can be very difficult, which can result in becoming very clinically focused. It is important to remember that although there are some immediate decisions and assessments to be made, how this is handled will have a lasting effect on everyone involved (see case study 16.1).

Case study 16.1

Joan is an 80-year-old lady with chronic obstructive pulmonary disease (COPD). She has been prescribed antibiotics by her GP for a recent chest infection. Joan is on the palliative care register as she is entering the end phase of her life, and has an advance care plan, which states that she wants to stay at home, as well as a DNACPR. However, she is breathless, confused and incoherent, so her anxious family has called an ambulance.

Consider how you might approach this situation: how might you interact with Joan and her family to ensure her needs and wishes are met and that, despite Joan's confusion, she is treated as a person and can remain at home?

Some key practical tips to help for end-of-life care

- **Consider the person:** try to establish something about the person that recognises them as a unique individual. People often try to cope with their illness by maintaining a sense of normality. Talking to the person or family about them while undertaking vital assessments helps them to feel more like a person than a patient. Sometimes there are clues in a person's home which help: photographs, trophies, pets, anything that might help make a connection.
- **Recognise their importance:** remember that the person you are treating is a significant and important individual to members of their family. This is why care needs to be compassionate and communication needs to be honest and clear.
- **Personhood:** life-threatening illness can erode a person's sense of identity; they can suffer a variety of losses and changes. Illness affects how they look physically and how they are able to fulfill their roles in their family and society. Any interaction with a healthcare professional can have an impact on their self-esteem and feelings of self-worth, so all aspects of communication need to be person-centred.

BREAKING BAD/SIGNIFICANT NEWS

There are several models that can help guide difficult conversations, an example of which is the SPIKES model (Baile et al., 2000). SPIKES focuses on the delivery of significant news and the factors that influence how this news is given. It guides the information giver to consider the setting where the news is given and what is already understood, and encourages information to be given in small chunks so that understanding can be assessed. It is important to consider how news might be received and the emotional responses people may have, such as denial, anger and distress, all of which should be respected and supported. Finally, the model encourages the discussion of next steps, ensuring no one is left uncertain of what will happen, for example the attendance of a police officer or funeral director, or admission to hospital.

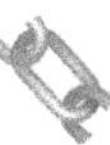

Chapter 1 for other models of communication that may be useful and **Chapter 2** for the power of reflection in such difficult situations.

Reflection: points to consider

Reflect on an occasion when you had to give some difficult or significant news to a patient or relative. What went well? What would you do differently and how did you feel?

CONCLUSION

This chapter has introduced you to the policies and frameworks underpinning end-of-life care. The delivery of high-quality end-of-life care can be a challenging part of the role of the paramedic or ambulance clinician. It requires multidisciplinary working and the successful implementation of the identified policies and initiatives to meet the needs of patients at the end of life. The GSF factsheet for paramedics (2019) suggests the following points for consideration before transporting a patient:

- Is there an advance care plan which may include information for DNACPR or where the patient wants to be cared for?
- Is there a decision to refuse treatment?
- Can you access the information you need?

- Can you use other options to avoid unnecessary admission?
- Is admission appropriate or could other services help?
- Can you avoid transporting a patient who is in the last weeks/days of their life when they wish to die in their home or care home?

Chapter key points:

- An understanding of the policies and frameworks underpinning end-of-life care will inform your practice.
- Multidisciplinary working is key to ensuring patients' needs are met.
- Too few people die at home or in their place of choice.
- Initiating discussions about preferences for end-of-life care is essential.
- Everyone is involved in end-of-life care.

REFERENCES AND SUGGESTED READING

Baile, W., Buckman, R., Lenato, R. et al. (2000) SPIKES: a six step protocol for delivering bad news – application to the patient with cancer, *The Oncologist*, 5 (4): 302–11.

Brady, M. (2014) Challenges UK paramedics currently face in providing fully effective end-of-life care, *International Journal of Palliative Nursing*, 20 (1): 37–44.

Care Quality Commission (CQC) (2021) *Protect, respect, connect – decisions about living and dying well during COVID-19. CQC's review of 'do not attempt cardiopulmonary resuscitation' decisions during the COVID-19 pandemic*, Final report. Available at: https://www.cqc.org.uk/sites/default/files/20210318_dnacpr_printer-version.pdf (accessed 12 April 2024).

Clark, D., Small, N., Wright, M. et al. (2005) *A Bit of Heaven for the Few? An Oral History of the Modern Hospice Movement in the United Kingdom*. Lancaster: Observatory Publications.

Coleman, J.J., Botkai, A., Marson, E.J. et al. (2020) Bringing into focus treatment limitation and DNACPR decisions: how COVID-19 has changed practice, *Resuscitation*, 155: 172–79.

Department of Health (DH) (2005) *Mental Capacity Act Code of Practice*. Available at: www.dca.gov.uk/legal-policy/mentalcapacity/mca-cp.pdf (accessed 12 April 2024).

Department of Health (DH) (2007) *Promoting innovative end of life care practice within Ambulance Trusts*. London: DH.

Department of Health (DH) (2008) *End of life care strategy: Promoting high quality care for all adults at the end of their life*. Available at: https://www.gov.uk/government/publications/end-of-life-care-strategy-promoting-high-quality-care-for-adults-at-the-end-of-their-life.

Department of Health (DH) (2010) *End of life care strategy: Second annual report.* Available at: https://www.gov.uk/government/publications/end-of-life-care-strategy-second-annual-report.

Department of Health (DH) (2013a) *More care, less pathway. A review of the Liverpool Care Pathway.* Available at: https://assets.publishing.service.gov.uk/media/5a75153340f0b6397f35d87d/Liverpool_Care_Pathway.pdf.

Department of Health (DH) (2013b) *Advance decisions to refuse treatment: A guide for health and social care staff.* London: DH.

Department of Health (DH) (2015) *Long-term health conditions.* London: DH.

Etkind, S.N., Bone, A.E., Gomes, B. et al. (2017) How many people will need palliative care in 2040? Past trends, future projections and implications for services, *BMC Medicine*, 15: 102. Available at: https://bmcmedicine.biomedcentral.com/articles/10.1186/s12916-017-0860-2 (accessed 12 April 2024).

Gold Standards Framework (GSF) (2019) *The Gold Standards Framework QOF support pack April 2019: to enable GP practices and primary care networks fulfil the new 2019 EOLC QOF.* Available at: https://www.goldstandardsframework.org.uk/cd-content/uploads/files/Primaryper cent20Care/FINALper cent20GSFper cent20QOFper cent20Supportper cent20Packper cent20vs6.pdf (accessed 12 April 2024).

Higginson, I.J., Brooks, D. and Barclay, S. (2021) Dying at home during the pandemic, *British Medical Journal*, 373: n1437. Available at: https://doi.org/10.1136/bmj.n1437.

Hospice UK (2015) *Dying matters.* Available at: http://www.dyingmatters.org/ (accessed 12 April 2024).

House of Commons Health Committee (2004) *Palliative Care, Fourth Report of Session 2003–2004.* London: TSO.

Humber and North Yorkshire Health and Care Partnership (2023) *EPaCCS.* Available at: https://humberandnorthyorkshire.org.uk/epaccs-is-about-putting-the-wishes-of-the-patient-at-the-centre-of-care-and-supporting-people-approaching-the-end-of-life-their-families-carers-and-the-clinicians-that-look-after-them/ (accessed 12 April 2024).

Joint Royal Colleges Ambulance Liaison Committee and Association of Ambulance Chief Executives (JRCALC/AACE) (2022) *JRCALC Clinical Guidelines.* Bridgwater: Class Professional Publishing.

Keeley, M.P. and Generous, M.A. (2017) Final conversations: overview and practical implications for patients, families, and healthcare workers, *Behavioural Sciences*, 7 (2): 17. Available at: https://doi.org/10.3390/bs7020017.

Legislation.gov.uk (2005) *Mental Capacity Act 2005.* Available at: https://www.legislation.gov.uk/ukpga/2005/9/contents.

Marie Curie (2021) *A place for everyone – what stops people from choosing where they die ? A review of the barriers to good end of life care facing diverse groups in the UK*, Marie Curie. Available at: https://www.mariecurie.org.uk/policy/a-place-for-everyone (accessed 12 April 2024).

Milling, L., Kjaer, J., Binderup, L.G. et al. (2022) Non-medical factors in prehospital resuscitation decision-making: a mixed-methods systematic review, *Scandinavian Journal of Trauma, Resuscitation and Emergency Medicine*, 30: 24. Available at: https://doi.org/10.1186/s13049-022-01004-6.

Moffat, S., Fritz, Z., Slother, A.-M. et al. (2019) 'Do not attempt CPR' in the community: the experience of ambulance clinicians, *Journal of Paramedic Practice*, 11 (5): 198–204.

National Ambulance Service Medical Directors (NASMeD) (2014) *Future national clinical priorities for ambulance services in England*. Available at: http://aace.org.uk/wp-content/uploads/2014/05/Future-national-clinical-priorities-for-ambulance-services-in-England-FINAL-2.pdf (accessed 12 April 2024).

National Council for Palliative Care (2010) *End of life care manifesto*. Available at: https://www.ncpc.org.uk/sites/default/files/2010Manifesto.pdf.

National Council for Palliative Care (2015) *Every moment counts: A new vision for co-ordinated care for people near the end of life calls for brave conversations*. Available at: https://s42139.pcdn.co/wp-content/uploads/every_moment_counts.pdf.

National End of Life Care Intelligence Network (NELCIN) (2014) Available at: http://www.endoflifecare-intelligence.org.uk/home (accessed 12 April 2024).

National End of Life Care Programme (2007) *Promoting Innovative End of Life Care Practice Within Ambulance Trusts*. London: Department of Health.

National End of Life Care Programme (2008) *Advance Care Planning: A Guide for Health and Social Care Staff*. London: Department of Health.

National End of Life Care Programme (2013) *The Route to Success in End of Life Care: Achieving Quality for Ambulance Services*. London: Department of Health.

National Institute for Health and Care Excellence (NICE) (2021) *End of life care for adults*, Quality Standard QS13. Available at: https://www.nice.org.uk/guidance/qs13 (accessed 12 April 2024).

National Palliative and End of Life Care Partnership (2021) *Ambitions for palliative and end of life care: a national framework for local action 2021–2026*. Available at: https://www.england.nhs.uk/wp-content/uploads/2022/02/ambitions-for-palliative-and-end-of-life-care-2nd-edition.pdf (accessed 12 April 2024).

NHS England (2014) *Actions for end of life care: 2014–16*. Available at: https://www.england.nhs.uk/wp-content/uploads/2014/11/actions-eolc.pdf.

NHS England (2019) *NHS long term plan*. Available at: https://www.longterm-plan.nhs.uk/wp-content/uploads/2019/08/nhs-long-term-plan-version-1.2.pdf (accessed 12 April 2024).

NHS England (2022) *Universal principles for advance care planning (ACP)*. Available at: https://www.england.nhs.uk/wp-content/uploads/2022/03/universal-principles-for-advance-care-planning.pdf (accessed 12 April 2024).

NHS England (2023) *Palliative and end of life care*. Available at: https://www.england.nhs.uk/eolc/#:~:text=Itper cent20preventsper cent20andper cent20relievesper cent20suffering,theper cent20lastper cent20yearper cent20ofper cent20life (accessed 12 April 2024).

Northern Cancer Alliance (2022) *Deciding right*. Available at: https://northerncanceralliance.nhs.uk/deciding-right/ (accessed 12 April 2024).

Office for Health Improvement and Disparities (2023) *Palliative and end of life care profiles*. Available at: https://fingertips.phe.org.uk/profile/end-of-life/ (accessed 12 April 2024).

Office for Health Improvement and Disparities (2024) *Public health profiles*. Available at: https://fingertips.phe.org.uk (accessed 13 May 2024).

Office for National Statistics (ONS) (2022) *Deaths registered weekly in England and Wales, provisional*. Available at: https://www.ons.gov.uk/peoplepopulationand-community/birthsdeathsandmarriages/deaths/datasets/weeklyprovisionalfig-uresondeathsregisteredinenglandandwales (accessed 12 April 2024).

Public Health England (2018) *Atlas of variation for palliative and end of life care in England*. Available at: https://fingertips.phe.org.uk/profile/atlas-of-variation (accessed 12 April 2024).

Resuscitation Council UK (RCUK) (2016) *Decisions Relating to Cardiopulmonary Resuscitation: Guidance from the British Medical Association, the Resuscitation Council and the Royal College of Nursing*, 3rd edition. London: NHS Improving Quality.

Resuscitation Council UK (RCUK) (2023) *ReSPECT*. Available at: https://www.resus.org.uk/respect (accessed 12 April 2024).

Rosenberg, M., Lamba, S. and Misra, S. (2013) Palliative medicine and geriatric emergency care: challenges, opportunities, and basic principles, *Journal of Clinical Geriatric Medicine*, 29 (1): 1–29.

Saunders, C. (2005) *Watch with Me*. Lancaster: Observatory Publications.

Stone, S., Abbott, J., McClung, C.D. et al. (2009) Paramedic knowledge, attitudes and training in end of life care, *Prehospital and Disaster Medicine*, 24 (6): 529–34.

Watt, T., Raymond, A., Rachet-Jacquet, L. et al. (2023) *Health in 2040: Projected patterns of illness in England*, The Health Foundation. Available at: https://www.health.org.uk/publications/health-in-2040.

World Health Organization (WHO) (2020) *Palliative care fact sheet*. Available at: https://www.who.int/news-room/fact-sheets/detail/palliative-care (accessed 12 April 2024).

World Health Organization (WHO) (2023) *Palliative care fact sheet*. Available at: https://www.who.int/europe/news-room/fact-sheets/item/palliative-care (accessed 12 April 2024).

17 Leadership styles and their impact on practice

Kath Jennings

> **In this chapter:**
>
> - Introduction
> - Why is this relevant?
> - Leadership theory and leadership styles
> - What makes a paramedic a good leader?
> - Paramedic leadership within a multi-professional context
> - Conclusion
> - Chapter key points
> - References and suggested reading

INTRODUCTION

Leadership refers to the way a situation is approached. Leadership style is a leader's approach to a situation, which usually involves providing direction, motivating people and implementing plans. At an organisational or individual level, leadership is about being able to articulate/communicate an idea, vision or behaviour to others, in order to bring them along with you. It is about influencing people.

This chapter discusses the variety of leadership styles and the work of several eminent theorists in this field. The subject of leadership is discussed in relation to the pre-hospital environment and the unique work of paramedics.

WHY IS THIS RELEVANT?

Paramedic practice has developed to include skills needed for leadership and management. Clinical leadership is key to delivering high-quality patient care. There is a need for paramedics to recognise and develop their leadership potential, present in the everyday decisions made, whether responding to life-threatening calls or not. The Health and Care Professions Council (HCPC) states that paramedics must understand the qualities, behaviours and benefits of leadership, and recognise that leadership is a skill all professionals can demonstrate. They must identify and develop their own leadership qualities, behaviours and approaches, taking into account the importance of equality, diversity and inclusion (HCPC, 2023). The need for greater leadership in paramedic practice was highlighted as far back as the Bradley Report, 'Taking Healthcare to the Patient' (DH, 2005), which identified the need for reinforcing and developing clinical and managerial leadership to create well-led organisations made up of supported and empowered staff. Improving patient care and developing staff were fundamentally dependent upon improved leadership. More recently, the NHS Long Term Workforce Plan (NHS England, 2023) links leadership to staff retention and inclusivity in teams. Well-documented high-profile failures in leadership led to catastrophic consequences for patients in the Bristol Royal Infirmary, Mid-Staffordshire, Morecambe Bay, and Shrewsbury and Telford hospital trusts. It is hoped that the content of this chapter will impact on your future patient care.

LEADERSHIP THEORY AND LEADERSHIP STYLES

As well as referring to the way situations are approached, leadership is a complex process by which a person influences others to accomplish a mission, task or objective. It is a role which is implicit in paramedic practice. From leading the coordinated approach in a multiple-casualty situation, to working with a colleague and assuming control of the situation, the philosophy of leadership is similar.

This section will examine leadership theory, including several models and provide a brief overview of the development of leadership theories over time.

Lewin's power relationships

Known as the 'father of social psychology', Kurt Lewin identified three different types of leadership styles based on power relationships.

- **Authoritarian:** with an authoritarian style, the dominant power base lies with the boss/leader while employees/team members hold a non-dominant power base.
- **Participative:** both the boss/leader and employees/team members hold a dominant power base with this style of leadership.
- **Delegative:** the power base of dominance lies with employees/team members and the non-dominant power base is held by the boss/leader.

While it is inevitable that one style will dominate behaviour, a good leader can adopt all three approaches and be able to change their approach to suit the situation. This is frequently seen within paramedic practice during patient care episodes. However, there are certain factors which will determine the style to be used, including:

- Resources available, i.e. time, financial, equipment.
- Basis of relationships, i.e. trust, distrust.
- Who holds the information: you, the employees, both?
- Knowledge and skills of you and your team.
- Internal dynamics of the team.
- Positive and negative stress levels.

Authoritarian

Also known as autocratic leadership, this style of leadership does not seek the advice of followers; rather, it is used when the leader tells followers what they want done and how they want it done. This is most commonly used when all the information to solve the problem is available, employees are well motivated and time is of the essence. There is no room for negotiation within the decision. This could be an approach to be used in resuscitation, as in this situation, the leader is very much in command. From the didactic approach of resuscitation courses, all members of the team will know their role. The leader must assess the problem quickly, work out a management plan and then give clear orders to the rest of the team. Although the leader will listen to suggestions from the members of the team, most of the direction and orders will come from the leader. Here the needs of the individual team members are of a low priority, while the key objective of saving the patient's life is paramount.

Although one can understand the reasons why this style is adopted in this situation, a good leader will recognise that the casualty of this style of leadership is the follower. This style can be used when working with a non-registered practitioner who is new to the job and needs direction and firm guidance. However, it must be noted that taking such an inflexible approach does not allow the followers to develop problem-solving skills for themselves and limits individual growth; this is acceptable if, in the whole scheme of the work scenario, it is tempered with periods of participative styles of leadership.

Participative

Also known as democratic leadership, this style of leadership involves team participation in the decision-making process. With this style, although one or more followers are involved in the decision-making process, the leader remains the final decision-making authority; this is a sign of strength that teams will respect. This is normally used when some key information is known to the leader and members of the team know other key parts. It is inclusive and acknowledges that everyone has a valuable contribution to make when shaping the service within which they work. This style sends the message that the leader cannot be expected to know everything and that skilful and knowledgeable colleagues are respected. This style may be adopted when working with an experienced crew that knows their job well. The leader knows the problem and the team members know their job and can offer advice on how to solve it.

Delegative (free rein)

Also known as laissez-faire leadership, this style of leadership means that the decisions are made solely by the team, but the leader still carries the responsibility. This is used when followers are able to analyse the situation and determine what needs to be done and how to do it. This style is best used when full trust and confidence is held in the people around the leader, as risk is shared among the team. In a clinical scenario, although one team may have been first on scene and assumed overall command of the situation, if a crew arrived to assist that had been in the same situation before, then leadership would be delegated to the other team. Delegative leadership can be abused by leaders offering little or no guidance to their team, and can lead to poorly defined roles and lack of motivation. However, they work well when team members are highly motivated, highly skilled and knowledgeable.

The example in case study 17.1 demonstrates paramedic leadership, team working, communication and delegation skills in the provision of advanced life support to a patient experiencing an out-of-hospital cardiac arrest. The systematic management of an out-of-hospital cardiac arrest may lead to this being interpreted as an example of authoritarian leadership by paramedics. However, in step with the evolution of theory and practice, the skills demonstrated in the case study are more demonstrative of situational leadership.

Case study 17.1

A paramedic crew respond to a 56-year-old male in cardiac arrest. After initiating basic life support, they are assisted by a second ambulance crew. Immediately on their arrival, an the crews exchange names and roles, and a handover is given without interruption to chest compressions. The lead paramedic delegates tasks and responsibilities associated with advanced life support, checking for understanding and confirming actions. Upon return of spontaneous circulation, a reversible cause is established and the crew work together under the leadership and delegation of the lead paramedic to haemodynamically stabilise the patient, before preparing him for transfer to an appropriate receiving facility.

Development of leadership theories over time

Although Machiavelli wrote on leadership in 1513 that it was better for leaders to be feared than loved, it was from the mid-nineteenth century that leadership theories were developed. They are broadly categorised as focusing on personality, power relations, behaviours, situations, actions, transaction, transformation and distribution. Table 17.1 traces the development of well-known leadership theories over time, and their associated theorists. It is not an exhaustive list and other leadership styles may be identified in literature.

Table 17.1   The historical development of leadership theories

Theory	Date	Ideas
Traits theory, Great Man theory	Mid-nineteenth century: T. Carlyle	Great leaders were born, not made and had certain traits or characteristics based on their physicality, abilities or personalities
Authoritarian Participative Free rein	1930s: K. Lewin	Influential early research identified three types of leadership styles
Behavioural theory	1960s: R.R. Blake and J. Mouton	Looks at the behaviour of leaders, who may be people-orientated or task-focused
Situational theory	Late 1960s: P. Hersey and K. Blanchard	Leadership can be temporarily changed depending on the strengths and limitations within a team. Successful leadership in one environment does not always translate to another
Action-centred leadership	Late 1970s: J. Adair	Three circles model, based on Task, Team and Individual, highlights three elements that leaders must consider
Transactional theory	1980s: B.M. Bass	Involves managing resources and systems within existing structures on a transactional basis
Transformational theory	1980s: J.V. Downton and B.M. Bass	Involves strategy and people management. The leaders share their goal as a vision, bringing people together to achieve it
Distributed theory	1990s: E. Hutchins	The cascade of leadership from above creates new leaders. Networking and widening participation in leadership are key to this theory

Adair and action-centred leadership

John Adair, a military tutor by background, developed his 'action-centred leadership' model while lecturing at Sandhurst Royal Military Academy. He helped change the accepted perception of management to encompass leadership and is well published on the subject. Adair (2020) asserts that there are core functions of leadership which can be applied in any situation:

- *planning* – seeking information, setting aims, defining tasks;
- *initiating* – briefing, task allocation, setting standards;
- *controlling* – maintaining standards, ensuring progress, ongoing decision-making;
- *supporting* – monitoring and rewarding individuals' contributions, encouraging team spirit, morale boosting, reconciling;
- *informing* – clarifying tasks and plans, updating, receiving feedback, interpreting;
- *evaluating* – feasibility of ideas, performance, enabling self-assessment.

The core of Adair's philosophy on action-centred leadership is the three circles model, recognising that there are three elements to effective leadership which require attention from individuals in a leadership position. These are Task, Team and Individual.

In this model, Adair represents the three areas as circles and the point where all three circles overlap (see Figure 17.1) he considers to be where effective leadership is occurring and all three elements are in perfect balance. The action-centred leadership model is simple and easy to remember,

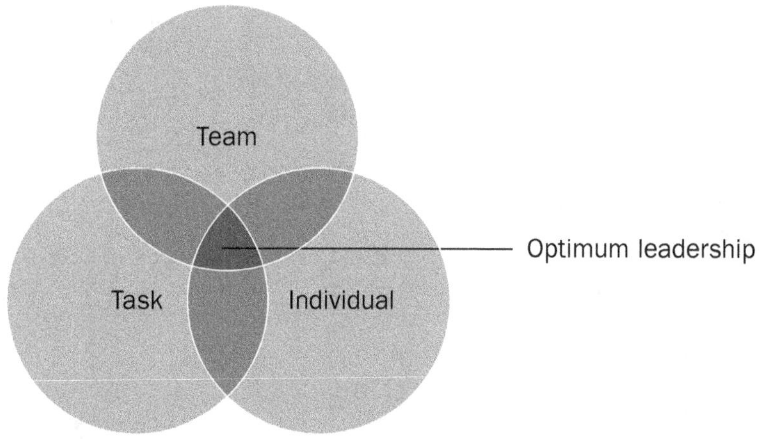

Figure 17.1 Example of overlapping circles

straightforward to apply in clinical practice in relation to both leadership and management, and can help leaders to quickly respond to changing circumstances. It is part of an integrated approach and although the three elements are collectively dependent, they are also independently crucial. Adair maintains that good leaders should have full control of the three main areas and that being able to do all these things and keep the balance right gets results by developing the team, increasing productivity, building moral and enhancing quality; this is the mark of a successful manager and leader.

Within each domain, there are certain factors for the leader to consider and achieve (see Table 17.2). In the clinical arena, all of these factors occur simultaneously and are rarely analysed in any great depth. For example, when managing a multiple-casualty event, the focus will be on the task – that is, the prioritisation of care and safe transfer to definitive facilities.

Table 17.2 Elements of Adair's leadership model that require completion

Task	Team	Individual
Define the task	Resolve conflict	Assist and support individuals
Identify resources	Develop team working	Agree to individual responsibilities
Create the plan	Encourage the team to achieve the task	Give recognition and praise
Establish the responsibilities	Give feedback to the group	Develop individual freedom and autonomy
Set the standards	Understand the team members	
Control and maintain the activities		
Monitor overall performance		
Review, reassess and adjust plan		
Establish standards of performance and behaviour		
Monitor and maintain discipline and integrity		

The leader of a patient care episode will need to determine and communicate who does what and when, including the request for additional resources, possibly from other agencies such as the fire service and police. The allocation of individual tasks therefore is different but related to the task management of the whole scene (Collen, 2019). While responsibilities need to be established across a team, a task must only be delegated to team members who have the knowledge, skills and experience necessary to carry it out safely and effectively (HCPC, 2024). In emergency services, this is typically identified by rank indicated by sliders worn on uniforms. In other healthcare areas, it may be different coloured uniforms, so seniority can be seen at a glance and is also clearly obvious to patients/families too.

The leader needs to maintain an overview of the care episode rather than be deeply involved in any single element such as airway management or placing a canula, so that the leader can always be aware of what has been done and what needs to happen next. Activities should be controlled and maintained by the leader and regular progress reports should be imparted to the team. The leader should recognise the individual variants in terms of personality, skills, strengths and needs. The team members should be given recognition for their achievements and support when they need guidance or tuition. This should be embedded in all teams for them to function at a productive level; however, the leader should recognise extraordinary contributions to the team and reward these appropriately.

While early leadership theories focused on personal attributes, more recent ones have looked at interactions between leaders and followers (Northouse, 2019). One problem with focusing on the characteristics of leaders is that the people who will be doing the work to deliver the plan are left out. Modern leadership theory emphasises the actual and potential leadership of the whole team. Distributing leadership across teams and organisations allows for opportunities to arise for people who may have previously been overlooked, hence it has an impact on equality, diversity and inclusion.

Transformational leadership and other theories broke away from the idea that leadership was about the characteristics of the leader, and whether they were a great person or demonstrated particular behaviours. Two of these theories are summarised below.

Transformational leadership

The transformational leadership style incorporates the softer side of leadership, which can be equally successful in paramedic practice as an authoritarian approach. The transformational approach to leadership challenges the autocratic unilateral leadership style of former years. It strives to elevate the needs of followers that are harmonious with their own goals and objectives, and it achieves this through charismatic people management, strategy and individual consideration. The transformational leader is characterised as a visionary or catalyst for change who crucially can motivate and energise followers to pursue mutual goals, share vision and create an empowering culture. With transformational leadership, both the leader and the follower have the same purpose and they raise one another's levels of performance. It also relies on mutuality, cooperation rather than competition, networking rather than hierarchy, and the empowerment of all employees. It recognises individuals' potential and will go further to satisfy higher-level needs such as self-esteem and achieving their full potential (Giltinane, 2013). The results of such an approach are that of increased work satisfaction and a low staff turnover. Workers are more likely to stick with an organisation that values their ideas and thoughts, and which creates an empowering culture. In a meta-analysis of newer leadership styles, many were found to have a high correlation with the characteristics of transformational leadership, suggesting organisations should focus resources on developing this style of leadership (Deng et al., 2023).

Distributed leadership

Distributed leadership in health care is the idea that due to the increased complexity in health systems, traditional leadership approaches are not fit for healthcare purposes. The three main reasons for this are: systems having a linear process, a lack of awareness of organisational culture and an inability to innovate (Northway, 2021). Complexity relates to the number of parts that constitute a system together with the level of interrelatedness of the parts. Healthcare systems are impacted by and impact upon other systems in society, and as such, are not linear. Non-linearity is a key feature of complexity theory and the theory of complex adaptive systems.

As well as healthcare systems becoming more complex, patients too have become more complex; many are living longer with long-term conditions, co-morbidities and require multiple medications (polypharmacy). There has, in turn, been an impact on the organisation of health systems, including ambulance services. Primary, secondary and pre-hospital systems have evolved to meet the demands of patients within new systems. Hence the role of the paramedic has changed from being predominantly *scoop and run* to a highly skilled role requiring degree entry to the HCPC register with a wide range of career opportunities within the profession.

Distributed leadership involves placing leaders in formal and informal roles throughout systems, not just in specific roles at the top. It places the focus on organisational connectedness. As such, it is a more fluid approach to leadership, giving individuals the opportunity to develop their own career interests. Aversion to this can be seen in the rotational paramedic role. The fluid nature of the leadership approach is intended to flow throughout the organisation. Technological innovation continues to influence the organisation of work, for example the increase in 'hear and treat' and remote decision-making.

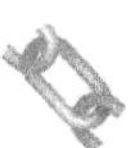 **Chapter 19** for more on remote decision-making.

Clinical care episodes within increasingly complex systems call for effective leadership, with clear communication and good task management. One factor affecting a leader's ability to execute good task management is cognitive task load, sometimes referred to as bandwidth or flow state. These terms all refer to the amount of brain power available for tasks. Its fluctuating nature is why pre-hospital systems routinise knowledge in the form of guidelines. In this way, therapeutic action is not delayed, and some bandwidth is available for complex tasks, or for application to a dynamic situation. Table 17.3 shows key ideas in the evolution of our understanding of cognitive task management in relation to leadership.

Csikszentmihalyi, one of the founders of positive psychology, described flow as being absorbed in a challenging but doable task. A state of flow is achieved by setting goals and obtaining feedback. Tasks should be

Table 17.3 Three models of coping with task management

Flow state model (Csikszentmihalyi, 1975)	Bandwidth (Staal, 2004)	Cognitive task load (Grootjen et al., 2006)
Control	Low arousal/	Vigilance
Relaxation	stimulation	Underload
Boredom	(30 per cent	Optimal
Apathy	bandwidth used)	Overload
Worry	Optimal arousal/	
Anxiety	stimulation	
Arousal	(80 per cent	
Flow	bandwidth used)	
	Overload (100 per	
	cent bandwidth	
	used)	

set at the right level of stretch, and feedback should ideally be instant, since the goals are reachable in a relatively short time (Csikszentmihalyi, 1975). Staal (2004) used a computer analogy to explain how brain power can become overloaded, leading to malfunction – or error in human terms. Similarly, the cognitive task load model (Grootjen et al., 2006) identified four workload states, one optimal and three suboptimal states (vigilance, underload and overload).

Reflection: points to consider

What style of leadership do you think best describes you? Is this how others see you? How do you manage your tasks?

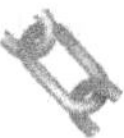

Chapter 1 for more in-depth information about communication theory and **Chapter 6** for detail on Human Factors.

WHAT MAKES A PARAMEDIC A GOOD LEADER?

Personal views of leadership may be shaped by one's previous experiences of it; even the birth order in our families may affect the experience of leadership and who would be expected to take what roles. We have all experienced good leaders, perhaps in a sports team, educators or college reps, and possibly have experienced poor leadership.

Developing leadership skills as a paramedic is part of developing as a person. Each of us approaches leadership with unique beliefs and assumptions about what makes us who we are. Understanding one's own values and being true to them is essential for becoming authentic (Kelly, 2023). Learning to be true to oneself demonstrates integrity and it is this that stands out as a leadership quality and as an example to others. Leadership skills therefore develop over time and can be developed by everyone. To lead people, paramedics need to determine if they are a good role model, competent and confident in their ability; able to collaborate effectively and develop trust between team members, and be open minded and able to bring out the strengths in others. Good leaders develop through a continuous process of reflection, education and experience. However, to provide effective leadership, you must have a clear understanding of your destination at the outset.

Followership, mentorship and emotional intelligence

All roles in paramedic practice involve aspects of mentorship and leadership in terms of influencing and engaging others (Dalrymple, 2019). Mentoring, the act of guiding or advising less experienced or learner paramedics, usually by a registrant, occurs through practice-based learning. From day one, demands are made on paramedics' capacity to engage with and influence others. Paramedics often begin as followers as the inexperienced look to the experienced for guidance on how to improve performance. Through learning to express themselves, paramedics become truer to themselves and less so to those whose example were once followed. Novice paramedics who exercise more awareness of their lack of experience will find it easier to grow than those who do not (Collen, 2019). The concept of followership may have negative connotations, but followership is a necessary component of team leadership. Barr and Dowding (2022) stipulate that without followers, there cannot be leaders and vice versa. Ambulance services are hierarchical organisations and those who do not lead may be considered to lack leadership capability or creativity. Effective followership requires self-discipline, respect for colleagues and the ability to accept instruction when necessary. Paramedics need to be able to move seamlessly between the leadership and followership roles, using experience gained as a follower to enhance their leadership skills (Rowland et al., 2021). Northouse (2019) claims that the degree to which followers have the competence and commitment necessary to accomplish a given task or activity is their developmental level. This implies ongoing learning through continuing professional development.

Reflection: points to consider

Think of examples where you have been a leader, a follower or a mentor. Which skills are required for each?

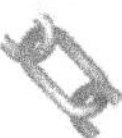

Chapter 20 for more information about practice-based learning and **Chapter 21** for more on continuing professional development.

Emotional intelligence (EI) is a key skill necessary for leadership. It involves having an awareness and understanding of the impact of one's actions on the emotions of others (Goleman, 1998). EI starts with self-awareness: the knowledge of one's own thoughts, feelings and motivations. Having the ability to objectively understand one's own emotional and behavioural reactions helps to recognise the effect that those reactions have on others, thus mitigating undesired effects. Emotional awareness then goes further in that it is the ability to pick up on others' reactions and analyse why they reacted in the way they did. Paramedic practice entails being in unpredictable situations, so developing the EI skill of self-regulation will facilitate the regulation of emotions in a variety of environments. Paramedics developing their leadership skills will also develop EI skills, self-management, motivation, social awareness and empathy to appreciate others' perspectives. These are key to becoming emotionally intelligent practitioners. Moreover, paramedics with high EI are more likely to stay calm under pressure, have more developed social skills and be able to resolve conflict quickly. According to Goleman (1998), the most effective leaders possess EI. Furthermore, he asserts that regardless of all other variables in leadership abilities, a leader will never be great without EI.

The psychology of EI is reflected within the *Standards of Proficiency for Paramedics* (HCPC, 2023), since paramedics are required to understand their own strengths and limitations, and to recognise their emotions and how they impact on others, including the impact of their own personal beliefs as biases. Paramedics are required to use self-awareness together with integrated skills to manage clinical challenges, to develop strategies for self-care and self-awareness, and to make a self-referral if necessary. Constructive reflection and feedback on professional practice provides opportunities to reconsider positive and negative experiences in a critical way.

Reflection: points to consider

Have you been in a situation where emotional leadership has been used? How can you ensure that you incorporate it into your leadership style?

Standards of leadership impact on patient care as well as relationships with colleagues, multi-agency partners and within organisational frameworks.

Leadership in the NHS

The history of clinical leadership in the NHS can be understood by following the evolution of leadership theory, already identified in this chapter. Snow and Benson (2023) identify four phases of health leadership: the pre-1940s, the 1940s to 1970s, the 1980s to 1990s and the 2000s to the present day. The evolution of healthcare leadership reflects a shift in understanding of leadership from being about the individual to being about individuals within teams. Early clinical leadership frameworks in the NHS focused on doctors; these were then widened to relate to all clinical staff via the NHS Leadership Academy, which sought to develop leadership behaviours among wider groups of individuals within large organisations rather than leave leadership matters to nominated or named persons. The Healthcare Leadership Model (NHS Leadership Academy, 2024) relates easily to those who identify themselves as working in teams and explicitly links leadership development with positive outcomes for both staff and patients. There are nine dimensions to the model designed to help individuals identify their own personal leadership qualities:

- inspiring shared purpose;
- leading with care;
- evaluating information;
- connecting our service;
- sharing the vision;
- engaging the team;
- holding to account;
- developing capability;
- influencing for results.

Leadership qualities can be summed up as inspiring, engaging, sharing, developing, influencing, collaborating, caring, evaluation and accountability. The Healthcare Leadership Model is one of a package of resources available nationally through the NHS Leadership Academy. All clinical staff, including paramedics, can access the Edward Jenner programme, taking budding leaders through their first steps on their leadership journey. A series of programmes follow, for clinicians through to senior leadership. The next section looks at paramedic leadership within a multi-professional context.

PARAMEDIC LEADERSHIP WITHIN A MULTI-PROFESSIONAL CONTEXT

Inter-professional collaboration involves two or more health professionals from various disciplines working together towards a common goal in which they understand and respect one another's roles (Hsiao et al., 2022). Despite being taught within specific unitary education programmes to the point of registration, paramedics, like other health professionals, will work in collaboration with and alongside other health professions during their careers. Multi-professional work requires all professionals to have a flexible approach in their attitudes and behaviours to value and respect the distinct contribution each profession makes. Via their collaboration with other health professionals, paramedics can grow their knowledge and abilities through discussion and feedback (Andersson et al., 2019). Furthermore, each inter-professional opportunity strengthens relationships between professions, builds personal relationships, improves learning and job satisfaction, and provides better patient care (Carney et al., 2019). In one study, as professional respect for colleagues increased, the willingness to exchange skills and knowledge also increased (Mulholland et al., 2019). Collaborative inter-professional working accommodates patients' needs when they extend beyond the limitations of the smaller paramedic team. This is how leadership demonstrated through collaborative inter-professional working enhances patient care.

Case study 17.2

Anne is a 65-year-old patient experiencing an acute episode of chronic obstructive pulmonary disease (COPD). She is tachypnoeic with shortness of breath and a wheeze on auscultation. Anne usually manages her condition well and has an emergency pack for such episodes but has not had it replaced since her last attack six months ago. Anne is reluctant to attend hospital.

The paramedic conducts a full assessment and begins to reverse the acute episode with medication. She then contacts Anne's respiratory nurse to discuss the episode and together with Anne they make a plan. The paramedic contacts Anne's GP to report the episode, share the plan and arrange a replacement emergency pack, which is available for collection at the local pharmacy. Anne's respiratory nurse calls back and brings forward her next home assessment.

In case study 17.2, the paramedic not only assesses and manages the presenting medical emergency but goes on to demonstrate leadership within a multi-professional context through her liaison with other stakeholders involved in the care of the patient. A shared decision is reached between the paramedic and the patient, thus empowering the patient. Key players in the successful patient interaction are the GP, the respiratory nurse and the pharmacist. There is recognition on the paramedic's part that appropriate, compassionate and patient-centred care cannot be met through intervention by a single profession.

Case study 17.3

Peter is a 59-year-old cardiac patient experiencing abdominal discomfort. After calling 999 for help, he is assessed by a paramedic who discovers that Peter is prescribed more than five different types of medication in tablet form to be taken per day. Peter collects his prescription boxes every two weeks from the pharmacy, returns home and then transfers all the tablets into one large jar. Each day he shakes a few out into the palm of his hand and swallows them with water. The paramedic ascertains that while Peter is able-bodied and self-caring, he has no idea what quantity of any drug he is taking each day but that he believes he is compliant with his medication regime. Peter agrees to be seen by a doctor that day but also requires better medicine management.

En route to hospital, the ambulance stops at Peter's local pharmacy and, with Peter's consent, the paramedic requests a blister pack for future dispensation of medications. The paramedic then communicates this decision to Peter's GP by telephone, while on the way to the hospital.

In case study 17.3, the paramedic demonstrates leadership skills by using joint decision-making to seek a more effective use of the existing services provided to the patient. He uses problem-solving, decision-making and communication skills, and cooperates with the patient and other stakeholders to improve quality of care.

CONCLUSION

It can be challenging for paramedics to recognise and develop their leadership potential, yet they must do so. Leadership skills take time to develop and require emerging leaders to be true to their values if they are to provide authentic leadership. It is useful to understand different styles of leadership and to be able to adapt to different styles when appropriate. Achieving great outcomes for patients through excellent leadership can be a transformative experience for those involved in the team. Appreciation gained for other health professionals through multi-professional working can build knowledge, relationships and even future careers. Leadership skills can be learned by everyone, and leadership is the responsibility of everyone within health and care organisations.

> **Chapter key points:**
> - Paramedics lead daily and have the potential to develop leadership skills.
> - Leadership skills can be learned by everyone to enhance relationships and improve patient care.

- Understanding leadership styles facilitates a greater understanding of decision-making.
- The NHS Leadership Academy has programmes for developing the leadership of all staff at all levels.

REFERENCES AND SUGGESTED READING

Adair, J. (2020) *The Best of John Adair on Leadership*, 2nd edition. London: Thorogood Publishing.

Andersson, U., Söderholm, H.M., Sundström, B.W., Hagiwara, M.A. et al. (2019) Clinical reasoning in the emergency medical services: an integrative review, *Scandinavian Journal of Trauma, Resuscitation and Emergency Medicine*, 27: 76. Available at: https://doi.org/10.1186/s13049-019-0646-y.

Barr, J. and Dowding, L. (2022) *Leadership in Health Care*, 5th edition. London: Sage.

Carney, P.A., Thayer, E.R., Palmer, R., Galper, A.B. et al. (2019) The benefits of interprofessional and teamwork in primary care ambulatory training settings, *Journal of Interprofessional Education and Practice*, 15: 119–26.

Collen, A. (2019) *Decision Making in Paramedic Practice*. Bridgewater: Class Professional Publishing.

Csikszentmihalyi, M. (1975) *Beyond Boredom and Anxiety*. San Francisco, CA: Jossey-Bass.

Dalrymple, R. (2019) Leadership and mentorship in paramedic practice, in S. Willis and R. Dalrymple (eds.) *Fundamentals of Paramedic Practice: A Systematic Approach*, 2nd edition. Oxford: Wiley-Blackwell.

Deng, C., Gulseren, D., Isola, C., Grocutt, K. et al. (2023) Transformational leadership effectiveness: an evidence-based primer, *Human Resource Development International*, 26 (5): 626–41.

Department of Health (DH) (2005) *Taking healthcare to the patient: Transforming NHS Ambulance Services.* Available at: https://ircp.info/Portals/11/Future/NHS%20EMS%20Policy%20Recommendation2005.pdf.

Giltinane, C.L. (2013) Leadership styles and theories, *Nursing Standard*, 270 (41): 35–39.

Goleman, D. (1998) The emotionally competent leader, *Healthcare Forum Journal*, 41 (2): 36–43.

Grootjen, M., Neerincx, M.A. and Veltman, J.A. (2006) Cognitive task load in a naval ship control centre: from identification to prediction, *Ergonomics*, 49 (12/13): 1238–64.

Health and Care Professions Council (HCPC) (2023) *Standards of Proficiency for Paramedics.* Available at: https://www.hcpc-uk.org/standards/standards-of-proficiency/paramedics/.

Health and Care Professions Council (HCPC) (2024) *Standards of Conduct, Performance and Ethics.* Available at: https://www.hcpc-uk.org/standards/standards-of-conduct-performance-and-ethics/.

Hsiao, C.-Y., Wu, J.-C., Lin, P.-C., Yang, P.-Y. et al. (2022) Effectiveness of interprofessional shared decision-making training: a mixed-method study, *Patient Education and Counselling*, 105 (11): 3287–97.

Kelly, L. (2023) *Mindfulness for Authentic Leadership: Theory and Cases.* Cham: Springer Nature.

Mulholland, P., Barnett, T. and Woodroffe, J. (2019) A grounded theory of interprofessional learning and paramedic care, *Journal of Interprofessional Care*, 34 (1): 65–75.

NHS England (2023) *NHS long term workforce plan.* Available at: https://www.england.nhs.uk/publication/nhs-long-term-workforce-plan/ (accessed 6 April 2024).

NHS Leadership Academy (2024) *Healthcare Leadership Model.* Available at: https://www.leadershipacademy.nhs.uk/healthcare-leadership-model/ (accessed 6 April 2024).

Northouse, P. (2019) *Leadership Theory and Practice*, 8th edition. London: Sage.

Northway, R. (2021) Context and the case for reconceptualising leadership in healthcare, in E. Curtis, M. Beirne, J.G. Cullen, R. Northway and S.M. Corrigan (eds.) *Distributed Leadership in Nursing and Healthcare: Theory, Evidence and Development.* London. Open University Press.

Rowland, M., Adefuye, A.O. and Vincent-Lambert, C. (2021) The need for purposeful teaching, learning and assessment of crisis resource management principles and practices in the undergraduate pre-hospital emergency care curriculum: a narrative literature review, *Australasian Journal of Paramedicine*, 18: 820. Available at: https://doi.org/10.33151/ajp.18.820.

Snow, S. and Benson, L. (2023) A brief history of healthcare leadership, in N. Chambers (ed.) *Research Handbook on Leadership in Healthcare.* Cheltenham: Edward Elgar.

Staal, M.A. (2004) *Stress, cognition, and human performance: A literature review and conceptual framework*, NASA/TM-2004-212824. Available at: https://core.ac.uk/download/pdf/10517392.pdf.

18   From instinct to protocol:
mastering paramedic decision-making
Liam Hamilton

In this chapter:

- Introduction and why this subject is relevant
- The changing landscape
- Foundations of paramedic decision-making
- Decision-making frameworks in paramedicine
- Decision-making models
- The value of experience
- Critical thinking
- Barriers to decision-making in paramedicine
- Conclusion
- Chapter key points
- References and suggested reading

INTRODUCTION AND WHY THIS SUBJECT IS RELEVANT

As an ambulance clinician, the decisions you make determine patient outcomes. You will treat hundreds, if not thousands, of patients throughout your career, without knowing which one you may be judged on, which is why it is important to make the right decision while navigating this landscape of uncertainty. This chapter delves into the intricate web of decision-making in paramedicine, exploring the fine balance between rapid assessments, critical thinking and the application of protocols in the face of uncertainty. From the pulse-pounding scenarios of practice to the structured frameworks guiding your actions, discover the art and science behind the pivotal decisions that define paramedic practice.

THE CHANGING LANDSCAPE

Over the last decade, the role of the paramedic has evolved from a largely protocol-driven practice to an autonomous practitioner with a broader scope of practice and greater responsibility. This transition blurred the lines as to how paramedics felt they were allowed to make decisions. In 2020, the COVID-19 pandemic fundamentally altered the landscape of paramedic decision-making, infusing each response with heightened precautions and considerations. Paramedics, once focused on a patient-centred approach, were confronted with a multifaceted challenge: navigating emergencies while assessing the risk of infectious exposure. The ever-changing, dynamic and meticulous personal protective equipment (PPE) protocols altered approaches to patient assessment, treatment and transport. Decisions became not only about clinical urgency but also about minimising potential transmission. COVID-19 prompted a paradigm shift, forcing the paramedic to make decisions in the absence of protocols and experience to protect both patients and providers amidst an unprecedented global health crisis. The fallout of the pandemic still resonates throughout the paramedic profession.

FOUNDATIONS OF PARAMEDIC DECISION-MAKING

Decision-making in paramedicine begins the moment you are assigned a call. What could be wrong with this patient? What kit should I take in? Krockow (2018) suggests that we could make up to 2,000 decisions an hour, so how many decisions could you make in the time spent with your patient and how do you make the decisions that could have a direct impact on the long-term outcome of your patient?

Paramedicine is unique in many ways. We tend to spend more time with our patients than most other healthcare professionals; we are commonly the first point of contact in their medical journey; and the environment in which we work largely dictates our decisions. These add another layer of complexity to the decisions you must make.

DECISION-MAKING FRAMEWORKS IN PARAMEDICINE

Decision-making frameworks offer a structured approach that bolsters the decision-making process in various ways. Their foremost strength lies in providing a systematic method for evaluating options, and enabling a comprehensive assessment of potential outcomes and risks associated with each choice. These frameworks also encourage a holistic consideration of factors, ensuring a more informed decision by incorporating diverse perspectives and relevant data. Moreover, they streamline complex decisions by breaking them down into manageable steps, enhancing clarity and reducing the chances of oversight or hasty judgements. Additionally, decision-making frameworks facilitate consistency, allowing individuals or teams to replicate successful decision-making processes in similar scenarios, promoting efficiency and reliability in decision-making across different contexts.

Decision-making and problem-solving are closely related but distinct processes. Decision-making involves selecting a course of action from several alternatives, focusing on choosing the best option based on available information and preferences; problem-solving, in contrast, is about identifying, analysing and resolving an issue or challenge. The latter encompasses understanding the root cause of a problem and devising strategies to address it effectively. While decision-making culminates in choosing one solution from multiple options, problem-solving involves a deeper investigation into the nature of the issue before determining the best course of action. Essentially, decision-making is about making a choice, while problem-solving is about finding solutions to specific challenges or obstacles.

In practice, however, it is sometimes difficult to separate the two, as our environment frequently presents us with problems that affect our decision-making. For example, the paramedic dealing with a violent patient may choose not to solve the root cause of the violent conduct, such as personality trait, or alcohol or drug intoxication or dependence. As an alternative, they may choose to utilise only decision-making skills to call for police assistance to facilitate removal of the patient to police custody. The paramedic has, therefore, made the decision to remove the problem (i.e. the violent patient) rather than examine the cause of the patient's behaviour and address that. This is not opting out of the situation; rather, it is identifying the resources available and utilising them to best advantage. Muoni (2012) advocates that before making any decision, one should evaluate all the information available about the problem, ensuring that informed decision-making becomes the norm.

Reflection: points to consider

Where could you look to find information that informs our decisions, particularly if the patient is unconscious or unable to communicate? How could you do this in a time-critical situation? What information would you prioritise?

What can help us make decisions?

Decisions can be classified into three types: routine, adaptive and innovative. Table 18.1 uses the example of a single patient to show how their circumstances can be categorised based on the three types. As the classification intensifies based on circumstance, the further the decision made moves away from procedure and towards experience.

Table 18.1 Classifications of decisions

Type	Description	Method	Example
Routine	Well-defined problems that are commonly seen in practice	Grounded in familiar policies and procedures, guiding a practitioner through a process, in order to make their decision	A patient has a potential C-spine fracture, so cannot move. Clinical Practice Guidelines would guide the practitioner through appropriate immobilisation and moving and handling
Adaptive	Decisions and solutions are less common and require a degree of adaptation as guidance is only partly applicable	Using some common sense and initiative to enable you to use the guidance	The position your patient is in means you are unable to immobilise your patient at first, so will have to overcome the problem by moving your patient into a more suitable position before being able to continue to immobilise
Innovative	Unusual and unclear problems that were previously unprecedented	Using experience, tools and resources you have at your disposal to come to your decision in the absence of policy or guidelines	Your patient is unable to lay flat due to injuries or pre-existing conditions, so you allow the patient to get into a position that is safe and comfortable but use blankets and padding to reduce unnecessary movements

DECISION-MAKING MODELS

There is no shortage of proposed decision-making models, the majority of which follow a very similar structure and contain the following elements:

- determine the goal;
- gather data carefully;
- generate many alternatives;
- think logically;
- choose and act decisively.

Box 18.1 details a model that is commonly applied in the healthcare arena (Marquis and Huston, 2012; Huston, 2023).

Box 18.1 Traditional problem-solving model

1. Problem identified
2. Data on causes and consequences gathered and analysed
3. Possible alternatives explored
4. Alternatives then evaluated
5. Solution then chosen to suit the situation (steps)
6. Solution then implemented
7. Results then evaluated and reflection occurs

Source: Marquis and Huston (2012).

With the traditional problem-solving model, the decision-making process does not begin until step 5 (Marquis and Huston, 2012; Huston, 2023). Although this could be construed as a weakness, it is important not to minimise the importance of examining the problem in full, in order to collect the maximum amount of information to enable informed decision-making. Furthermore, it could be said that the amount of time needed for proper implementation and the lack of initial objective setting does not always lend itself to use in a real-world setting. This model would be suited to a patient who is medically stable but has a complex social situation that requires safety-netting. It may take the paramedic some time to fully explore the options available to the patient, involving them or the family in the decision and making phone calls to engage community services if required.

Due to the variety of patient presentations and situations the paramedic may find themselves in, it is common for a different decision-making model to be utilised in order to come to a conclusion. Other decision-making models and their features are described below, together with examples of paramedic practice in which each might be the most appropriate model to use.

A model of decision-making supported by Ryan and Halliwell (2012) is the hypothetico-deductive model. This involves the paramedic assessing the impact of the information collected on the situation and then ruling in, or ruling out, bits of information as necessary to make an informed decision. An example of this is an oxygen saturation probe providing a significantly low reading in a patient who is not struggling for breath, does not appear cyanosed, does not have any pre-existing medical conditions and called 999 because they fractured their wrist.

Ryan and Halliwell (2012) assert that when making an informed decision, there are three important areas of reasoning:

1. The paramedic will make a *conscious* decision to rule in, or rule out, information by actively considering its significance.
2. The paramedic will understand the *evidence* that supports the decision and so follows best practice.
3. The paramedic will understand that their practice has to *stand up to the scrutiny* of the relevant stakeholder, patients, peers and the HCPC.

In the above example, the paramedic may consciously decide to withhold administering oxygen, despite an indication to do so, because the information collected does not fit the presentation of the patient or any other findings. However, the paramedic would have to justify their decision if it was questioned.

Ryan and Halliwell (2012) recognise the many attributes of intuitive decision-making and the hypothetico-deductive model. However, when they conducted a comparison of paramedics who followed an Institute of Health Care Development (IHCD) paramedic route and those who followed a university route, they found significant differences. They reported that those who followed the IHCD route were very confident in using intuitive mechanisms, whereas graduates had more confidence in following a template and relying on it, due to their lack of experience and confidence. These findings can also be applied to non-qualified colleagues who may have significantly more experience than direct-entry paramedics.

In order to overcome this, Ryan and Halliwell (2012) recommend a combined approach, using a model of decision-making while also incorporating the observational experience of the paramedic. This will ensure that they use all of the resources available to them. In the past few years, the introduction of the Newly Qualified Paramedic (NQP) pathway adopted by the Ambulance Service ensures NQPs work with a colleague with a certain amount of experience for a defined period when they qualify, to extend their exposure to the experience and intuition of senior colleagues.

Reflection: points to consider

What enables you to make decisions? Think of an example where you may not have agreed with policy and procedures. What difference could it have made to a patient outcome?

An old but personal favourite of mine is the Vroom-Yetton decision-making model (Vroom and Yetton, 1973). Frequently described as the most complex of the models with its basis in business leadership decision-making, it is particularly useful when working collaboratively as part of a team. It would be fair to say that some of the more time-critical or logistically complex patients find themselves in the hands of multiple clinicians or agencies with varying degrees of seniority. The model works as a flexible 'yes/no' decision-making tree, and takes into consideration time constraints and facilitates rationality in chaos.

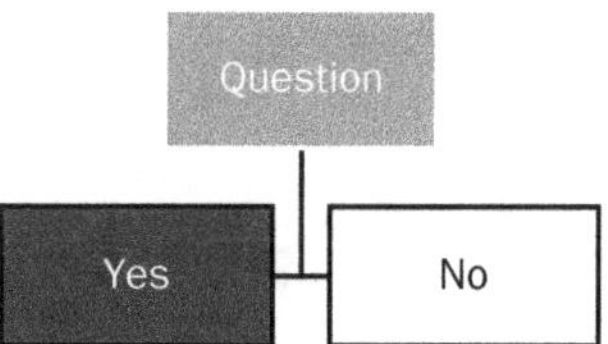

Figure 18.1   Visual representation of the Vroom-Yetton decision-making model (1973)

Case study 18.1

A good example of this model being used was reported by a facilitator during a student paramedic simulation of a chaotic road traffic collision (RTC) in which a child was hit by a car. The child was in an awkward position, to the extent the child could not be treated in the manner intended. The student paramedic knew what was needed, as they had previously discussed it, but were struggling to work out how. This student verbalised their decision-making to the group in the following way:

Paramedic: *Can we treat the child?*
Colleagues: *No.*
Paramedic: *So we need to either move the child or the car. Can we move the car?*
Colleagues: *No.*
Paramedic: *So we need to move the child?*
Colleagues: *Yes.*

This exchange instantly brought clarity and rational thought to a situation that was designed to reduce the bandwidth of a group of students with minimal exposure to practice. It also is an example of an adaptive form of decision-making, in that the students wanted to follow their protocols as they had been taught, as supported by Ryan and Halliwell (2012), but had to adapt before following their guidelines.

Decision-making is a complex cognitive process that is often described as 'choosing a particular course of action', implying that there are several courses of action that could be followed and that a considered judgement is required to decide which route to follow. Inherent within decision-making is the concept of 'critical thinking', defined as purposeful, goal-orientated thinking that is based on a body of knowledge derived from research and other sources of authenticated evidence (Ignatavicius, 2001). It is more complex than problem-solving and decision-making because it involves a higher level of reasoning and deductive thinking.

CRITICAL THINKING

Decision-making is heavily reliant on critical thinking skills. Heidari and Shahbazi (2016) maintain that to make competent decisions and maintain professional competence, critical thinking is key. Furthermore, they develop this concept and recommend that the best setting for teaching these higher-order skills is the clinical setting, in which authenticity and patient-centredness can be fostered. They argue that case-based lectures do not allow the learner to develop these skills due to the physical separation between student and teacher and the passive nature of learning in such a setting. As clinical education in higher education institutions continues to develop, the emergence of simulation as a learning tool lends itself perfectly to the student's ability to develop these critical thinking skills before qualifying, better preparing themselves for the role.

Sullivan and Garland (2013) describe critical thinking as the process of probing underlying assumptions, interpreting and evaluating arguments, imagining and exploring alternatives, and developing a sense of reflective criticism. This is in line with Marquis and Huston (2020), who affirm that critical thinking is related to evaluation, which is broader than decision-making and requires the skills of conceptualisation, analysis, synthesis and evaluation of information. It also supports Ryan and Halliwell (2012), who describe the conscious inclusion or exclusion of information based on the overall clinical picture. Box 18.2 lists six critical thinking skills reported by Ignatavicius (2001).

Box 18.2 Six critical thinking skills

- *Interpretation* – clarifying data
- *Analysis* – understanding data
- *Evaluation* – determining outcome
- *Inference* – drawing conclusions
- *Explanation* – justifying actions based on data
- *Self-regulation* – examining one's own practice

Source: Ignatavicius (2001).

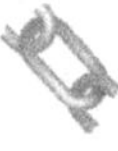 **Chapter 2** for more about reflection and thinking critically.

There are certain qualities that successful decision-makers possess. They need to be willing to take a risk, and have the sensitivity to react both to the situation and to the other members involved in the decision-making process, the energy to make things happen, and the creativity to develop new ways to solve problems. Such people have a lot of balls to juggle, as shown in Figure 18.2, but they possess a repertoire of skills that they can call on to assist them in the decision-making process.

Paramedics regularly work in stressful conditions, managing complex and dynamic cases in a time-critical manner. Moilanen (2015) proposes that in order to meet this challenge, paramedics require highly developed critical thinking skills in order to operate in the midst of chaos and make informed decisions in the moment.

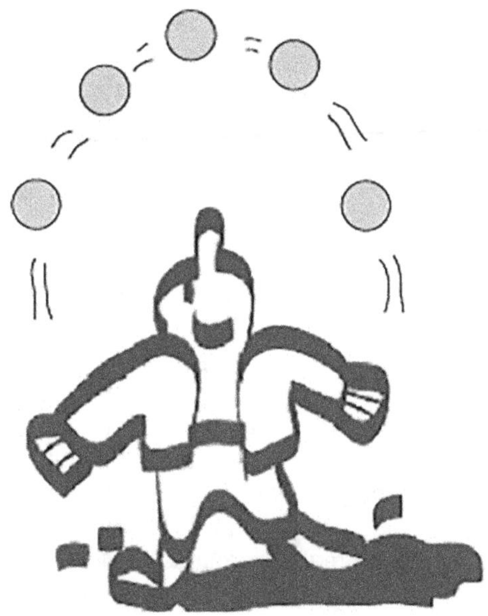

Figure 18.2 Characteristics of a critical thinker

Source: Marquis and Huston (2012).

 **Reflection: points to consider**

Do you possess any of the traits of a critical thinker? How might your personality traits make your working life more frustrating, if you feel constrained by your organization's policies/procedures?

THE VALUE OF EXPERIENCE

Within the process of decision-making, we use our life experiences to guide the way in which we act. Although dated, Cioffi (1997) remains the torch-bearer of this concept and defines it as intuitive knowing associated with past personal experiences, which she refers to as heuristics in her work. The more mature a person is, the greater the range of alternatives that they will be able to draw on. This is not 'maturity' in the traditional sense of age but of time spent in one's chosen career. Knowing the effects of past experiences and outcomes helps us to make decisions and guide our thinking. This is supported by Lyneham et al. (2008), who highlight the concept of intuition in their work. Furthermore, they claim that an expert will make decisions faster and with greater accuracy than an individual at any other stage of professional development. This could be attributed to the tacit knowledge that we all have, but is rarely acknowledged. Banning (2008) cites Benner (1984) when describing how the inexperienced practitioner will use procedures and guidelines to make decisions but as they become more experienced, decision-making becomes intuitive, drawing on past experiences to inform future actions.

Timmons (2009) compared the outcomes of decisions made by first responders and those of team-based decisions. He found that first responders tended to use heuristics in their decision-making process due to the need to make rapid decisions. Timmons deemed that people tend to favour this form of decision-making in high-pressure, unfamiliar circumstances as it requires less of a cognitive process to reach a decision, which ultimately reduces the amount of time it takes to begin treating a patient.

Looking further into heuristics as a decision-making process, while the benefit of quick decision-making allows treatment to get underway more quickly – something that is imperative in time-critical contexts – Tversky and Kahneman (1974) warned of the cognitive biases and predictable errors that could occur as a result of this form of decision-making. While this evidence is significantly outdated, it is considered pioneering and more recent studies have also looked into heuristics as a decision-making process to evaluate impact on performance and outcome, but the conclusions have largely been inconclusive in that the evidence is not robust enough yet and more work needs to be done.

In the context of paramedicine, while the concept of heuristics may be considered risky and affected by potential bias due to the lack of a framework, it is highly successful among solo responders, who do not have the luxury of utilising a more thorough, structured group decision-making tool such as the Vroom-Yetton model. It should further be acknowledged that it would be commonplace for a solo responder to be joined by colleagues at some point, thus allowing a different decision-making process to occur, thus neutralising some of the flaws inherent in heuristics. With this in mind, practitioners should not be afraid to use heuristics as an initial form of decision-making.

Whelehan et al. (2020) concluded that, on average, decisions made heuristically have more positive outcomes than negative ones; however, a lot of other factors come into play (e.g. experience, personality and situation), which can lead to a negative outcome. There is a suggestion that reflective practice may encourage the proper use of heuristics to improve positive outcomes and reduce negative outcomes.

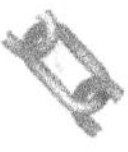

Chapter 2 for more on reflective practice.

There are some, however, who do not re-examine decisions that they have made and therefore do not learn from their experiences. It is always advisable to remember that we do not learn by doing, rather we learn by doing and then reviewing. Cioffi (1997) stated that intuitive, heuristic judgements are qualitative, critical, discriminating and associated with past experiences, and she identified six key aspects of heuristic decision-making, maintaining that they can be used as a part of complex decision-making (see Box 18.3).

Box 18.3 Heuristic decision-making

- *Pattern recognition* – recognition of patterns of responses presented by patients
- *Similarity recognition* – comparison of similar and dissimilar characteristics of past patients who have had similar conditions
- *Common-sense understanding* – understanding diversity from a selection of information, i.e. vital signs that give subtle trends/indications about a patient
- *Skilled knowhow* – that considers possibilities for each patient
- *Sense of salience* – perceptions about a patient that stand out as more important
- *Deliberative rationality* – selective attention of certain aspects/events

Source: Cioffi (1997: 205).

Reflection: points to consider

Have you ever been in a situation where you have felt pressured to conform to cultural norms. What could you do in future to manage this?

BARRIERS TO DECISION-MAKING

With any decision, there are individual variations that may affect the outcome. Any choices generated and made are affected by personal values and bias. These are moral and ethical codes socialised within us as part of our culture, exposure and experience. These include those instilled in us as children or those values that we have acquired through our workplace culture and customs.

When reviewing any decision, it is important not only to examine the component parts of the decision but also to look at the external factors that have influenced it. The impact of factors such as evidence-based practice, working culture and bias on decision-making cannot be underestimated.

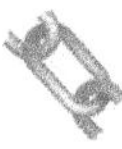

Chapter 5 for more theory on evidence-based practice.

Evidence-based practice (EBP) should be the cornerstone of contemporary clinical practice (AbuRuz et al., 2017). We no longer do things because we have always done them in a certain way but because the evidence demonstrates that the approach recommended works and has been proven to be beneficial through rigorous scientific testing and research; however, this is not always the case.

One of the reasons for this reluctance may lie in the theory of change management. Cork (2012) cogently argues that change is inevitable in any organisation, especially those following an EBP agenda. Practitioners who understand change are more likely to embrace, influence and accept it. However, in order to embrace change, we have to accept that what we are doing can be improved, and some paramedics will find this an uncomfortable position to be in. Nevertheless, it is unavoidable and in order to make decisions that are based on contemporary evidence, we need to ensure that the culture within which we work is conducive to change (Cork, 2012).

The *Oxford English Dictionary* (2023) defines culture as 'the ideas, customs and social behaviour of a particular people or society'. The ambulance service itself is a society with leaders, followers, rules and regulations, and based on legal frameworks, evidence-based practice, tradition, cultural norms and social influences.

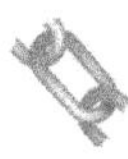

Chapter 9 for more on sociological theory.

Schöbel et al. (2016) conducted a study to explore social influences in sequential decision-making. They claim that individuals will often follow the behaviour of others and ignore their own opinions, even if the behaviour of others is misinformed. Parallels can be drawn in the paramedic world. As part of a team and working closely alongside crew members, individual practitioners, particularly newly qualified paramedics, are exposed to external opinions and pressures to conform to what is seen as the *cultural norm*. To step outside this can sometimes place the individual in an awkward position. However, in order to ensure that decisions reflect current clinical excellence, it is sometimes necessary.

A controversial but common example of this is driving to emergency calls without audible and visual warnings (lights and sirens). It was previously mandatory to respond to all emergency calls with visual and audible warnings. However, it has now emerged that a practitioner may deduce that the call does not require an emergency response, so will drive to scene under routine conditions. Policies and procedures differ and have changed over the years to allow clinicians more flexibility in deciding whether to use audible or visual warnings, but they must be able to justify their decision. It is largely for the driver of the vehicle to decide, based on road conditions and safety, as opposed to the needs of the patient. New members of staff often find themselves pressured by a colleague, not to use audible or visual warnings based on their assessment of the patient's details. This example perfectly demonstrates the 'authority influence hypothesis' (Schöbel et al., 2016: 5). This hypothesis predicts that an individual's position within the hierarchy of the organisation will influence their behaviour. Schöbel et al. (2016) state that the individual will often ignore their own opinions in favour of the opinions of senior colleagues, even when those senior colleagues are imparting inaccurate information.

Finally, individual biases must be acknowledged to ensure that decision-making is based on altruistic principles. Biases are a product of all of our experiences, learned either explicitly or implicitly in cultural contexts. These are often unconscious and not immediately apparent to us. Sporek (2015) states that although we may consider our decisions are based on facts, they are frequently influenced by hidden feelings and thoughts that we are not apparently aware of. An example could be attending a frequent caller who usually complains of chest pain, but on this occasion, complains of abdominal pain and the paramedic dismisses their symptoms due to previous experiences. This is supported by Marquis and Huston (2020), who maintain that value judgements will always be part of any decision, no matter how objective the criteria. Furthermore, they propose that the alternatives generated and the final choices are limited by the individual's value system. Stone and Moskowitz (2011) propose that in order to decrease the unintentional acts of discrimination, bias education should be a part of all healthcare programmes.

The implications of decision-making in line with cultural norms, rather than the evidence which supports it, is immense. As a registrant, the HCPC requires you to use your judgement to make informed and reasonable decisions and meet the HCPC Standards. In addition, they mandate that you must always be prepared to justify your decisions and actions (HCPC, 2024). You are also accountable, first and foremost, to your patients and they have the right to pursue this through the civil and criminal courts. All practitioners must be prepared to justify the decisions they make to an expert audience, if called upon to do so.

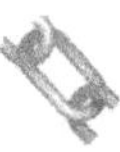

Chapter 4 for more on legal and ethical issues.

The high-stakes nature of the job, coupled with time constraints and unpredictable environments, creates several other hurdles that can impede decision-making ability. One significant barrier is the pressure of time. Paramedics often operate in time-critical situations where split-second decisions can have profound consequences. This time pressure can lead to stress and a narrowing of bandwidth, affecting a paramedic's ability to carefully weigh options and make the most appropriate decision. The urgency to act swiftly, especially in life-threatening situations, can sometimes overshadow a more thorough evaluation of available choices.

Furthermore, the lack of complete information poses a considerable challenge. In many emergencies, paramedics must make decisions based on limited or rapidly changing information. This uncertainty can hinder their ability to accurately assess the situation and choose the most suitable course of action. Factors such as not being able to access a patient's medical history, unclear patient presentation and chaos at the scene of an accident can obscure crucial details that would help inform decision-making. However, this shouldn't mean a decision can't be made, just that a decision must be made with the limited information at one's disposal. The heuristics decision model and Vroom-Yetton model might be useful in overcoming this problem.

Another significant barrier is the emotional and psychological toll of the job. Paramedics frequently encounter distressing scenes and traumatic events, which can impact their mental state. Emotional stress and fatigue from dealing with intense situations and night shifts may cloud their judgement or affect the decision-making process. Ganesan et al. (2019) found that alertness and performance were affected the most on consecutive night shifts, especially at the end of the last night shift, resulting in poorer outcomes.

Resource limitations present a practical challenge for paramedics. In some cases, insufficient or inadequate equipment, limited access to specialised care facilities or a shortage of personnel will limit the available options. These resource limitations can force paramedics into making decisions that may not align with the ideal standards of care or procedures. While the decision-making model in this context is situational-dependent, by classifying this type of decision as adaptive or innovative, it should facilitate a decision still being made as it acknowledges it is outside of the ideal situation.

Ethical dilemmas also pose significant barriers to paramedics' decision-making. Balancing the need to provide immediate care with respect for patient autonomy and ethical principles can present complex challenges. Decisions regarding consent, end-of-life care or situations involving moral or legal considerations can create dilemmas that hinder the decision-making process.

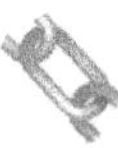

Chapter 1 to explore the value of communication and barriers to effective communication, and **Chapter 6** for further explanation of Human Factors affecting paramedic practice.

CONCLUSION

This chapter has introduced a range of decision-making models and highlighted the classifications each decision can take. It has highlighted the way paramedic decision-making has changed, and brought the 'grey areas' of paramedic practice to the forefront, to acknowledge that not every event you are called to will fit the narrative of a policy or procedure. It has shown how decision-making models can be used interchangeably, but may be more or less effective depending on the situation you find yourself in, but also act as a framework to help support you in justifying your decision when facing scrutiny.

Chapter key points:

- Understanding the component parts of the decision-making process enables a higher level of reflection.
- Every decision, whether made at an organisational, local or personal level, has consequences that should be considered before the decision is made.

REFERENCES AND SUGGESTED READING

AbuRuz, M.E., Hayeah, H.A., Al-Dweik, G. and Al-Akash, H.Y. (2017) Attitudes and practice about evidence-based practice: a Jordanian study, *Health Science Journal*, 11 (1): 485.

Association of Ambulance Chief Executives (AACE) (2016) *Annual report 2015–2016*. Available at: https://aace.org.uk/aace-annual-reports/.

Banning, M. (2008) A review of clinical decision making: models and current research, *Journal of Clinical Nursing*, 17 (2): 187–95.

Benner, P. (1984) *From Novice to Expert: Excellence and Power in Clinical Nursing Practice*. Menlo Park, CA: Addison-Wesley.

Chew, B. (2014) Exploring factors influencing the development and implementation of evidence-based healthcare practice in emergency care setting, *Singapore Nursing Journal*, 41 (2): 29–34.

Cioffi, J. (1997) Heuristics, servants to intuition, in clinical decision-making, *Journal of Advanced Nursing*, 26 (1): 203–8.

Cork, A. (2012) Change management theory and its usefulness to practice, in A.Y. Blaber (ed.) *Foundations for Paramedic Practice*, 2nd edition. Maidenhead: Open University Press.

Ganesan, S., Magee, M., Stone, J.E., Mulhall, M.D. et al. (2019) The impact of shift work on sleep, alertness and performance in healthcare workers, *Scientific Reports*, 9 (1): 4635. Available at: https://doi.org/10.1038/s41598-019-40914-x.

Health and Care Professions Council (HCPC) (2024) *Standards of Conduct, Performance and Ethics*. Available at: https://www.hcpc-uk.org/standards/standards-of-conduct-performance-and-ethics/.

Heidari, M. and Shahbazi, S. (2016) Effect of training problem-solving skill on decision-making and critical thinking of personnel at medical emergencies, *International Journal of Critical Illness and Injury Science*, 6 (4): 182–87.

Huston, C.J. (2023) *Leadership Roles and Management Functions in Nursing: Theory and Application*, 11th edition. Philadelphia, PA: Wolters Kluwer.

Ignatavicius, D.D. (2001) 6 critical thinking skills for at-the-bedside success: key ways to practice, nurture, and reinforce staff members' cognitive skills, *Nursing Management*, 32 (1): 37–39.

Joint Royal Colleges Ambulance Liaison Committee and Association of Ambulance Chief Executives (JRCALC/AACE) (2022) *JRCALC Clinical Guidelines*. Bridgwater: Class Professional Publishing.

Krockow, E. (2018) How many decisions do we make each day?, *Psychology Today*. Available at: https://www.psychologytoday.com/us/blog/stretching-theory/201809/how-many-decisions-do-we-make-each-day (accessed 6 April 2024).

Lyneham, J., Parkinson, C. and Denholm, C. (2008) Explicating Benner's concept of expert practice: intuition in emergency nursing, *Journal of Advanced Nursing*, 64 (4): 380–87.

Marquis, B.L. and Huston, C.J. (2012) *Leadership Roles and Management Tools for the New Nurse*, 7th edition. Philadelphia, PA: Lippincott, Williams & Wilkins.

Marquis, B.L. and Huston, C.J. (2020) *Leadership Roles and Management Functions in Nursing: Theory and Application*, 10th edition. Philadelphia, PA: Wolters Kluwer.

Moilanen, J. (2015) Intuitive decision making: The wisdom of tacit knowing-in-action, in C.J. Boden-McGill and K.P. King (eds.) *Developing and Sustaining Adult Learners*. Charlotte, NC: Information Age Publishing.

Muoni, T. (2012) Decision-making, intuition, and the midwife: understanding heuristics, *British Journal of Midwifery*, 20 (1): 52–56.

Oxford English Dictionary (OED) (2023) *Oxford English Dictionary*. Oxford: Oxford University Press.

Rice, D.T., Nudell, N.G., Habrat, D.A., Smith, J.E. et al. (2016) CPR induced consciousness: sedation protocols for this special population, *British Paramedic Journal*, 1 (2): 24–30.

Ryan, L. and Halliwell, D. (2012) Paramedic decision-making: how is it done?, *Journal of Paramedic Practice*, 4 (6): 343–51.

Schöbel, M., Rieskamp, J. and Huber, R. (2016) Social influences in sequential decision making, *PLoS ONE*, 11: e0146536. Available at: https://doi.org/10.1371/journal.pone.0146536.

Sporek, P. (2015) Unconscious bias, *British Journal of Midwifery*, 23 (12): 910.

Stone, J. and Moskowitz, G. (2011) Non-conscious bias in medical decision making: what can be done to reduce it?, *Medical Education*, 45 (8): 768–76.

Sullivan, E. and Garland, G. (2013) *Practical Leadership and Management in Healthcare*. London: Pearson.

Timmons, R. (2009) *Sensory overload as a factor in crisis decision-making and communications by emergency first responders*, Dissertation, University of Texas at Dallas, Richardson.

Tversky, A. and Kahneman, D. (1974) Judgment under uncertainty: heuristics and biases, *Science* (NS), 185 (4157): 1124–31.

Vroom, V.H. and Yetton, P. (1973) *Leadership and Decision Making*. Pittsburgh, PA: University of Pittsburgh Press.

Whelehan, D.F., Conlon, K.C. and Ridgway, P.F. (2020) Medicine and heuristics: cognitive biases and medical decision-making, *Irish Journal of Medical Science*, 189 (4): 1477–84.

19
Remote assessment consultation and clinical decision-making

Mike Brady

In this chapter:

- Introduction
- Why is this relevant?
- Who undertakes remote clinical decision-making?
- What is visualisation?
- Working with computer decision support tools and video
- Video consultation
- Keeping safe
- Special considerations in remote clinical decision-making
- Inclusive remote assessment
- Health technology in remote assessment
- Conclusion
- Chapter key points
- References and suggested reading

INTRODUCTION

The term 'remote clinical decision-making' (RCDM), within the context of this chapter, refers to a clinician's role and responsibility in consulting, triaging and/or making any decisions about the outcome and/or onward referral of a patient in the absence of a face-to-face patient–clinician interaction. RCDM is also known as 'virtual care' to better reflect the broader range of technologies, communication methods and clinical skills used in practice (such as video consultations, online consultations, remote monitoring, virtual wards and wearable technologies) (Brady and Harry, 2023). RCDM is an established strategy used within primary, urgent and emergency care to assess patients and better manage the increasing patient demand. While historically, there have been differing views surrounding the best definition of RCDM

(Brady and Northstone, 2017), various studies have demonstrated a high degree of patient safety associated with its use (Dale et al., 2004; Meer et al., 2010; Huibers et al., 2011; Payne et al., 2023; Brady et al., 2024b). The COVID-19 pandemic saw numerous health services increasingly transitioning to remote consultations as a safety measure to reduce transmission (Snooks et al., 2021); however, the practice is much older. Since its invention in 1876, the telephone has been used as a tool for delivering health care, and – while it is not the only method of remote communication now – by the 1970s, the telephone was described as having become as much a part of standard medical equipment as the stethoscope (Car and Sheikh, 2003).

This chapter explores the use of RCDM and covers important areas for paramedics and other clinicians to consider when practising, such as safety and risk stratification.

WHY IS THIS RELEVANT?

 **Reflection: points to consider**

Have you ever assessed a patient with your eyes closed? When was the last time you asked a patient if their lips or fingernails were blue, or if their skin was cold, mottled or clammy to the touch, or if their abdomen was distended?

Many professionals undertake RCDM, including nurses, paramedics, midwives, doctors and psychiatrists. The goal of RCDM depends on the context of its use but from a paramedic's perspective, RCDM has predominantly involved the enhanced triage of patients calling 999/911/112. More recently, paramedics have undertaken RCDM in settings such as NHS 111, out-of-hours services and urgent primary care settings. RCDM, however, can mean much more than undertaking a remote clinical assessment and can involve providing remote senior clinical support to face-to-face colleagues and remote colleagues in different bases, advising ambulance dispatch staff, providing support and supervision to non-medically trained call handlers or community responders, validating newly qualified colleagues' outcomes, reviewing online symptom checker uses, and monitoring call/response queues.

These responsibilities involve making decisions about the outcome and/ or onward referral of patients without a face-to-face patient–clinician interaction; however, one cannot practise remotely like one does face-to-face.

Such is the difference between face-to-face and remote practice, the topics covered in this chapter are increasingly relevant to more paramedics working in various clinical settings.

In Box 19.1, the objective of the building brick communication comparison is to build a model as close to the instructions provided as possible – why not give it a try?

Box 19.1 The building brick communication comparison

Two people sit back-to-back or in different rooms and take verbal instructions from a third person acting as a facilitator. Whoever finishes with a model closest to that of the facilitator wins.

What you will find, however, is that two people (medically trained or not) will hear different things, take instructions in different ways, understand words, colloquialisms, shades of colours, orientation of shapes and placements of bricks in entirely different ways.

There is an art to communicating remotely – both in receiving and delivering information. Whilst a fun game to play, imagine if the model you were trying to build involved instructions on how to stem a bleed, assess skin turgor or describe how responsive a young child was over the phone.

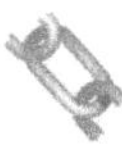

Chapter 1 for more on various means of communication.

WHO UNDERTAKES REMOTE CLINICAL DECISION-MAKING?

Table 19.1 sets out the range of clinicians who work remotely and the vast array of settings in which they work. Paramedics work across a range of settings but often not in isolation. It is useful to know who might be able to provide support, guidance and shared decision-making.

Holmström (2007) describes remote decision-making as a highly complex process, which is neither mechanical nor linear, but rather a highly skilled, knowledge-intensive specialty. There has always been an emphasis on the knowledge derived from systematic, scientific and empirical data to inform clinical decisions. However, working remotely from a patient often means that

Table 19.1 Range of clinicians who work remotely and their clinical settings

Practitioner	Remote role example
Paramedics	General practice, out-of-hours services, NHS 111, ambulance service contact centres, forensic units, prisons, police station cover
Nurses, general	General practice, out-of-hours services, NHS 111, ambulance service contact centres, forensic units, prisons, police station cover
Nurses, other	District nurses, sexual health nurses, diabetes nurses, critical care nurses, dental nurses
Cancer/palliative care nurse specialists	Cancer and palliative care nurse specialists (in addition to the district nurses) operate many cancer care helplines where they assess patients remotely
Midwives	Midwives operate maternity advice lines and remote clinics
Approved mental health practitioners	Crisis teams, early intervention teams, assertive outreach teams. Some also use remote video software to assess patients
Practitioner psychologists	Clinical psychologists, forensic psychologists, counselling psychologists, educational psychologists, sport and exercise psychologists, health psychologists, occupational psychologists
Speech and language therapists	Speech and language therapists work remotely using remote video software to assess patients and undertake therapy sessions
Public health practitioners/ consultants	Public health practitioners/consultants offer a range of remote advice and situational assessments to other clinicians, often in acute and emergency roles
Dietitians	Dietitians work remotely over the phone using remote video software to assess patients and undertake intervention sessions
Pharmacists	Pharmacies, general practice, out-of-hours services, NHS 111, ambulance service contact centres
Optometrists	Optometrists work remotely in their clinical practice to offer patients support, advice and often assessment of a minor ophthalmological nature
Physician associates	General practice, out-of-hours services, a wide range of other clinical settings

such systematic and scientific data is not always available to the clinician, or the method of capturing it should be used with caution (personal wearable devices). The expert skills derived from face-to-face clinical practice must be transferred to this alternative way of working. Thus, if one has not gained expertise in face-to-face practice, it will be difficult to practise remotely.

McHugh and Lake (2010) describe clinical experts as distinguishable from their colleagues by their often-intuitive ability to efficiently make critical clinical decisions while grasping the whole nature of a situation. Such knowledge is acquired through experience gained in special domains and is linked closely with experience-guided working (Herbig et al., 2001). There is some evidence to indicate that length of clinical experience has an impact on RCDM in emergency and out-of-hour care settings (Varley et al., 2016). For example, a somewhat dated study of 60,794 calls managed by 296 NHS Direct nurses reported a positive relationship between years of nursing experience and call disposal patterns. Nurses with less than 10 years of clinical experience were less likely to arrive at self-care dispositions than nurses with more than 20 years of experience (O'cathain et al., 2004).

There is a lack of up-to-date research on remote confidence, competence and correlation to years of qualification or experience. Caution should be exercised when introducing newly qualified, junior or back-to-practice clinicians to remote practice who have not received prolonged positive supervision and support. Thompson (2015), referring to face-to-face practice, proposed that whilst newly qualified paramedics, for example, have clinical knowledge and application, they lack confidence in their abilities due to lack of exposure and experience. They rely on the support given to them by colleagues, peers and preceptors in the early stages of their careers.

Other forms of knowledge have been widely recognised as having an impact on how decisions are made in clinical practice (Chinn and Kramer, 2011), such as tacit or intuitive knowledge. Polanyi's (1967) seminal work defined tacit knowledge as occurring when something is known only by relying on an awareness of it for attending to a secondary activity.

# Reflection: points to consider

Listen to that gut feeling. That gut feeling is your tacit knowledge. A gut feeling is a collection of many different experiences, patient encounters, stories listened to, cases reviewed, audits received, all telling you that something is happening – even if you can't articulate it. *Don't ignore it!*

Marsden (1999) states that it is widely accepted that tacit knowing and intuitive knowing are integral to expert decision-making, including RCDM, where systematic, scientific and empirical data is often unavailable. Thus, it is reasonable to assert that a clinician cannot be considered an expert unless they have developed tacit knowledge of their clinical area. Considering that tacit knowledge is integral to RCDM, it is reasonable to assert that only experts should undertake this highly complex way of working. Working remotely is so inherently different from working face-to-face that despite the clinician's experience and expertise, some clinical decisions will require further support.

WHAT IS VISUALISATION?

Unlike face-to-face clinical practice, RCDM involves working with limited senses. For example, the clinician is, effectively, wearing a blindfold. Even video assessment is fraught with complexities related to lighting, skin colour, skin opacity, camera angle and picture quality. Clinicians normally rely explicitly and implicitly on what is communicated non-verbally and what they physically see during a consultation. An experienced clinician can see an ashen-coloured patient or feel the cold clamminess of the patient when taking a pulse, often without conscious effort. Working remotely means not being able to see the home environment, or the patient's colour or condition, or to palpate the patient or provide the therapeutic physical contact normally provided to emotionally upset patients and family. In addition, clinicians are unable to smell any overt urinary infection, the odour of diabetic ketoacidosis or alcohol on a patient's breath. RDCM clinicians must therefore devise methods of gathering information that would otherwise be readily accessible to them and transfer their face-to-face skills, built up through many years of practice, to working remotely.

Pettinari and Jessopp (2001) consider the process of picture-building, of visualisation of the patient and the situation, to be a recognised strategy in RCDM. They explain that clinicians develop skills to manage the interaction

Case study 19.1

Eliza is a 90-year-old lady who has pressed her alarm system at 05:00 because she needs some help getting out of her living room chair. She cannot get her shoes on to help her get up.

When assessing Eliza remotely, it might be thought the call is mobility related or due to a care package breaking down. Some clinicians may be able to visualise Eliza. They have met Eliza hundreds of times before. They think the following:

1. Why is Eliza in her living room chair at this time of the morning?
2. Has Eliza slept in her living room chair?
3. For how long has Eliza been sleeping in her living room chair?
4. Is Eliza using pillows or cushions?
5. Is Eliza unable to reach her shoes or do they not fit her anymore?
6. Are Eliza's legs, ankles and feet swollen?
7. Is this really a mobility issue or carer breakdown, or is Eliza actually in heart failure?

Try visualising Eliza yourself.

with callers to compensate for the patient not being visible to them. Such skills involve using non-biased, non-leading, open and closed questions to determine various aspects of the patient's condition. A recent evaluation of a postgraduate module on RCDM by Brady et al. (2018) noted how participants could link existing knowledge to remote practice through the course content – which possibly increased their confidence. This training in linking existing knowledge to visualise the patient, described as the co-application of knowledge, is important.

Reflection: points to consider

Refresh your visualisation and picture-building skills with regular hands-on, face-to-face clinical practice or observations in clinical settings. Practise your mental picture of how your patient may be presenting.

Whilst knowledge is not a static concept and is regularly renewed, validated and challenged in different ways, it is best practice to 'top up' one's visualisation skills by frequently seeing patients in face-to-face (non-video) hands-on practice. Greenhalgh et al. (2024) believe that the knowledge needed to deliver high-quality remote consultations to diverse patient groups is often complex. They identify the vital role of non-didactic training in ensuring this quality: joint clinical sessions, case-based discussions and in-person, whole-team, on-the-job training. This mix should also include regular face-to-face observation or hands-on clinical shifts. More research is needed to explore the concept of visualisation in remote consultation. This process of picture-building, visualisation and information gathering can be challenging and can be affected by human factors. Remote consultations are often facilitated and aided by consultation frameworks and clinical decision support software.

WORKING WITH COMPUTER DECISION SUPPORT TOOLS AND VIDEO

Remote clinicians often use clinical decision support tools, both formal and informal, to support their practice (Payne et al., 2023). Digital clinical support software helps clinicians guide, structure and record their assessments, providing clinical assessment and advice in an auditable, evidence-based way. Brady et al. (2024a) note that many services employing paramedics and other clinicians use digital tools to augment remote/virtual decision-making. Examples in the UK and internationally include NHS Pathways (NHS Digital, 2023), Manchester Triage Tool (Marsden et al., 2023), Odyssey TeleAssess (OneAdvanced, 2024) and the Emergency Communication Nurse System™ in LowCode™ (Priority Solutions, 2024).

Clinical decision support software (CDSS) allows remote clinicians to ask questions to which the answers would be obvious if they were working in face-to-face clinical practice, and thus might be forgotten. Such systems prompt the clinician to ask questions in ways that gather information that their hands-on visual care might have previously done.

Clinicians need to consider the use of questions and prompts, especially if new to RCDM. However, it is also important not to sound robotic or scripted, as this may undermine the patient's confidence in the clinical consultation – although more research is required to validate this. This communication skill takes time and practice to achieve and is one in which informality, without the loss of systematic questioning, can help – this process is known as the 'ums and ahs' (see Box 19.2). Whilst 'ums and ahs' in public speaking or lecturing can at times be annoying, adding them occasionally to otherwise scripted questions and other filler statements can be helpful when using CDSS to maintain the patient's confidence in the consultation.

It is important to ask questions singly, in a non-leading way, and in a way that does not change the question's meaning or the information you are trying to get. However, by exploring the concept of the 'ums and ahs' (perhaps with your clinical supervisor, training or education team), the consultation may feel less robotic or scripted.

> ## Box 19.2 The 'ums and ahs'
>
> *Robotic example:* Have you had any of the following symptoms: (A) crushing central chest pain, (B) pain in the neck or shoulder, (C) tightness in the chest?
>
> *Ums and Ahs example:* Tell me, have you had any crushing central chest pain? … [*pause for answer*] … What about any pain in the neck or shoulder? … [pause for answer] … um, have you had any tightness in your chest at all? … [*pause for answer*].

Whilst there are benefits associated with the use of CDSS, such as a reduction in errors, standardisation of assessment and efficiency of workload (Islam et al., 2021), it is important for remote clinicians not to rely entirely on it. CDSS cannot assess and plan for every clinical eventuality and cannot replace the nuances of clinical experience. Remote clinicians are more likely to override CDSS recommendations if they have detailed knowledge of the health problem under consideration, and rely more on CDSS for conditions about which they have limited clinical knowledge (O'cathain et al., 2004). Warner (2008), however, explains that if remote clinicians err slavishly on the side of caution, they effectively become receptionists and not clinicians. If they stick rigidly to established algorithms, they could spend a quarter of an hour consulting with a patient with a pimple on his chin, while a potential heart attack or stroke case might still be in the queue. If they skim over a triage encounter, lose concentration, get interrupted or forget to ask a vital question, a patient could ultimately die. These tools are decision-support tools, not decision-making tools, and clinicians are required to use their critical thinking skills when deciding to follow – or not follow – recommended outcomes and not allow the system to tell them what they ought to do, whilst also not ignoring the often highly evidence-based systems. Warner's (2008) narrative continues to be an apt description of the complexity of RCDM and outlines how challenging working without one's senses can be in clinical practice.

Sahota and colleagues' (2011) systematic review of the literature found that most CDSS demonstrate improvements in the process of patient care; however, there remains a lack of evidence that the use of CDSS leads to positive patient outcomes. A later systematic review of the literature concluded that whilst efforts have been made to understand more about CDSS and how its use may vary across settings in general, the evidence base remains limited (Islam et al., 2021). Further research is needed to determine whether the benefits based on historical research are still valid.

Reflection: points to consider

CDSS outcomes assume that responses are available, clinics are open or appointments are available. Remember to consider service and clinician availability when determining the most appropriate outcome.

VIDEO CONSULTATION

The COVID-19 pandemic led to the widespread implementation or increase in the use of video consultation in many primary, urgent and emergency care settings (Tang et al., 2020; Bell et al., 2021); however, there has been an interest in its use in health care for some time. Greenhalgh et al. (2018) report that what research has been done shows such consultations to be acceptable, safe and effective for patients deemed clinically eligible for a range of conditions, including adult and teenage diabetes, but that some authors have questioned whether video consultations might be less reliable, less safe and less cost-effective than traditional encounters. Bell et al. (2021) evaluated video triage for low-acuity calls in a single NHS Ambulance Trust. They concluded that video triage for low acuity calls appeared to be safe, with low rates of re-contact and high levels of patient and clinician satisfaction compared to standard telephone triage, albeit there was only a small number of studies in similar settings across the UK. In a systematic review, Campbell et al. (2023) demonstrated that virtual consultations, including video, may be as effective as face-to-face care and have a potentially positive impact on the efficiency and timeliness of care; however, there is a considerable lack of evidence on the impacts on patient safety, equity and patient-centredness. This lack of evidence is particularly apparent for the use of video consultation in urgent and emergency care settings, and at the time of writing, individual clinicians should use such consultations with care.

Despite currently low levels of video use in a range of clinical settings, its use will likely increase over time; as such, clinicians need to remember that just because you can see the patient, a video consultation is not the same as conducting one face-to-face (see Box 19.3).

Box 19.3   Video consultation

Considerations include:

- What can you still not see, hear or smell?
- Is video one-way or two-way – can the patient see you? Does this imbalance affect rapport and communication?
- Do you or the patient have a bias which is accentuated through the use of video?
- How can lighting affect how a patient may appear?
- How can camera quality affect how a patient may appear?
- How do you assess different skin colours differently through video? Or do you not?
- Do you still ask all your questions when using video, or are some things so obvious that you do not need to?
- Do you need video to assess your patients, or can skilled questioning over the telephone be equally as effective?

It would be wrong to assume that training is not required for video consultation. Leach et al. (2023) helpfully outline some areas of focus for clinicians undertaking remote consultation, including:

- preparation;
- specific communication techniques;
- examination using video;
- assessment of the environment;
- gesturing;
- what happens if the patient hangs up or the connection is lost;
- encountering an unexpected person on the screen or in the background;
- whether anything is missing.

Recent small-scale research, typically in primary care, has shown that video consultation can be used as an adjunct to telephone assessments and is useful for bringing others into the consultation – either to assist with a physical examination or to get specialist advice for the patient (Payne and Clarke, 2023). However, ensuring clinicians receive suitable training, education, audit and supervision in video consultation is vital.

KEEPING SAFE

Clinicians must always know what is needed to do a good job and how to protect patients and themselves from harm, distress and professional risk. Keeping safe differs fundamentally from being risk-averse, which some remote settings have been known to be (Standing et al., 2016; Phillips, 2020).

 **Reflection: points to consider**

Have you ever said, 'Oh the patient didn't tell me that!!' Could it be that:

- you did not ask the patient the right question(s)?
- the patient was not qualified to understand what you enquired about?
- you made an assumption, instead of taking a more thorough history?

Risk aversion, also known as over-triage, happens when patients receive a higher level of care than needed (Simonson et al., 2022). Whilst such approaches have sometimes been thought to be safe in the past (better to be safe than sorry), over-triage can have significant financial implications for health systems, contribute to poor patient flow and poor capacity, and increase mortality and patient harm, as those who require help most urgently have care delayed (Simonson et al., 2022). Highly skilled, autonomous clinicians can reach clinically appropriate outcomes while remaining safe.

Safety in remote practice is achieved through three main means: (1) adequate communication, (2) adequate documentation and (3) adequate escalation.

See Box 19.4 for something to be mindful of, both in your own practice and the practice of colleagues.

Box 19.4   The three hellos – 'hello, hello, hello!'

Be aware of the sudden rapid deterioration of a remote patient. Listen out for new or junior colleagues who you hear entertaining the 'three hellos'.

The patient may have collapsed or gone into cardiorespiratory arrest. Would you know what do to? Saying 'hello' one more time is not going to help. *You need to act fast!*

In a multi-method qualitative study, Payne et al. (2023) explored safety incidents in remote triage and consultation from a primary care perspective. They concluded that safety incidents are extremely rare, although they usually involve various clinical, communicative, technical and logistical issues, sometimes in extremely busy and understaffed settings. Table 19.2 is adapted from Payne et al. (2023) and can be used to support safe remote practice.

Table 19.2 Safety incidents in remote triage and consultation

Is a face-to-face assessment needed?	• Acute chest or abdominal pain • Breathing difficulties • New psychosis • Diabetes review where eye or foot examination is needed • Persistent or progressive skin lesion • Acute history that does not make sense
Presentations leading to a need for a face-to-face assessment	• Condition has not resolved as expected • Escalating parental concern • Acute condition complicated by complex illness
Patient characteristics that make remote assessment more difficult	• Extremes of age • Care home residents if on-site staff are not confident in undertaking observations • Language disconcordance • Impairment (e.g. deafness) • Conditions that may complicate communication (e.g. autism)
Effective safety netting	• Determine what to do if things worsen and what action to take if expected care (e.g. a call-back) does not happen • Make all points explicit; do not assume the patient knows • Fully document what safety-netting advice has been given • Back up verbal advice with text, email or leaflet • Ask the patient/family member/carer to repeat safety-netting instructions
Organisational factors	• Adequate staffing and appropriate mix • Protocol for times of extreme stress (absence, high demand) • Reduce distractions • Provide training for all staff (not just in the technology)

Adapted from: Payne et al. (2023).

Poots (2024) used a Delphi study approach to explore contributory factors to safety incidents in remote consultation, with the intention of developing a framework for investigation and system change. Poots concluded that there is a paucity of literature about telephone triage and consultation safety. Whilst many frameworks of contributory factors for investigating incidents exist, they are often intended for face-to-face care and may miss latent system factors contributing to safety, specifically in telephone triage.

Table 19.3 can be used to support safe remote practice, and is particularly helpful for those clinicians starting in remote consultation.

Reflection: points to consider

Be wary of being 'sold' a patient! There will be occasions when referring clinicians or staff try to 'sell' you a patient, by only offering the clinical history, observations and information that suits the narrative for you to accept their care. This practice is often born out of clinical bias but can be difficult to challenge. For example:

- Only relaying the best observations – until asked
- Not relaying symptoms that might make you question their suitability for the service – until asked
- Reiterating an irrelevant point to sway decision-making: 'Oh they only live round the corner from your clinic'.

Ask everything you want of anyone trying to refer a patient into your care.

Understanding the key areas of risk and common pitfalls clinicians experience when practising remotely is important. This, together with an appreciation of tacit knowledge and being able to visualise effectively, will help keep the consultation safe. However, certain specialist areas of remote practice should be considered especially complex.

SPECIAL CONSIDERATIONS IN REMOTE CLINICAL DECISION-MAKING

This text is a foundation of paramedic practice, and as such does not address highly specialised areas of clinical practice in detail, for which there will be specific training. Clinicians should explore different, in-depth remote assessment textbooks or speak to their local education and training team for further support. Indeed, working remotely is as much about applying existing clinical practice to a remote setting as it is being adept at working remotely. Areas of practice to consider are set out below Table 19.3.

Table 19.3 Themes and considerations for remote consultation

Theme	Considerations
Tools and technological factors	• Using the CDSS incorrectly could cause safety incidents
Internal environment	• Temperature, noise, lighting • Distractions • Physical proximity to team members for support
Organisational factors	• Inadequate communication in the organisation could affect safety performance • Organisational culture could affect safety outcomes • Organisational resources (e.g. staffing) should be sufficient for safety performance
Task factors	• Clear communication is important for safety • Multiple demands • Task complexity
External factors	• Availability of follow-up services is important • Collaboration and information-sharing between organisations • External, conflicting pressures could affect safety

Adapted from: Poots (2024).

Assessing autistic people and those with learning disabilities

Autistic people and those with learning disabilities generally have poorer outcomes than people without such diagnoses. Both groups may experience different but multiple barriers to effective remote consultation and should have a lower threshold for being seen face-to-face. Autistic people and those with learning disabilities may have very different signs of deterioration; for example, changes in mental state or behaviour might indicate distress, discomfort or even pain (higher levels of anxiety, changes in vocal noises, poor appetite, changes in bowel movements). It is important to note that some CDSS does not consider how autistic people or those with learning disabilities might present, and good critical thinking is often needed.

Depending on the setting, the barriers that autistic people and those with learning disabilities face may differ. Barriers include:

- Clinical bias – do not assume a disability causes the presentation.
- Lack of adaptation of assessment techniques – allow longer appointments.
- Traditional styles of communication are difficult to understand.
- Non-adapted technology (email, video call) is challenging if not supported well or if not enough preparation is made.

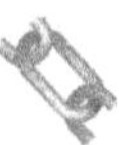

Chapters 7 and 8 for more on children with learning needs.

Reflection: points to consider

Verbal cues and affirmative body language *does not* confirm understanding. Someone may say 'yes' or 'okay', or nod and smile, or even remain silent when spoken to. This does not confirm understanding or retention of information. Adapt your style to ensure the patient or family friends and carers truly understand your questions, advice and action request.

High-frequency users

High-frequency users, sometimes called frequent or repeat callers, are some of the most complex and vulnerable patients who access services. Multiple assessments, distrust of healthcare systems, unusual reactions or overreactions to simple triggers, frustration and often confusion can create a complex and, at times, increasingly risky context for remote assessment and consultation.

Frequent use is not always inappropriate use

The UK Ambulance Service Frequent Caller National Network (FreCaNN, 2022) defines high-frequency users as:

> *An individual aged 18 or over who makes 5 or more emergency calls relating to individual episodes of care in a month or 12 or more emergency calls related to individual episodes of care in three months.*

High-frequency users are often perceived to be violent and aggressive towards healthcare staff; however, there is little evidence to support this misconception. It is common for clinicians to become frustrated and feel a lack of value when caring for high-frequency users, given the high number of calls they make and their perceived lack of compliance. It is important not to allow that frustration to affect clinical assessment and not create or enable unhelpful coping mechanisms. Some top tips in assessing high-frequency users are addressed in Box 19.5.

Box 19.5   Tips for assessing high-frequency users

- Many high-frequency users have alert markers and support plans which contain helpful information.
- Remote assessment is a good method for the initial assessment of high-frequency users but should not preclude a face-to-face assessment if needed.
- Initial clinical assessment should be the same as for any other patient, and helps control bias.
- Make a clear plan with the patient and involve others if needed.
- Do not forget to update high-frequency users' notes and plans.

INCLUSIVE REMOTE ASSESSMENT

Clinicians have a responsibility and moral imperative to provide high-quality care to patients that is effective, safe, evidence-based and personalised to their needs and their families if appropriate. People are different. Clinicians and health providers should not 'treat everyone the same'. People's differences often define their individual needs, perspectives and beliefs, and there are some whose health outcomes and experiences are often poorer than most – sometimes made worse by remote assessment and the removal of face-to-face interactions. Clinicians should regularly challenge themselves to reflect on any bias they may have, which might be identified through patient feedback or clinical call audits.

Reflection: points to consider

In your physical assessment and/or remote assessment education and training, did you cover how to assess those with black and brown skin?

Groups such as the homeless, asylum seekers and those perceived to be on the margins of society, such as sex workers, will have very individual healthcare needs that need to be considered. Characteristics such as gender, age, race, religion, sexual orientation and disability need to be considered when assessing and managing someone's care remotely, and adapted to ensure the most appropriate and safest outcomes are reached.

Much of the medical education in the western world has historically been based on caring for those with white skin. Increasing evidence suggests the need for educational institutions to address equality and diversity to ensure that future clinicians can effectively treat people of all backgrounds (Mukwende et al., 2020), which includes how we ask clinical questions. How do you assess skin tone, pallor or even signs of cyanosis in non-white patients? How do you assess rashes, anaemia or jaundice in patients with black and brown skin?

For example, asking a patient or caller if their complexion or that of their family member is normal is a good way to illicit useful information. Asking open-ended questions, such as 'In what way are they looking different today?' can help the clinician build a fuller picture and a link to a possible differential diagnosis.

Being aware of your own possible biases, trying to make care as individualised as possible and considering how to adapt your remote assessment to get the most out of the interaction, be that for religious reasons, reasons of gender reassignment, age or race, and asking questions in different ways can all contribute to a positive patient experience and outcome. If you have not received specific training in how to assess patients who do not have white skin, reach out to your education and training team and ask for some.

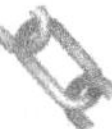

Chapters 6 and **Chapter 10** for more on the complexities of health care.

HEALTH TECHNOLOGY IN REMOTE ASSESSMENT

Recent technological developments, partly as a result of the COVID-19 pandemic, mean that many more people are utilising various types of health technology. The list of available products has increased dramatically, and remote clinicians must consider how useful the data from such devices is – should it be considered, or should it be ignored? Indeed, calls to clinicians are sometimes driven by changes in data that the patient can view (a run of tachycardia, for example) or the anxiety created by the over-monitoring of signs historically not seen unless you were in a clinic or hospital, not your own home.

Smartphones, personal wearable devices and dermal monitors can capture and record pulse rate, oxygen saturation, electrocardiograms, blood pressure, blood glucose, weight and even UV exposure whilst passing information back to personal applications or even directly to health providers, personal trainers and dietitians.

Such devices can differ dramatically from those considered medical devices, especially if bought on the cheap from an online retailer. The accuracy of data captured from such devices will often depend on the user's compliance with the manufacturer's instructions, environmental variables, battery quality and signal strength.

Whilst the landscape of such devices is increasingly complex, they will definitely play a larger part in healthcare assessment and delivery in the coming years. Virtual wards and remote monitoring schemes are already being used worldwide to tackle increases in demand, reductions in hospital capacity and geographical challenges, as well as to allow more patients to remain closer to home and in control.

 **Reflection: points to consider**

Devices can create false readings and false alerts. They can also help a clinician build a richer clinical picture and history and should be used to augment robust clinical questioning.

When presented with information or data from a personal wearable device or remote monitoring device, remote clinicians should consider it, as they would all other information. Listen to what the patient is saying and why they think the information is important for you to hear. If the patient is not calling from a recognised virtual ward or a remote monitoring scheme that your organisation is managing, then enquire what type of device they have, why they have it and what they use it for. Is it a well-known, recognised brand – possibly used in healthcare settings – and have they discussed their data with other clinicians? Consider extremes of data, such as low blood glucose readings in a worried diabetic patient or tachycardia in an otherwise fit and healthy person.

It is important to assess your patient and not only their screen. Remote consultation has remained safe for many years without such devices through careful and robust clinical questioning. Such devices can augment such questioning and be used safely and successfully to build a better remote picture and history. However, they cannot replace the need for robust and thorough clinical assessment.

CONCLUSION

This chapter has explained remote assessment consultation and decision-making and why it is increasingly relevant to paramedics and other clinicians. It has explained how unique and specialised this type of practice is, and how clinicians can visualise the patient and keep safe during consultations – either over the phone or by video link. It has briefly covered special considerations in remote assessments that the reader should explore in more depth and has provided useful tactics and tips.

> **Chapter key points:**
>
> - The goal of RCDM differs depending on the context of its use, but from a paramedic perspective, RCDM has predominantly involved the enhanced triage of patients calling 999/911/112.
> - One cannot practise remotely in the same way as one does face-to-face.
> - A gut feeling is a collection of many experiences: patient encounters, stories listened to, cases reviewed, audits received, all telling you something is happening. Even if you cannot articulate it, do not ignore it.
> - Remember, intimate examinations should *not* be conducted by video.

REFERENCES AND SUGGESTED READING

Bell, F., Pilbery, R., Connell, R., Fletcher, D. et al. (2021) The acceptability and safety of video triage for ambulance service patients and clinicians during the COVID-19 pandemic, *British Paramedic Journal*, 6 (2): 49–58.

Brady, M. and Harry, E. (2023) What effects did home working have on 999 clinician practice from one UK ambulance service during the COVID-19 pandemic?, *International Journal of Emergency Services*, 12 (3): 343–58.

Brady, M. and Northstone, K. (2017) Remote clinical decision-making: a clinician's definition, *Emergency Nurse*, 25 (2): 24–28.

Brady, M., Jackson, J. and Northstone, K. (2018) Remote clinical decision making: evaluation of a new education module, *Nurse Education in Practice*, 29: 150–58.

Brady, M., Fivaz, M.C., Noblett, P., Olola, C. et al. (2024a) Emergency Communication Nurse System outcomes of advanced medical priority dispatch codes in a UK ambulance service: a descriptive analysis, *Annals of Emergency Dispatch and Response*, 12 (1): 11–18.

Brady, M., Fivaz, M.C., Noblett, P. Scott, G. et al. (2024b) 999 telephone triage: a comparison of UK ambulance nurse and paramedic case mix, outcomes and audit compliance, *International Journal of Emergency Services*. 13 (1). Available at: https://doi.org/10.1108/IJES-08-2023-0033.

Campbell, K., Greenfield, G., Li, E., O'Brien, N. et al. (2023) The impact of virtual consultations on the quality of primary care: systematic review, *Journal of Medical Internet Research*, 25: e48920. Available at: https://doi.org/10.2196/48920.

Car, J. and Sheikh, A. (2003) Telephone consultations, *British Medical Journal*, 326 (7396): 966–69.

Chinn, P.L. and Kramer, M.K. (2011) *Integrated Theory and Knowledge Development in Nursing*, 8th edition. St Louis, MO: Elsevier.

Dale, J., Williams, S., Foster, T. and Higgins, J. (2004) Safety of telephone consultation for 'non-serious' emergency ambulance service patients, *Quality and Safety in Health Care*, 13 (5): 363–73.

Frequent Caller National Network (FreCaNN) (2022) *Frequent Caller National Network (FreCaNN) – written evidence*, AES0008. Access to emergency services, UK Parliament Inquiry. Available at: https://committees.parliament.uk/written-evidence/113035/pdf/#:~:text=Launched%20in%202013%20the%20Frequent,frequently%20make%20emergency%20calls%20to.

Greenhalgh, T., Shaw, S., Wherton, J., Vijayaraghavan, S. et al. (2018) Real-world implementation of video outpatient consultations at macro, meso, and micro levels: mixed-method study, *Journal of Medical Internet Research*, 20: e150. Available at: https://doi.org/10.2196/jmir.9897.

Greenhalgh, T., Payne, R., Hemmings, N., Leach, H. et al. (2024) Training needs for staff providing remote services in general practice: a mixed-methods study, *British Journal of General Practice*, 74 (738): e17–e26. Available at: https://bjgp.org/content/74/738/e17.

Herbig, B., Büssing, A. and Ewert, T. (2001) The role of tacit knowledge in the work context of nursing, *Journal of Advanced Nursing*, 34 (5): 687–95.

Holmström, I. (2007) Decision aid software programs in telenursing: not used as intended? Experiences of Swedish telenurses, *Nursing and Health Sciences*, 9 (1): 23–28.

Huibers, L., Smits, M., Renaud, V., Giesen, P. et al. (2011) Safety of telephone triage in out-of-hours care: a systematic review, *Scandinavian Journal of Primary Health Care*, 29 (4): 198–209.

Islam, F., Sabbe, M., Heeren, P. and Milisen, K. (2021) Consistency of decision support software-integrated telephone triage and associated factors: a systematic review, *BMC Medical Informatics and Decision Making*, 21: 107. Available at: https://doi.org/10.1186/s12911-021-01472-3.

Leach, H., Payne, R., Hanson, I. and King, K. (2023) Video consulting for GP trainees, *InnovAiT: Education and Inspiration for General Practice*, 17 (3): 113–17.

Marsden, J. (1999) Expert nurse decision-making: telephone triage in an ophthalmic accident and emergency department, *NT Research*, 4 (1): 44–52.

Marsden, J., Newton, M., Windle, J. and Mackway-Jones, K. (eds.) (2023) Manchester Triage Tool, in *Emergency Triage: Telephone Triage and Advice*, Version 1.7. Chichester: Wiley Blackwell.

McHugh, M.D. and Lake, E.T. (2010) Understanding clinical expertise: nurse education, experience, and the hospital context, *Research in Nursing and Health*, 33 (4): 276–87.

Meer, A., Gwerder, T., Duembgen, L., Zumbrunnen, N. et al. (2010) Is computer-assisted telephone triage safe? A prospective surveillance study in walk-in patients with non-life-threatening medical conditions, *Emergency Medicine Journal*, 29(2): 124–28.

Mukwende, M., Tamony, P. and Turner, M. (2020) *Mind the Gap: A Handbook of Clinical Signs in Black and Brown Skin*. London: St George's, University of London. Available at: https://www.blackandbrownskin.co.uk/mindthegap (accessed 7 April 2024).

NHS Digital (2023) *NHS Pathways*. Available at: https://digital.nhs.uk/services/nhs-pathways (accessed 7 April 2024).

O'cathain, A., Nicholl, J., Sampson, F., Walters, S. et al. (2004) Do different types of nurses give different triage decisions in NHS Direct? A mixed methods study, *Journal of Health Services Research and Policy*, 9 (4): 226–33.

OneAdvanced (2024) *Odyssey TeleAssess: Clinical decision support*. Available at: https://www.oneadvanced.com/products/clinical-decision-support/ (accessed 7 April 2024).

Payne, R., Clarke, A., Swann, N., van Dael, J. et al. (2023) Patient safety in remote primary care encounters: multimethod qualitative study combining Safety I and Safety II analysis, *BMJ Quality and Safety*. Available at: https://doi.org/10.1136/bmjqs-2023-016674.

Payne, R.E. and Clarke, A. (2023) How and why are video consultations used in urgent primary care settings in the UK? A focus group study, *BJGP Open*, 7: 25. Available at: https://doi.org/10.3399/BJGPO.2023.0025.

Pettinari, C.J. and Jessopp, L. (2001) 'Your ears become your eyes': managing the absence of visibility in NHS Direct, *Journal of Advanced Nursing*, 36 (5): 668–75.

Phillips, J.S. (2020) Paramedics' perceptions and experiences of NHS 111 in the South West of England, *Journal of Paramedic Practice*, 12 (6): 227–34.

Polanyi, M. (1967) *The Tacit Knowledge Dimension*. London: Routledge & Kegan Paul.

Poots, J. (2024) *Investigating human-system interactions to improve patient safety outcomes in integrated urgent care telephone triage*, Unpublished doctoral thesis, Leeds Beckett University.

Priority Solutions (2024) *Emergency Communication Nurse System: LowCode software*. Available at: https://prioritysolutionsinc.com/lowcode/#:~:text=LowCode%20includes%20a%20series%20of,an%20appropriate%20Recommended%20Care%20Level (accessed 7 April 2024).

Sahota, N., Lloyd, R., Ramakrishna, A., Mackay, J.A. et al. (2011) Computerized clinical decision support systems for acute care management: a decision-maker-researcher partnership systematic review of effects on process of care and patient outcomes, *Implementation Science*, 6: 91. Available at: https://doi.org/10.1186/1748-5908-6-91.

Simonson, R.J., Keebler, J.R., Fernandez, R., Lazzara, E.H. et al. (2022) Over triage: injury classification mistake or hindsight bias?, *Proceedings of the International Symposium on Human Factors and Ergonomics in Health Care*, 11 (1): 7–12.

Snooks, H., Watkins, A.J., Bell, F., Brady, M. et al. (2021) Call volume, triage outcomes, and protocols during the first wave of the COVID 19 pandemic in the United Kingdom: results of a national survey, *Journal of the American College of Emergency Physicians Open*, 2 (4): e12492. Available at: https://doi.org/10.1002/emp2.12492.

Standing, C., Standing, S., McDermott, M.-L., Gururajan, R. et al. (2016) The paradoxes of telehealth: a review of the literature 2000–2015, *Systems Research and Behavioral Science*, 35 (1): 90–101.

Tang, S., Brady, M., Mildenhall, J., Rolfe, U. et al. (2020) The new coronavirus disease: what do we know so far?, *Journal of Paramedic Practice*, 12 (5): 193–201.

Thompson, S. (2015) The perceived concerns of newly qualified paramedics commencing their careers: a pilot study, *Journal of Paramedic Practice*, 7 (2): 74–78.

Varley, A., Warren, F.C., Richards, S.H., Calitri, R. et al. (2016) The effect of nurses' preparedness and nurse practitioner status on triage call management in primary care: a secondary analysis of cross-sectional data from the ESTEEM trial, *International Journal of Nursing Studies*, 58: 12–20.

Warner, J. (2008) Telephone triage requires high-quality nursing skills, *Nursing Times*. Available at: https://www.nursingtimes.net/archive/telephone-triage-requires-high-quality-nursing-skills-08-09-2008/ (accessed 7 April 2024).

20

Practice-based learning
Vince Clarke

In this chapter:

- Introduction
- Why is this relevant?
- The history of paramedic practice-based learning
- Theory, practice and paramedic praxis
- Approaches to practice-based learning
- Getting the most from practice-based learning
- Conclusion
- Chapter key points
- References and suggested reading

INTRODUCTION

Practice-based learning is an integral part of all student paramedics' educational programme. This often takes the form of placements on frontline emergency ambulances, although placements in a wide range of healthcare settings have been part of the development of paramedics for many years and continue to be used in a variety of ways across different educational programmes. Learning in and from practice goes beyond initial pre-registration education and should be considered a lifelong skill, one that registered paramedics need to engage in throughout their careers. This professional expectation is set out by the Health and Care Professions Council (HCPC) in their guidance on continuing professional development (CPD) and the associated standards of CPD (HCPC, 2018).

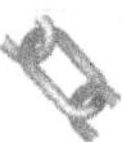

Chapter 21 for more detail on continuing professional development and your responsibilities.

The HCPC also recognises the importance of registered paramedics support-ing learners in their development of both clinical and professional standards, with standard of proficiency 4.8 stating that paramedics must be able to:

> *understand the need for active participation in training, supervision and men-toring in supporting high standards of practice, and personal and professional conduct, and the importance of demonstrating this in practice. (HCPC, 2023: 9)*

WHY IS THIS RELEVANT?

Understanding how practice-based learning can be approached better pre-pares learners for the challenges that the clinical environment can sometimes present. Being aware of the theories that support practice-based learning will help ensure that learners do not perceive a detrimental 'theory–practice gap'. Such a perception can have a significant, often detrimental, impact on learn-ing experiences and development as a registered healthcare professional who appreciates the importance of lifelong learning. Understanding practice-based learning also better prepares learners for their later role as a practice educator and/or preceptor or mentor. See Box 20.1 for a quick who's who guide.

Box 20.1 Who's who?

- A *practice educator* is generally considered to be the individual who directly supports a learner in practice during their initial educational programme.
- A *preceptor* is someone who supports a newly qualified and registered healthcare professional in their transition from edu-cation to professional practice, an opportunity often referred to as the 'preceptorship period'.
- A *mentor* is someone who offers peer-to-peer support to a col-league of the same, or a lower, clinical level. Mentorship can be used to support transitions to new roles within an organisa-tion or to support individuals who are new to an organisation at a non-entry level position.
- In some organisations, the above terms may be used inter-changeably, and learners may find themselves supported by a 'mentor' rather than a practice educator. In most cases, this does not make a material difference and the learner is appro-priately supported.
- A *link tutor* is responsible for ensuring that the relationships between the education provider, the practice setting, the learner and the practice educator are functioning well, and all parties are fully aware of the needs and expectations of the others.

THE HISTORY OF PARAMEDIC PRACTICE-BASED LEARNING

Paramedics have always undertaken some kind of practice-based learning, although it has not always been referred to as such. In the early days of the profession, from the late 1980s to the late 1990s, paramedics were members of the existing workforce who undertook additional training. A period of supervised practice was completed following initial emergency medical technician (EMT) training. After a period working as an EMT, a pre-dominantly skills-based paramedic course lasting around six to eight weeks was undertaken before paramedic placements were completed in hospital operating theatres and emergency departments. The focus of these place-ments was psychomotor skill consolidation, which included completing a set number of endotracheal tube insertions, canulations, intravenous giving set preparations and so on. The core objective of these placements was to hit the required number of interventions, often meaning running between operating theatres when there was a chance of intubating a patient!

There was limited support given to paramedics following the completion of their hospital placement, although some ambulance services did provide a period of mentorship to newly qualified paramedics. Alongside the evolution of the paramedic role away from that of a pre-hospital emergency clinician, tasked with conveying patients to hospital, and towards the out-of-hospital practitioner, managing a range of undifferentiated urgent and emergency presentations, was the development of higher education paramedic degree programmes.

The additional expectations of paramedics, including seeking to avoid unnecessary hospital admissions and instead making robust decisions regarding appropriate care pathways for service users, has increased the importance of robust approaches to practice-based learning. Develop-ing the cognitive skills to identify the most appropriate care pathway for patients, whilst also managing the unpredictable – and sometimes danger-ous – out-of-hospital environment, requires a level of self-awareness and cognition that was, arguably, not previously addressed in approaches to practice placements.

These changes in the role of the paramedic have been addressed by advances in paramedic education, with all new entrants to the HCPC regis-ter, since 2021, needing to have qualified with the equivalent of a bachelor of science degree qualification.

As the role of the paramedic further expanded, and the amount of theo-retical teaching increased significantly, the balance between classroom teaching and placement time shifted significantly in favour of the class-room. This required greater consideration being given to the nature of placements and their role within undergraduate paramedic education. It was concluded that, rather than 'placements', where the role and expectations of students were often unclear to all parties, practice-based learning would be approached from a position more aligned to the academic modules taken by the students – that is, explicitly clear learning outcomes were to be associated with placements, and the focus moved towards the achievement of these learning outcomes rather than the simple accrual of hours on placement.

Contemporary paramedic programmes should be expected to have robust practice-based learning systems underpinned by explicit learning outcomes and clear communication between the education provider and the place-ment provider to ensure that everyone knows exactly what is expected from the learner on placement.

THEORY, PRACTICE AND PARAMEDIC PRAXIS

The theory–practice gap

In general terms, the theory-practice gap can be defined as a discrepancy between what is taught in a classroom setting – the theoretical aspects of the role – and what is experienced on clinical placement – the reality of prac-tice. Recently, the existence of a theory–practice gap has been discussed in the context of various professions, including teaching, engineering, accounting, clinical medical practice, midwifery, nursing and physiotherapy, as well as paramedic practice (Michau et al., 2009; Donaghy, 2010; Armit-age, 2011; Edwards, 2011; Clarke, 2020).

To avoid theory being perceived as a 'utopia' or an 'ivory tower' position, that is not grounded in the lived experience of day-to-day practitioners, edu-cators are expected to ensure that taught theory accurately reflects the realities of practice while continuing to make theory input relevant to current practice in the professional setting (Corlett et al., 2003).

Although there is a general acceptance of the existence of a 'gap' between theory and practice, cited by both practitioners and theorists, the forms in which it is considered to emerge, and approaches to addressing it, differ. Concepts and theories such as boundary crossing (Engeström, 2000; Tsui and Law, 2007), social practice theory (Lave, 1996; Bourdieu, 2000), the the-ory of reflective practice (Schön, 1983) and cultural-historical activity theory (CHAT) (Cole and Engeström, 1993; Roth and Lee, 2007) all view the theory–practice gap differently.

Wortham (2010) considers that there is a gap but one between different domains of activity, holding the view that, when exploring how theory gets translated into practice, the use of a decontextualised, non-activity-based sense of knowledge has the potential to generate a 'gap' between theory and practice. However, as knowledge is always embedded in activities, there can be no such gap when knowledge is applied to practice. Wortham (2010) considers that the beliefs, habits and capacities of academic researchers differ from those of practitioners, with each having a distinct repertoire of practice, which, whilst they do overlap, are fundamentally different.

Using Wortham's position, it could be argued that university-based academics are more likely to build conceptual arguments and analyse data, while paramedic practice educators support their students to become more competent when participating in practice-based activities with a view to 'changing the world' (i.e. undertaking actions that have an external effect). That is not to lessen the role of either party but to determine that there are – and we should expect there to be – differences in the way in which academics and practitioners approach both theory and practice. If there were not such differences, then the value of undertaking practice-based learning as a core component of a paramedic programme, or any other professional programme, would be significantly reduced.

The theory–practice relationship

Clarke (2018) explored several considerations in the literature related to the perceived importance of theory, practice and knowledge. He identified a range of positions, including a hierarchical structure where theory underpins, leads and informs practice, in contrast to the position that practice takes 'precedence' and is more important than the idealised world view considered to be presented by theory (Clarke, 2018). Clarke's conclusions were that perceptions of the theory-practice relationship are less straightforward, with the relationship between theory and practice not so clearly delineated, or so obviously hierarchical in structure, supporting Carr's (1995) and Misawa's (2011) views of the inseparability of theory and practice.

Such a position informed the concept whereby theory and practice, being closely integrated entities, are of equal import with each continually informing the other; a concept described by Misawa (2011: 694) as 'interpenetrating'. This representation is considered by Clarke (2018) to be one of a 'healthy' theory–practice relationship. Clarke further considered that the interrelation and integration of theory and practice is a continuously iterative process that is only formalised during focused feedback and reflection-on-action. Such a view informed the model presented below: the overlap

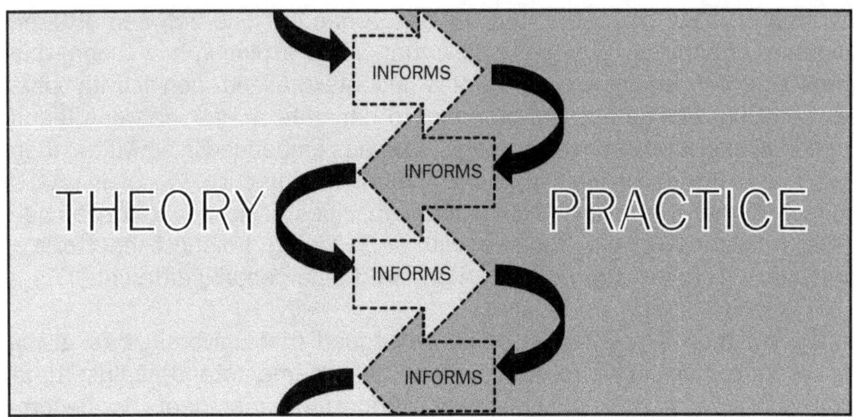

Figure 20.1 The theory–practice relationship

Source: Clarke (2018).

between theory and practice represents the cyclic nature of the relationship where both theory and practice continuously interact to develop 'paramedic praxis'. This concept can be seen to align with that described by Misawa (2011: 695) as 'intertwined and shifting', and the view of Carr (1995), Rolfe (1996) and Misawa (2011) of the distinction between theory and practice being an unhelpful one.

Within the overlap between theory and practice falls the very important educational tool of simulation (see Figure 20.1). Simulation provides an effective link between the theory of a practical activity and the physical application of that activity, an application that can take place in the safety of the educational setting prior to engaging with service users during practice-based learning.

Paramedic praxis

Clarke (2018, 2020) proposes an alternative to the concept of a theory–practice gap in the form of 'paramedic praxis'. Rolfe (1996) proposed a model of nursing praxis which he considered to facilitate the 'dissolution' of the theory–practice gap considered to exist within nursing education at the time. Clarke (2018) deconstructed Rolfe's model and rebuilt it based on the findings of research specific to paramedic undergraduate practice-based learning. The resultant model can be considered to represent a theory-of-practice (McIntyre and Murphy, 2016), a model which develops consideration of the theory–practice *relationship* rather than focusing on the negativity associated with a theory–practice gap.

The notion of a 'healthy' theory–practice relationship is considered to be an appropriately balanced relationship between theory and practice. That is not to say that theory and practice should always be considered equally balanced at all times and in all situations, rather that the degree to which one is reliant on the considerations of either element will depend on the circumstances and situation in which one finds oneself.

One way of viewing this notion would be to consider the student who is preparing for an upcoming written examination in pathophysiology. It would be expected that, in their approach to this task, considerations of formal theory would heavily outweigh considerations of practice, although components of such formal theory may well have been reinforced and consolidated by previous exposure to case examples whilst experiencing practice-based learning. When the same student subsequently undertakes treating a patient in the practice setting, the balance of their consideration will shift towards situated practice, whilst still being supported by the theory previously engaged with when focusing on the written examination.

In this respect, a 'healthy' theory–practice relationship can be seen to be one where the component elements presented within the praxis model are not necessarily drawn upon simultaneously or considered in all situations. Paramedic praxis is, therefore, a considerably broader construct than the two overarching components of 'theory' and 'practice', incorporating as it does reflection and knowledge as inseparable components of the theory–practice relationship.

It is, therefore, the ability to consider all the circumstances surrounding a particular, individual situation, including a commitment to human wellbeing and respect for others, which distinguishes the informed, committed action of praxis.

Clarke's simplified model of paramedic praxis is represented by the zip analogy (Clarke, 2018, 2020). In the zip analogy, theory and practice are presented as two sides of a zipper, with the teeth of the zip representing individual components of the taught curriculum on one side (i.e. the 'theory') and experiences gained in practice-based learning, or simulation, represented by the teeth on the other side (i.e. the 'practice') (see Figure 20.2). The learner is the 'slider' of the zip, the part that brings together the two aspects of theory and practice into a single element, that of paramedic praxis. The learner is the only individual to experience both the theory of the education setting and the practice of practice-based learning. As such, they are responsible for robustly linking both concepts and experiences to develop their personal professional practice, ideally by making effective use of facilitated reflection.

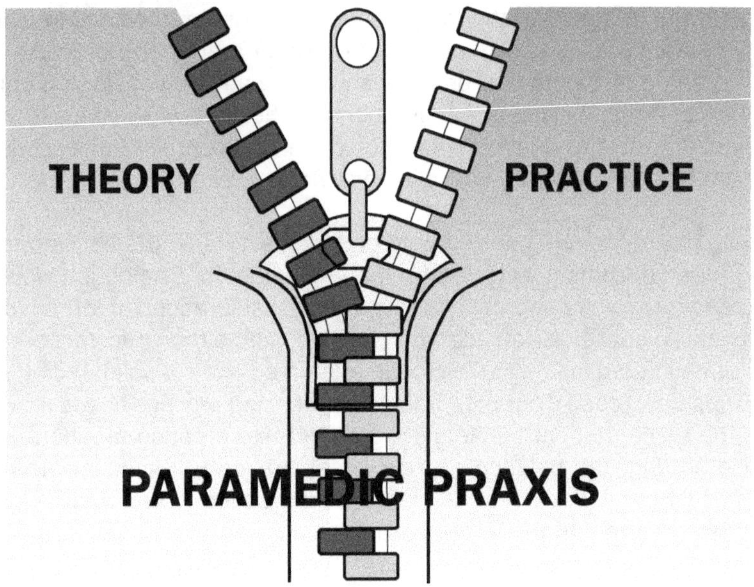

Figure 20.2 Paramedic praxis: the zip analogy

Source: Clarke (2018).

The 'pull-tab' of the zip, the part that is attached to the slider, and makes the doing up of the zip considerably easier, represents the practice educator, whose role is to facilitate learning. An effective learning relationship between the learner and the practice educator enhances the bringing together of the theory and practice components of the educational pathway.

APPROACHES TO PRACTICE-BASED LEARNING

Communities of practice

Practice placements allow students many opportunities to develop as clinicians. As well as being able to practise their clinical skills, students begin to develop a professional identity while increasing their knowledge base and transferring classroom knowledge to the clinical setting (Kirkpatrick et al., 1991; Wills, 1997; Atack et al., 2000), becoming part of what Wenger describes as a community of practice (Wenger, 1998; Wenger et al., 2002). This is a group of people who interact on a regular basis, united by a shared interest or profession and the value that they place on learning in that area.

The student body and the ambulance service practice educators could be considered to represent separate communities of practice, with an overlap of membership during periods of practice placement. The wider ambulance service could also be representative of a community of practice; however, it could be questioned whether all members of that wider community place value on learning (Wenger, 1998). During practice placement, student paramedics' social interactions with, and contributions to, the community of practice go towards constructing their professional identity, a process termed 'situated learning' (Lave and Wenger, 1991). When students are placed with multiple practice educators, they are exposed to a diverse range of previous experiences. A key challenge is how the student can best utilise such diversity for the development of their own knowledge and, therefore, their own subsequent practice, without perceiving 'mixed messages' or potentially conflicting viewpoints.

Lane (2014) discusses how the one-on-one practice educator model required in the ambulance service setting may lead to students placing significant emphasis on developing a good working relationship with their practice educator. The very nature of the paramedic role, where student and practice educator are in very close physical proximity as well as sharing the inherent emotional challenges presented by the situations in which they find themselves, lends itself to the forming of very strong emotional links (Williams, 2013). By comparison, students in other healthcare professions are generally supported in a wider team context and can form different relationships with different team members, depending on their needs and wants at the time. The student paramedic does not have the same range of options available to them during ambulance service practice-based learning, although this may be possible in other settings.

Being aware of the potential challenges within the learner–practice educator relationship can help both parties avoid the development of a toxic learning relationship and focus on establishing a healthy learning relationship, where boundaries are clear and respected. It is also important for learners to remember that their practice educator's focus in relation to the theory–practice relationship may be different to their own. A practice educator supports learners in the practice setting, where behaviour, skills and attitude may be considered of greater importance than overt demonstrations of theoretical knowledge.

The practice educator

Practice educators can be considered facilitators of learning, rather than teachers. Bentley (1994) highlighted the difference between teaching and facilitating learning, in that facilitators concentrate on providing the resources and opportunities for learning to take place, rather than managing and controlling learning. The majority of NHS Ambulance Trusts in the UK provide their practice educators with some degree of formal training, often developing partnerships with universities to deliver such programmes. One key aim of delivering such training is to attempt to provide student paramedics with a standardised approach to their placements, regardless of who their practice educator is. Unfortunately, despite this formal training, poor practice placement experiences still occur. Being well prepared for practice-based learning can help learners to reduce the chances of a poor experience.

Working with your practice educator

The nature of paramedic practice-based learning is such that the learner is often supported by a paramedic practice educator when working on a front-line ambulance service resource, such as an ambulance or a rapid response car. In these situations, the learner–practice educator relationship is key to ensuring a healthy and effective learning environment. In cases where the relationship is not productive and conducive to learning, the learner will not progress as effectively, and the practice educator will likely become disengaged from facilitating learning. As a learner, it is important to remember that your practice educator's primary role is to deliver patient-centred care to service users. As such, they may not be able to facilitate learning or to fully engage you in every aspect of every patient encounter. Being mindful of the hierarchy of priorities for the practice educator can help the learner to plan for their learning and to make the most of their experiences at the most opportune time.

One of the key methods of achieving a healthy learning environment is for the learner to be proactive in identifying how they will work with the practice educator to facilitate learning. These principles can be applied to all practice-based learning environments, especially those in which paramedics are less frequently employed. In the first instance, there should be an initial meeting at the very beginning of the placement or, if possible, before the first shift, between the learner and the practice educator. This initial meeting should be used by the learner to introduce themselves and set out their needs for the upcoming practice-based learning experience (see Box 20.2). Learners should remember that practice educators will be responsible for supporting a range of students from different education providers, different professional groups and at different stages of their programme. It would be unrealistic for learners to expect their practice educator, amongst their everyday responsibilities as a paramedic/healthcare professional, to know all about the learner's individual circumstances and/or the exact remit of their placement.

> ## Box 20.2 Initial learner/practice educator meeting checklist
>
> - Introduction and background
> - Identify learning outcomes
> - Identify strengths
> - Clarify scope of practice
> - Identify specific, individual areas for focused development
> - Agree on approaches to coaching, direction and feedback
> - Agree on how and when documentation will be completed
> - Agree on how the learner can raise concerns with the practice educator
> - Confirm support systems for both the learner and practice educator

Clearly setting out the learning outcomes of the placement, alongside any individual areas of development identified by the learner, or their previous practice educators, is essential in preparing both parties for the placement. Explicitly identifying the scope of practice of the learner at the earliest opportunity is also key to success. Again, this is most important in settings considered less traditional for paramedics and the remit of the paramedic learner may not be well understood by all. The expectations of a practice educator in relation to a final-year student on their final placement can be reasonably expected to differ to their expectations of a first-year student on their first placement.

Planning for feedback

Feedback is essential for development. Having the external, objective observations of your practice educator enables you to better engage in effective reflection.

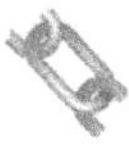 **Chapter 2** for more detail on reflection and reflective frameworks.

Discussing approaches to feedback before there is any feedback given is important in establishing an effective learning environment and an effective learning relationship. Feedback can be given before, during or after a patient encounter, or a combination of all three. Agreeing on parameters for discussion about feedback is also important. There may be circumstances where the practice educator's priority for patient care requires them to be very directive in their approach to the learner, telling them what to do and not having an opportunity to discuss the whys and wherefores of what they are instructing. On other occasions, the practice educator can take a more facilitative approach to learning, whereby the learner can be coached through a patient encounter by in-action feedback and prompting, to enable the learner to actively engage in delivering care while simultaneously ensuring that the patient is the focus of the encounter. Having a clear understanding of which approach is to be adopted, and when, can make both the learner and the practice educator more comfortable when giving and receiving feedback.

Receiving feedback

Everyone's considerations around feedback are different. Some learners crave positive comments, others can be hypercritical of their own performance; some dread feedback, others love it. Feedback is your opportunity to develop.

Sometimes feedback can be overwhelming! In some cases, practice educators may have a list of every aspect of a patient encounter that could have been approached differently by the learner. As a learner, having such a list presented to you can be very disheartening. This is where feedback in-action can reduce the amount of feedback given on the conclusion of an incident, with the opportunity then given for key learning points to be focused on and explored in greater depth.

As a learner, you must be receptive to feedback and accept it in the spirit in which it is given – that is, to develop you to the level required to register as a paramedic. You must also be mindful of your approach and reflect, honestly, on your performance. There can be a tendency to become defensive when reviewing aspects of one's own practice-based experiences. Having the maturity and insight to consider the feedback offered is key in developing the skills required for continued reflective practice and professional behaviours.

Feedback is given by practice educators, and others, to learners with the aim of enabling reflection and subsequent development of the learner. It is difficult for learners to not take feedback personally, but it is important to separate the person from the performance. Consider your approaches to service users as your 'performance', in the same way that an athlete will undertake an event and their performance will be reviewed and fed back to them by their coach/trainer. The feedback is about what was done, and not done, and should be presented as an objective perspective of performance.

Feedback is not a personal assault on the learner as an individual. The learner's personality and psyche are not being evaluated – their performance is. As a learner, preparing yourself for objective, factual feedback, and being able to accept that feedback, is important for moving forward and developing.

GETTING THE MOST FROM PRACTICE-BASED LEARNING

Practice-based learning can be very challenging for a wide variety of reasons. Learners have their own challenges outside of their educational programme which may impact on their ability to fully demonstrate their competence in practice. One of the most important things a learner can do is *be open* with their practice educator. Sharing concerns, challenges and self-identified areas for development helps build a trusting learning relationship between the learner and the practice educator. Similarly, practice educators have a range of responsibilities above and beyond supporting a learner in practice, and this needs to be appreciated by all.

There will be times, however, when the relationship between the learner and the practice educator is not developing well and the learner's experience is significantly impacted by it. In a high proportion of cases, this is down to poor communication, either between the learner and the practice educator, or between the two of them and the education provider. Expectations on all sides need to be realistic and achievable. Where a practice educator expects a learner to be able to undertake a full clinical assessment of a patient, but the learner has yet to cover all the relevant areas in their training, the practice educator may consider the learner to lack competence, which would not be a fair assessment of the reasonably expected level of the learner and may tarnish the practice educator's perception of the learner's ability.

All placement providers will have some sort of support mechanism in place for learners. It is vitally important to access these mechanisms as early as possible if there are any potential problems identified (see Box 20.3). Support can be broadly categorised into 'pastoral' and 'academic'.

Pastoral support

Pastoral support is that which is offered to ensure the physical and emotional welfare of the recipient. In the case of education providers, this support is generally provided at a programme level (e.g. module leads and/or personal tutors) and at an institutional level (e.g. student wellbeing, occupational health, student counselling services). When studying, learners should be

---

> ## Box 20.3 Tip for practice – seek support early
>
> Learners should seek support from their lecturers and/or link tutors at the earliest opportunity. If there is a miscommunication or a perception of unrealistic expectations, a meeting between the learner, the practice educator and the link tutor/lecturer can help to clear up any issues and support both the learner and the practice educator to move forward. There is often trepidation on the part of learners to 'report' any issues with their practice educator as they perceive that this would be 'rocking the boat'. Learners should feel supported and welcomed in whatever practice-learning setting they enter. The organisational culture and individual attitudes among some staff may make learners feel uncomfortable. If this is the case, do not be afraid to discuss the situation with your link tutor/lecturer.

able to access these services through the processes of their education provider. During practice-based learning, these mechanisms, whilst still available, may be less immediate than the support mechanisms in place within the placement provider organisation. Most placement agreements between education providers and ambulance services include a provision for the immediate pastoral care provided to staff to be extended to learners. Examples of this include 'hot debriefs' of incidents as well as opportunities to discuss experiences with peer counsellors. Learners should make sure that they are clear as to what immediate provision they can access from the placement provider to prevent delays in accessing support through other mechanisms.

Practice educators are important in the pastoral care of learners. It is often the practice educator who first notices that a learner is struggling or has problems (see Box 20.4). Support structures should clearly identify how practice educators can raise their concerns over a learner's wellbeing with the education provider. This is where the link tutor role is vital in supporting both the learner and the practice educator in their support of the learner.

Academic support

Learners sometimes lose sight of the fact that practice-based learning is a core component of their academic progression to registered status, perhaps seeing it as an add-on to their degree rather than being integral to it. The meeting of learning outcomes in practice can be considered to fall under the 'academic' umbrella and, as such, appropriate support should be sought by learners and practice educators alike. Box 20.5 provides some guidance regarding practice assessment documentation. As with pastoral support, there

---

Box 20.4 Triggering incidents

Some organisations identify circumstances, or patient presentations, which, when attended by staff, would automatically trigger a referral for a wellbeing check very soon after the incident. Examples include paediatric cardiac arrests, hangings, road traffic collisions resulting in fatalities, etc. It is important to remember that seemingly routine encounters, not like those identified above, may be triggers for individuals based on their own circumstances at the time. Do not be afraid to seek support simply because it is not immediately offered.

---

should be clearly defined mechanisms for learners and practice educators to access academic support, with link tutors again being key to the successful application of such mechanisms. Learners may need support in practice when they realise that their knowledge and understanding of a concept or process is not at the required level. See box 20.6 for details on developmental action plans. It may be too onerous for the practice educator to seek to address the identified learning need, whereas their liaising with link tutors and academic staff would go towards the facilitation of learning opportunities which could run alongside practice-based learning to augment learning. In this respect, learners must not be afraid to report back to their education provider, via their link tutor, if they are having any difficulties when in a practice-based learning setting. Support can only be given if those responsible for arranging it are fully aware of the learner's needs.

Box 20.5 Tip for practice – keep on top of practice assessment documentation

Practice educators are, first and foremost, paramedics who are responsible for delivering patient care. Part of their role as a practice educator is to support learners and evaluate their development, record meetings and complete documentation as required. Learners *must*, however, take full responsibility for getting their practice educator to complete any practice assessment documentation. The learner will always be more familiar with their education provider's documentation than their practice educator, whether it be a paper-based system or an electronic one. As such, the onus is on the learner to approach the practice educator throughout their placement to ensure that documentation is completed in a timely fashion. It is unfair, and unreasonable, to wait until the last day of a placement block/period before presenting documentation for completion.

Learning differences

Some learners will have been diagnosed with a developmental condition, such as dyslexia, dyspraxia and/or autistic spectrum disorder (ASD). The Equality Act 2010 (not applicable in Northern Ireland) recognises these conditions, meaning that it is against the law for individuals with these conditions to be treated unfavourably, either by employers or by educators. Under the legislation, employers and education providers have a duty to make 'reasonable adjustments' to ensure that such individuals are not discriminated against. For education providers, such changes might include providing extra support, additional time for assessments or aids, such as computers or recording devices for revision. Making the same adjustments in the practice-based learning environment is sometimes not so straightforward.

Some learners may require their practice educator to adapt their teaching approach. This can only be accomplished if the practice educator is made aware of the specific needs of the individual learner. Education providers generally produce study needs agreements, in conjunction with their learning support team, that should be used to enable discussion between the learner, the practice educator and, if necessary, the link tutor/lecturer.

Challenges in practice-based learning

One of the most reported challenges experienced by learners is that of the practice educator 'stepping in' and taking over the patient encounter when the learner was 'just about' to move on to the next stage of their assessment/treatment. The main reason why this occurs is that the practice educator, through their experience and tacit understanding of the situation, is several steps ahead of the learner in their thinking. The perspective of the learner is that they are going through their procedures in a step-wise, methodical way. The perception of the practice educator is that the learner should have already reached the end of the process. These different approaches to thinking are summarised in Figure 20.3 (Clarke, 2018).

In the figure, the practice educator's decision pathway, 'A', is much shorter than the learner's, 'A' to 'E'. In practice, this may be only a matter of several seconds, but differing perceptions can adversely impact on the practice educator's ability to 'hold back' and let the learner think through the situation. A great technique for avoiding any confusion in this type of situation is for the learner to present a verbal commentary on their actions and thoughts, an approach which not only keeps the practice educator informed, but also goes to improve communication with the service user and others on scene.

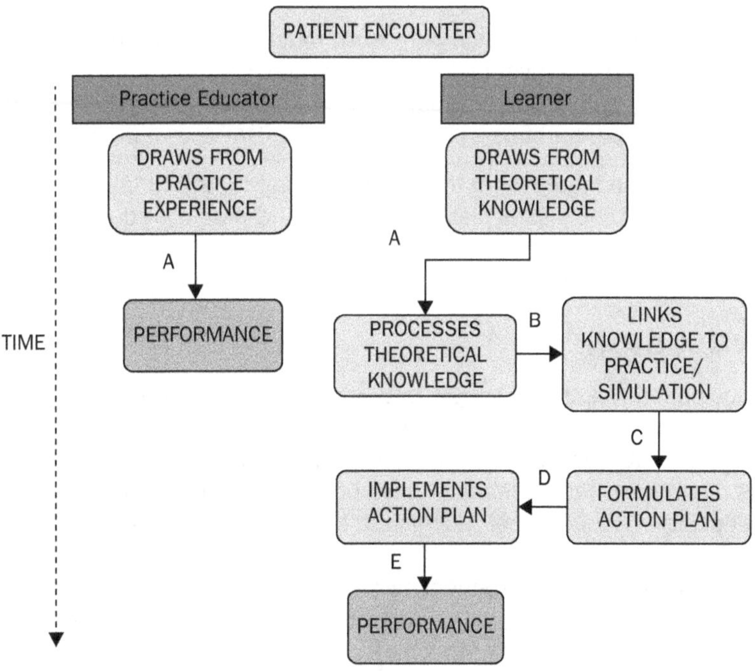

Figure 20.3 Practice educator and learner – the application of theory to practice

---

Box 20.6 Tip for practice – developmental action plans

Developmental action plans (DAPs) are used by practice educators to clearly identify which aspects of a learner's performance, knowledge, understanding or behaviour do not yet meet the required standard. Unfortunately, DAPs tend to be associated with a negative perspective and are rarely welcomed by learners. DAPs should not be viewed as a punishment, or a notification of failure; rather they are a tool for clearly setting out which areas of practice the learner needs to develop. DAPs should follow the SMART principles:

- **S**pecific: identify exactly what behaviour, skill or area of understanding needs to be developed.
- **M**easurable: the area being developed must be able to be objectively observed to have improved.
- **A**chievable: the area being developed must be within the expected scope of the learner at the current stage of their programme.

- **R**elevant: the development need must be relevant to the learner's achievement of success.
- **T**ime-limited: a review point, where the remit of the DAP will be reviewed, must be set at the time the DAP is put in place.

Learners should make sure that their DAPs follow the SMART principles and, if they do not, seek clarification from the practice educator or link tutor.

CONCLUSION

Practice-based learning is an essential aspect of a learner's development. It can be daunting, challenging, exhilarating, rewarding and exhausting! It is your opportunity to bring together all of your learning and apply it to service users. Learners should embrace the experience and work closely with practice educators to direct their learning in a way that suits them.

Relating practice-based experiences directly to the learning undertaken in the classroom is key to the development of effective reflective practice and should be undertaken throughout one's career.

Chapter key points:

- Effective practice-based learning is reliant on the learner's full engagement and immersion in learning.
- Practice educators are responsible for facilitating learning.
- Maintaining documentation is key.

REFERENCES AND SUGGESTED READING

Armitage, E. (2011) Role of paramedic mentors in an evolving profession, *Journal of Paramedic Practice*, 2 (1): 26–31.

Atack, L., Comacu, M., Kenny, R., LaBelle, N. et al. (2000) Student and staff relationships in a clinical practice model: impact on learning, *Journal of Nursing Education*, 39 (9): 387–400.

Bentley, T. (1994) *Facilitation: Providing Opportunities for Learning.* Maidenhead: McGraw-Hill.

Bourdieu, P. (2000) *Pascalian Meditations.* Stanford, CA: Stanford University Press.

Carr, W. (1995) *For Education: Towards Critical Educational Enquiry.* Buckingham: Open University Press.

Clarke, V. (2018) *The theory-practice relationship in paramedic undergraduate education*, Unpublished doctoral thesis, University of Hertfordshire, Hatfield. Available at: https://uhra.herts.ac.uk/handle/2299/21089.

Clarke, V. (ed.) (2020) *Paramedic Practice-Based Learning: A Handbook for Practice Educators and Facilitators*. Bridgwater: College of Paramedics.

Cole, M. and Engeström, Y. (1993) A cultural historical approach to distributed cognition, in G. Salomon (ed.) *Distributed Cognitions: Psychological and Educational Considerations*. Cambridge: Cambridge University Press.

Corlett, J., Palfreyman, J.W., Staines, H.J. and Marr, H. (2003) Factors influencing theoretical knowledge and practical skill acquisition in student nurses: an empirical experiment, *Nurse Education Today*, 23 (3): 183–90.

Donaghy, J. (2010) Equipping the student for workplace changes in paramedic education, *Journal of Paramedic Practice*, 2 (11): 524–28.

Edwards, D. (2011) Paramedic preceptor: work readiness in graduate paramedics, *The Clinical Teacher*, 8 (2): 79–82.

Engeström, Y. (2000) Activity theory as a framework for analyzing and redesigning work, *Ergonomics*, 43 (7): 960–74.

Health and Care Professions Council (HCPC) (2018) *Standards of Continuing Professional Development*. Available at: https://www.hcpc-uk.org/standards/standards-of-continuing-professional-development/.

Health and Care Professions Council (HCPC) (2023) *Standards of Proficiency for Paramedics*. Available at: https://www.hcpc-uk.org/standards/standards-of-proficiency/paramedics/.

Kirkpatrick, H., Byrne, C., Martin, M. and Roth, M. (1991) A collaborative model for the clinical education of baccalaureate nursing students, *Journal of Advanced Nursing*, 16 (1): 101–7.

Lane, M. (2014) Student perceptions in relation to paramedic educator (PEd) roles, *Journal of Paramedic Practice*, 6 (4): 194–99.

Lave, J. (1996) Teaching, as learning, in practice, *Mind, Culture, and Activity*, 3 (3): 149–64.

Lave, J. and Wenger, E. (1991) *Situated Learning: Legitimate Peripheral Participation*. Cambridge: Cambridge University Press.

Legislation.gov.uk (2010) *Equality Act 2010*. Available at: https://www.legislation.gov.uk/ukpga/2010/15/contents.

McIntyre, M.L. and Murphy, S.A. (2016) The theory of practice and the practice of theory, *Industry and Higher Education*, 30 (2): 109–16.

Michau, R., Roberts, S., Williams, B. and Boyle, M. (2009) An investigation of theory-practice gap in undergraduate paramedic education, *BMC Medical Education*, 9: 23. Available at: https://doi.org/10.1186/1472-6920-9-23.

Misawa, K. (2011) The Hirst-Carr debate revisited: beyond the theory-practice dichotomy, *Journal of Philosophy of Education*, 45 (4): 689–702.

Rolfe, G. (1996) *Closing the Theory-Practice Gap*. Oxford: Butterworth Heinemann.

Roth, W.M and Lee, Y.J. (2007) Vygotsky's neglected legacy: cultural-historical activity theory, *Review of Educational Research*, 77 (2): 186–232.

Schön, D.A. (1983) *The Reflective Practitioner*. London: Temple Smith.

Tsui, A.B.M. and Law, D.Y.K. (2007) Learning as boundary-crossing in a school-university partnership, *Teachers and Teacher Education*, 23 (8): 1289–1301.

Wenger, E. (1998) *Communities of Practice: Learning, Meaning and Identity*. Cambridge: Cambridge University Press.

Wenger, E., McDermott, R. and Snyder, W.M. (2002) *Cultivating Communities of Practice: A Guide to Managing Knowledge*. Boston, MA: Harvard Business School Press.

Williams, A. (2013) The strategies used to deal with emotion work in student paramedic practice, *Nurse Education in Practice*, 13 (3): 207–12.

Wills, M. (1997) Link teacher behaviours: student nurses' perceptions, *Nurse Education Today*, 17 (3): 232–46.

Wortham, S. (2010) Redefining the gap between theory and practice: should anthropologists try to change the world?, *Anthropology News*, 51 (6): 31–32.

21 Continuing professional development pre- and post-registration

Graham Harris and Bob Fellows

In this chapter:

- Introduction
- Why is this relevant?
- Pre-registration and the role of the HCPC
- Post-registration and the role of the HCPC
- What is continuing professional development?
- Standards for CPD
- The HCPC audit
- Examples of types of CPD activity
- The purpose of each part of the profile
- What happens to your completed CPD profile?
- Conclusion
- Chapter key points
- References
- Useful websites

INTRODUCTION

This chapter incorporates the appropriate and updated information from the third edition of the text. It includes and differentiates between continuing professional development (CPD) for the pre-registered student and the registrant paramedic on their CPD requirements. From the perspective of the regulatory body the Health and Care Professions Council (HCPC), there are differing CPD requirements for a pre-registered student and the registrant paramedic who needs to maintain registration as a paramedic and continue to practise safely and effectively by maintaining their skills and knowledge in their field of practice.

WHY IS THIS RELEVANT?

Whether you are a student on a HCPC-approved programme of education leading to eligibility to apply to the register, or an existing qualified and registrant paramedic with the HCPC, we all as health professionals need to maintain a continuous and accurate record and be able to demonstrate that on request as part of our own CPD.

PRE-REGISTRATION AND THE ROLE OF THE HCPC

To be eligible to register with the regulatory body and use the protected title of 'paramedic', the student paramedic needs to successfully complete a pre-registration programme of education and training that meets the requirements of the registrant body, currently the Health and Care Professions Council. A programme which meets the *Standards of Education and Training* (SETs) (HCPC, 2017a) allows a student who successfully completes that programme to meet the *Standards of Proficiency for Paramedics* (HCPC, 2023). They are then eligible to apply to the HCPC for registration. To enable an education provider – a higher education institute (HEI) or university – to deliver such a programme, they must apply to the HCPC for the programme to be approved. The pre-registration programme curriculum would be mapped against and meet the following standards:

- College of Paramedics (CoP) *Paramedic Curriculum Guidance*, 5th edition (2019);
- Quality Assurance Agency (QAA) Subject Benchmark Statement for Paramedics (2019);
- HCPC Standards of Education and Training (2017a);
- HCPC *Standards of Proficiency for Paramedics* (2023).

As a student on such a programme, you will be expected to adhere to the *Guidance on Conduct and Ethics for Students* (HCPC, 2016), and aspire to the *Standards of Conduct, Performance and Ethics* (HCPC, 2024). You will need to compile and maintain a continuous 'portfolio of evidence', which will provide confirmation of your CPD throughout your education and training. Successful completion of such a programme entitles you to be eligible to apply for registration with the HCPC as a paramedic. Once registered, you should continue CPD and lifelong learning throughout your career, as it is a significant part of the re-registration process undertaken by registrant paramedics every two years.

POST-REGISTRATION AND THE ROLE OF THE HCPC

The regulatory body requires all registrants to meet their *Standards of Continuing Professional Development* (HCPC, 2017b). To assist registrants to meet these standards, the regulatory body published information for registrants in the document entitled *Continuing Professional Development and Your Registration* (HCPC, 2017c). The HCPC carries out an audit each time a professional renews their registration – every two years – to make sure that their standards are being met. This requires the paramedic to sign a 'professional declaration' as part of the re-registration process (HCPC, 2017d). Signing the declaration confirms that the paramedic has:

- continued to practise their profession since the last registration, or
- not practised their profession since the last registration, but has met the 'Returning to Practice' (HCPC, 2017e) requirements.

They are also confirming that:

- they continue to meet the HCPC *Standards of Proficiency for Paramedics.*
- since the last registration, there has been no change relating to their good character (this includes any conviction or caution that they are required to disclose), or any change to their health that may affect their ability to practise safely and effectively.
- they continue to meet the HCPC *Standards of Continuing Professional Development.*
- they either have a professional indemnity arrangement in place which provides appropriate cover, or they are not practising at the time of their renewal, but understand the requirement to have a professional indemnity in place which provides appropriate cover, and will have this in place when they practise.

To stay registered, you will need to ensure that you continue to meet all of the above standards and can sign the professional declaration on your renewal form. Bear in mind that if you come off the register, you will not be able to use the title 'paramedic' to refer to yourself or to your work. You should also consider that you may need to update your skills to come back onto the register at a future date. The regulatory body's document stipulates their requirements for individual registrants to update their knowledge and skills before returning to practice as follows (HCPC, 2017e: 8):

- *0 to 2 years out of practice – no requirements*

- *2 to 5 years out of practice – 30 days of updating*

- *5 or more years out of practice – 60 days of updating*

In the 'days' requirements above, we consider one day to be equivalent to seven hours.

For the purpose of registration renewal, the HCPC defines 'practising your profession' as 'drawing on your professional skills and knowledge in the course of your work'. Therefore, if you work in education, leadership and management, or research and development, the HCPC regards this as practising your profession. If you have moved to a non-clinical area of work but wish to stay on the register, you need to ensure that you keep up to date with your professional skills and knowledge and that you stay within your scope of practice. If you return to clinical work or change your scope of practice, then you may need to update your skills.

When you are planning or undertaking your CPD, you will need to make sure that it is relevant to your current or future role in your work. Similarly, to stay registered, you need to make sure you keep within the 'scope of your practice'. This refers to the particular area in which you are trained to practise – lawfully, safely and effectively in a way that meets the HCPC Standards and does not present any risk to patients, the public or to yourself. Scope of practice may vary between paramedics and will relate to job role, experience and training. For example, two paramedics both met the *Standards of Proficiency for Paramedics* (HCPC, 2023), but then went on to develop in different areas. If they were then to perform one another's role without training, they may be practising outside their scope of practice, as their lack of experience in the different area may lead to unsafe practice, or pose a risk to patients or to themselves.

The *Standards of Proficiency for Paramedics* are the standards which every registrant paramedic must meet in order to be registered and must continue to meet in order to stay on the register. They set out the required knowledge, understanding and skills for the practice of paramedics. Registrants must also read and agree to abide by the HCPC's *Standards of Conduct, Performance and Ethics* (HCPC, 2024) and adhere to the confidentiality guidance for registrants (HCPC, 2017f).

If someone is no longer fit to practise their profession and does not remove themselves voluntarily, the HCPC can take action using the 'fitness to practise' process. If you feel that for any reason, you no longer meet the HCPC Standards, then you should seriously consider coming off the register. This is known as professional self-regulation, which means that you (the registrant) are in the best position to judge your ability to practise safely and lawfully. It is your responsibility to stay on the register, or to decide if you need to come off for any reason. Likewise, you need to inform the HCPC of any changes in your circumstances which may affect your ability to practise safely. It is felt that as an accountable registered professional, you are in the best position to make professional judgements of this nature and the HCPC trusts you to do so.

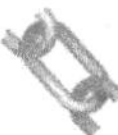 **Chapter 4** for more detail on fitness to practise and professional regulation.

WHAT IS CONTINUING PROFESSIONAL DEVELOPMENT)?

The HCPC defines continuing professional development as follows: 'CPD is the way in which registrants continue to learn and develop throughout their careers, so they keep their skills and knowledge up to date and are able to practise safely and effectively' (HCPC, 2017c: 5). The Interprofessional CPD and Lifelong Learning UK Working Group define CPD as: 'The way in which you continue to learn and develop throughout your career. CPD is essential. It adds to your skills, knowledge, professional identity, and ways of thinking so that you stay up to date and practise safely and effectively, now and in the future' (Broughton and Harris, 2022: 4). Quite simply, CPD is not only about undertaking formal courses but any activity from which you learn and develop, and can include work-based learning, professional activity, formal education and self-directed learning.

Why do I need to record my CPD?

In addition to being linked to your HCPC registration, CPD is an essential part of your development as a professional. Recording your CPD is as valuable as doing your CPD in the first place. However, without the evidence of the value of your CPD, how will you be able to demonstrate and show how it really was worthwhile to your service, personal development and patient care? In essence, if you do not have an up-to-date continuous record of your CPD, you cannot demonstrate that you have grown professionally and maintained your own development.

STANDARDS FOR CPD

Paramedic registrants must do the following (HCPC, 2017c: 5):

1 *maintain a continuous, up-to-date and accurate record of their CPD activities [Note: Registrant assessors would expect no unaccounted gaps of 3 months or more];*

2. *demonstrate that their CPD activities are a mixture of learning activities relevant to current or future practice;*

3. *seek to ensure that their CPD has contributed to the quality of their practice and service delivery;*

4. *seek to ensure that their CPD benefits the service user; and*

5. *upon request, present a written profile (which must be their own work and supported by evidence) explaining how they have met the Standards for CPD.*

Additional guidance is available on the College of Paramedics website.

THE HCPC AUDIT

To assist registrants who are selected to submit a CPD profile as part of the re-registration audit process, the regulatory body published 'How to Complete Your Continuing Professional Development Profile' (HCPC, 2017g). In 2021, the HCPC published its latest paramedic CPD audit, which included the CPD audit statistics for the 2019–21 renewal cycle (HCPC, 2021). A total of 649 paramedics were asked to present their CPD profile. Of these, 525 (80.9 per cent) were accepted, 72 (11.1 per cent) deferred, 29 (4.5 per cent) did not renew their registration, 16 (2.5 per cent) voluntarily deregistered, none were removed from the register and 7 (1 per cent) were still awaiting (4 of the latter 7 audits were awaiting 'fitness to practise' outcomes – CPD on hold).

If you are audited, the HCPC will give you a form to fill in – the CPD profile. In it, you must write a statement which informs them how your CPD has met the standards. When you return this, you must also provide supporting evidence from your personal CPD record. You need to complete your CPD profile honestly and accurately. If you provide false or misleading information in your CPD profile, the HCPC could begin the process to bring a fitness to practise charge. This could lead to you being struck off the register, meaning that you could no longer practise.

EXAMPLES OF TYPES OF CPD ACTIVITY

The following are activities that the HCPC suggests might make up your CPD profile (HCPC, 2017c: 19).

Work-based learning
- Learning by doing
- Case studies
- Reflective practice
- Coaching from others
- Audit of service users
- Peer review
- Discussions with colleagues
- Gaining and learning from experience
- Involvement in the wider, profession-related work of your employer (e.g. member of a committee)
- Job rotation
- Journal club
- In-service training
- Expanding your role
- Project work or project management
- Secondments
- Supervising staff or students (practice educator)
- Filling in self-assessment questionnaires
- Significant analysis of events
- Work shadowing

Professional activity
- Being a national assessor
- Being a tutor
- Being an external examiner
- Being an expert witness
- Organising journal clubs or other specialist groups
- Giving presentations at conferences
- Involvement in your professional body (special interest group or other group)
- Lecturing or teaching
- Maintaining or developing specialist skills (e.g. musical skills)
- Mentoring or coaching new staff (preceptor or practice educator)

- Organising accredited courses
- Supervising research or students

Formal/educational
- Attending conferences (e.g. College of Paramedics National Conference, UK Student Paramedic Conference, Life Connections, Emergency Services Show) – note that attendance is not enough; registrants would also need to show what learning took place
- Courses accredited by your professional body (College of Paramedics)
- Distance or online learning
- Further education
- Going to seminars
- Planning or running a course
- Research and audit
- Writing or editing a chapter in a book
- Writing articles or papers

Self-directed learning
- Keeping a file of your progress
- Reading journals/articles (e.g. *British Paramedic Journal, Emergency Medicine Journal*)
- Reviewing books or articles
- Updating knowledge through the internet or TV

Other
- Public service
- Voluntary work

THE PURPOSE OF EACH PART OF THE PROFILE

The CPD profile has four parts:

- summary of practice history (up to 500 words);
- statement of how you met the standards (up to 1,500 words);
- dated list of the CPD activities you have carried out since you last renewed your registration;
- supporting evidence.

First, the summary of your practice history should help to show the CPD assessors how your CPD activities are linked to your work and practice. This part of the CPD profile should help you to show how your activities are relevant to your current or future work.

Second, your statement of how you have met the HCPC Standards should clearly show how you believe you meet each of the standards, and should refer to all the CPD activities you have undertaken and the evidence you are submitting to support your statement.

Third, your dated list might be something you produce as a result of the audit, looking at your personal CPD record, or it may be something you can produce automatically if you use an electronic record-keeping system.

Finally, the supporting evidence you submit to the HCPC on request will reinforce the statements you make in your CPD profile. It should demonstrate that you have undertaken the CPD activities you have referred to, and should also show how they have improved the quality of your work and benefited service users. The evidence you provide should include a summary of all your CPD activities, as this will show that you meet Standard 1. From this, the CPD assessors should also be able to see how your CPD activities are a mixture of learning activities and are relevant to your work (and therefore meet Standard 2).

Writing the summary of your practice

Your summary should describe your role and the type of work you do. The summary should identify the people you communicate and work with the most, and identify the specialist areas you work in, including your main responsibilities, such as your job description if appropriate.

When you have written your statement about how you meet the HCPC standards for CPD, you may find it helpful to go back over your summary of work, to make sure that it clearly explains how your CPD activities are relevant to your future or current work.

Writing your statement

When you write your statement, the HCPC expect you to concentrate and focus on how you meet Standards 3 and 4 – how your CPD activities have improved the quality of your work and the benefits to service users. One way to complete your statement is to choose four to six CPD activities you have carried out and for each one you should describe:

- what the activity was;
- what you learnt;
- how you think the activity improved the quality of your work and benefited your service users.

You can choose to tell the HCPC about the activities which you think benefited you the most and for which you have some supporting evidence. Writing your statement like this can be a clear and simple way of showing the HCPC how you have met the standards. However, there is more than one way of completing your statement, including using your professional development plan or similar (if you have one), or structuring your statement around each of the CPD standards.

Not all paramedics have a personal development plan or review their role or performance – you may be self-employed, or your employer may not work in this way. But if you do have a personal development plan, you will find it helpful to use this as a starting point for writing your statement.

CPD and competence

There is no automatic link between your CPD and your competence. This is because it would be possible (although unlikely) for a competent paramedic not to undertake any CPD and yet still meet the HCPC Standards for their skills and knowledge. Equally, it would be possible for a paramedic who was not competent to complete a lot of CPD activities but still not be fit to practise. Box 21.1 explains how HCPC Standards 1–5 can be demonstrated in your CPD profile.

Box 21.1 How HCPC Standards 1–5 can be demonstrated within your CPD profile

Standard 1 – A registrant must maintain a continuous, up-to-date and accurate record of their CPD

You can keep a record of your activities in a way that is most convenient for you. However, the evidence you submit should include a summary page or sheet of all your CPD activities, which must be accurate, continuous and up to date, and concentrate on the CPD you have undertaken in the previous two years. (For paramedics, it is usually 1 September year one through to the beginning of the new registration period, so nearly two years.)

The simplest way to prove that you have kept a record of your CPD is to send the HCPC, as part of your evidence, a list in date order of all of your CPD activities since your previous registration.

This could be in any format you choose, but it is suggested that it might be a simple table which includes the date and 'type' of each activity.

Standard 2 – A registrant must demonstrate that their CPD activities are a mixture of learning activities relevant to current or future practice

You *do not* need to undertake or log a certain number of hours or days. This is because different people will be able to dedicate different amounts of time to CPD, and also because the time spent on an activity does not necessarily reflect the learning gained from it.

To comply with this standard, your CPD must include a mixture of learning activities, so you should include different types of learning activities in your CPD record. The CPD might be a mixture of what is relevant in your current job and activities that are helping to prepare you for a future role. Or you may choose to concentrate most – or all – of your CPD on the new area of work you will be moving into. This means that your CPD may be very different from that which your colleagues undertake, even though you are from the same profession. For example, if you manage a team, your CPD may be based around your skills in appraising your team, supporting their development and financial planning. *It might not even include dealing with, treating or caring for clients/patients/ service users.*

Standard 3 – A registrant must seek to ensure that their CPD has contributed to the quality of their practice and service delivery

You should aim for your CPD to improve the way you work. Your learning activities should lead you to make changes to how you work, which improve the way you provide your service. This might mean that you continue to work as you did before but you are more confident that you are working effectively.

You do not necessarily have to make drastic changes to how you work to improve the quality of your work and the way you provide your service. You may meet this standard by showing how your work has developed as your skills and knowledge have increased as a result of your learning. In meeting this standard, you should be able to show that your CPD activities are part of your work, contribute to your work and are not separate from it.

Standard 4 – A registrant must seek to ensure that their CPD benefits the service user

You will meet this standard as long as you have demonstrated that your CPD has benefited your service users.

Where you work will dictate who your service users are; for many, this will be patients. However, if you work in education, your service users may be your students or the team of educationalists you oversee. Similarly, if you work in management, your service users may be your team, or other teams that you are part of. If you work in research, your service users may be the people who use your research. So, in this standard, 'service user' means anyone who is primarily affected by your work.

Standard 5 – A registrant must, upon request, present a written profile (which must be their own work and supported by evidence) explaining how they have met the standards for CPD

If you are selected for audit, the HCPC will send you a CPD profile. Under this standard, you must complete the profile, including details of how you have met the standards for CPD. You must return the profile to them, with evidence to support it, by the deadline set.

CPD can and does take many forms; it does not, however, set down exactly how or what paramedics should learn. Paramedics may already be taking part in activities through which they learn, and which develop their work, but they may not call these activities CPD.

Many people think of CPD as being formal education only (e.g. going on courses). The HCPC standards take account of the fact that a course may not be the most useful kind of CPD for all health professionals, and some health professionals may not have access to courses, or be able to gain funding support or study time. Different registrants will have different development needs, and their CPD activities may be very different. However, the HCPC does stipulate that the CPD profile should be both the registrant's own work and a true reflection of their CPD activity. It is worth noting your CPD is your 'responsibility' and *not* that of your employers. So being busy at work is *not* CPD and not an excuse for failing to undertake it. However, gaps in CPD can be accounted for by long-term illness or maternity and paternity leave in support of a new child.

The following are examples of CPD:

Paramedic registrant working in a clinical role

- Attending a short course on new laws affecting your work
- Appraising an article with a group of colleagues
- Giving colleagues a presentation on a new technique

Paramedic registrant working in education

- Member of learning and teaching committee
- Review for a professional journal
- Studying for a formal teaching award

Paramedic registrant working in management

- Member of an occupational group for managers
- Studying management modules
- Supporting the development and introduction of a national or local policy

Paramedic registrant involved in research

- Presentation at a conference
- Member of a local ethics research committee
- An article for a scientific journal

Two years' registration

The HCPC will only audit registrants who have been registered for more than two years (HCPC, 2017b). They believe that all registrants should undertake CPD throughout their careers; they also believe that registrants should be allowed at least two years on the register to build up evidence of their CPD activities before they are audited. This means that if you are a recent graduate, and you renew your registration for the first time, you will not be chosen for audit. Similarly, if you have had a break from work, and you have just come back onto the register, you will not be chosen for audit the first time you renew your registration.

WHAT HAPPENS TO YOUR COMPLETED CPD PROFILE?

The HCPC will ask CPD assessors to assess your CPD profile. At least one of these assessors will be a paramedic. While your profile is being assessed, and during any appeal that takes place, you will stay on the register and can continue to work. There are three possible outcomes at this point:

- *Your profile meets the standards* – you will stay on the register. The HCPC will write to you and let you know that the profile met all five standards.
- *More or further information is needed* – the HCPC will write to you and let you know what information the assessors need to decide whether you meet the standards of CPD. You will stay on the register while you send more information to the assessors.
- *Your profile does not meet the standards* – if this is the case, the CPD assessors will decide whether or not to offer you more time (up to an extra three months) to meet the standards. The HCPC will normally ask you for more information without extra time allocated before making this decision.

The CPD assessors will decide whether to offer you an extra three months by considering whether:

- you have made a reasonable attempt to provide a complete CPD profile;
- you have met some of the standards;
- with extra time, it would be possible for you to meet the standards.

If you do not meet the standards, the HCPC will consider removing you from the register. However, whatever decision they reach, they will advise you of it and the reasons for making it.

Finding out more

Published example profiles can be seen on the HCPC website (see www.hcpc-uk.org/). These profiles, which were put together in partnership with the College of Paramedics, are intended to show how health professionals can prove that their CPD activities have met the standards and how they can write a statement that can evidence this.

For further information about the CPD audit, read the document *Continuing Professional Development and Your Registration* (HCPC, 2017b). This is a helpful publication, and more details about CPD and the audit process can again be found on the HCPC website.

CONCLUSION

CPD is fundamental to the development of all health and social care practitioners, and registrants must seek to ensure that their CPD benefits the service user. Professional bodies and organisations campaign for greater support and recognition of your CPD activities, from your employers and other organisations. As the UK professional body for paramedics, the College of Paramedics provides its members with access to its online *British Paramedic Journal*, together with CPD activities that include regional CPD events throughout the UK, e-learning CPD and a CPD Hub which contains a large collection of videos, podcasts and links to courses, details of which can be found on their website.

Chapter key points:

- This chapter has provided an explanation of the role and value of continuing professional development (CPD).
- It has addressed the HCPC's CPD standards and discussed the associated documentation.
- Examples have been provided of CPD activity for inclusion in your profile.
- Each of the relevant standards are discussed and ideas are provided about how you can meet the standards within your written profile.
- An explanation of what will happen to your completed profile is given, along with advice about how to obtain further information and guidance.

REFERENCES AND SUGGESTED READING

Broughton, W. and Harris, G. (eds.) (2022) *Principles for Continuing Professional Development and Lifelong Learning in Health and Social Care*. On behalf of the Interprofessional CPD and Lifelong Learning UK Working Group. Bridgwater: College of Paramedics.

College of Paramedics (CoP) (2019) *Paramedic Curriculum Guidance*, 5th edition. Available at: https://collegeofparamedics.co.uk/COP/ProfessionalDevelopment/Paramedic_Curriculum_Guidance.aspx (accessed 9 April 2024).

Health and Care Professions Council (HCPC) (2016) *Guidance on conduct and ethics for students*. Available at: https://www.hcpc-uk.org/resources/guidance/guidance-on-conduct-and-ethics-for-students/ (accessed 9 April 2024).

Health and Care Professions Council (HCPC) (2017a) *Standards of Education and Training*. Available at: https://www.hcpc-uk.org/standards/standards-relevant-to-education-and-training/set/ (accessed 9 April 2024).

Health and Care Professions Council (HCPC) (2017b) *Standards of Continuing Professional Development*. Available at: https://www.hcpc-uk.org/standards/standards-of-continuing-professional-development/ (accessed 9 April 2024).

Health and Care Professions Council (HCPC) (2017c) *Continuing Professional Development and Your Registration*. Available at: https://www.hcpc-uk.org/resources/guidance/continuing-professional-development-and-your-registration/ (accessed 9 April 2024).

Health and Care Professions Council (HCPC) (2017d) *How to renew your registration*. Available at: https://www.hcpc-uk.org/globalassets/resources/guidance/how-to-renew-your-registration.pdf?v=637145224790000000 (accessed 9 April 2024).

Health and Care Professions Council (HCPC) (2017e) *Returning to practice*. Available at: https://www.hcpc-uk.org/globalassets/resources/guidance/returning-to-practice.pdf (accessed 9 April 2024).

Health and Care Professions Council (HCPC) (2017f) *Confidentiality: Guidance for registrants*. Available at: https://www.hcpc-uk.org/resources/guidance/confidentiality--guidance-for-registrants/ (accessed 9 April 2024).

Health and Care Professions Council (HCPC) (2017g) *How to complete your continuing professional development profile*. Available at: https://www.hcpc-uk.org/globalassets/resources/cpd/how-to-complete-your-cpd-profile.pdf (accessed 9 April 2024).

Health and Care Professions Council (HCPC) (2021) *Paramedic CPD audit (2021): CPD audit statistics for the 2019–2021 renewal cycle*. Available at: https://www.hcpc-uk.org/about-us/insights-and-data/cpd/cpd-audit-statistics-2019-2021/cpd-audit-statistics-2018-2020-pa/ (accessed 9 April 2024).

Health and Care Professions Council (HCPC) (2023) *Standards of Proficiency for Paramedics*. Available at: https://www.hcpc-uk.org/standards/standards-of-proficiency/paramedics/ (accessed 9 April 2024).

Health and Care Professions Council (HCPC) (2024) *Standards of Conduct, Performance and Ethics*. Available at: https://www.hcpc-uk.org/standards/standards-of-conduct-performance-and-ethics/ (accessed 9 April 2024).

Quality Assurance Agency (QAA) (2019) *Subject benchmark statement: Paramedics*. Available at: https://www.qaa.ac.uk/docs/qaa/subject-benchmark-statements/subject-benchmark-statement-paramedics.pdf?sfvrsn=7735c881_4 (accessed 9 April 2024).

USEFUL WEBSITES

College of Paramedics: https://collegeofparamedics.co.uk/
Department of Health and Social Care – England: https://www.gov.uk/government/organisations/department-of-health-and-social-care
Health and Care Professions Council: www.hcpc-uk.org/
Health and Care Professions Council – What activities count as CPD?: https://www.hcpc-uk.org/cpd/your-cpd/cpd-activities/
Health and Social Care Northern Ireland: https://www.hscni.net/
NHS England eLearning for Health (elfh) Hub: https://portal.e-lfh.org.uk/
NHS Scotland: https://www.scot.nhs.uk/
NHS Wales: https://www.nhs.wales/

Index

Page numbers in *italics* are figures; with 't' are tables.

TOP 7

REASONS WHY YOU SHOULD BE A MEMBER:

01

Discounts on a range of products and services, including books and medical supplies

02

Access to over 500 conference videos on the CPD Hub

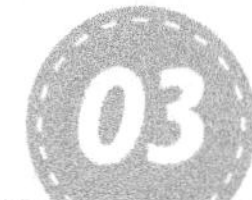

03

A quarterly membership magazine 'Paramedic INSIGHT', packed with interesting features, news and advice

04

Free subscription to the College of Paramedics' very own quarterly electronic research journal, the 'British Paramedic Journal' (BPJ)

05

A regular email news digest, keeping you informed of what's going on within the College and the profession

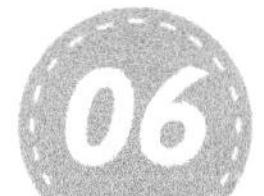

06

Access to our national network of CPD events, discounted for members

07

£5 million medical malpractice and public liability insurance for elective placements and good Samaritan Acts
(T's & C's Apply)

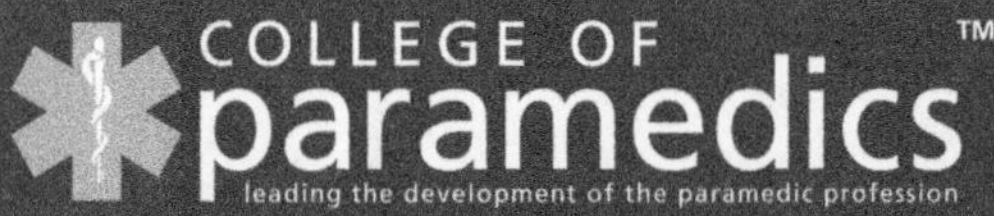

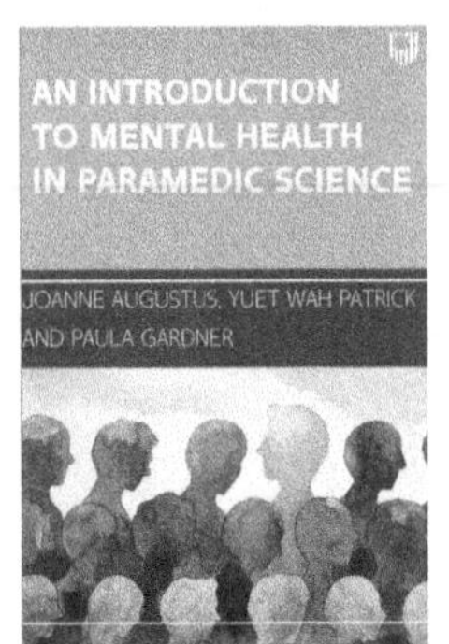

An Introduction to Mental Health in
Paramedic Science

**Joanne Augustus, Yuet Wah Patrick,
Paula Gardner**

ISBN: **9780335249930** (Paperback)
eISBN: 9780335249947

2022

An Introduction to Mental Health for Paramedic Science explores
how mental health problems impact on the individual in the context
of emergency medicine, covering the critical areas that students and
practitioners need to know, such as:

- **The key characteristics of mental health problems**
- **How mental health problems relate to the assessment performed in the community**
- **Referral pathways**
- **Treatment following referral**
- **Transition to registration**

Taking key concepts of mental health, including person-centred care, as
the framework Mental Health for Paramedic Science includes guidance
on:

- **Multidisciplinary working**
- **Principles and practical applications of legislation**
- **Evidence based bio-medical approaches**
- **Trauma informed care**

Written by experienced paramedic educators this new book is the go-
to guide for students and practicing paramedics wanting to explore
mental health treatments as encountered in paramedic settings.

www.mheducation.co.uk

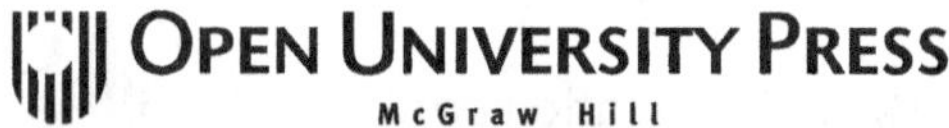

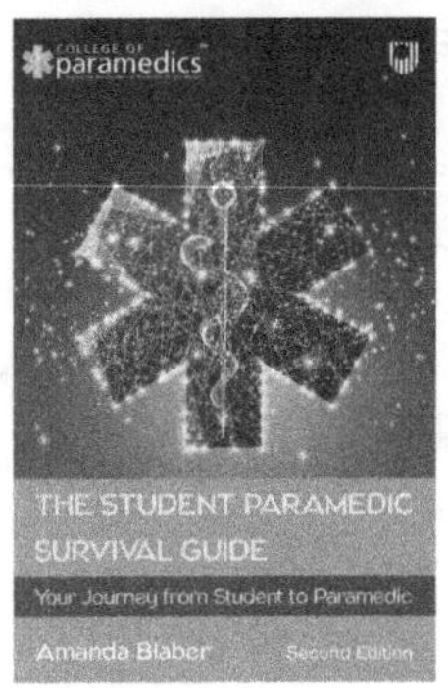

The Student Paramedic Survival Guide: Your Journey from Student to Paramedic

Amanda Blaber

2nd Edition

ISBN: **9780335251926** (Paperback)
eISBN: 9780335251933

2023

The second edition of the bestselling *The Student Paramedic Survival Guide 2e* gives vital information and advice to help you succeed in your education and become a registered paramedic. The book prepares you to make the transition into your first paramedic job by following a clear and helpful 5-part structure:

- **Is this the right career for me?**
- **Preparing to apply**
- **Making the most of your academic study**
- **Placement: preparing for it and making the most of it**
- **Transition to registration**

To equip you with insights into what studying to be a paramedic is really like, the book is packed full of comments and case studies from students, paramedics, practice educators, academics and brand new to this edition – family members. Their expertise and experience will be invaluable as you study and prepare for practice.

The book also includes advice on making the most of your preferred learning style and guidance on how to look after yourself when you encounter traumatic events.

www.mheducation.co.uk

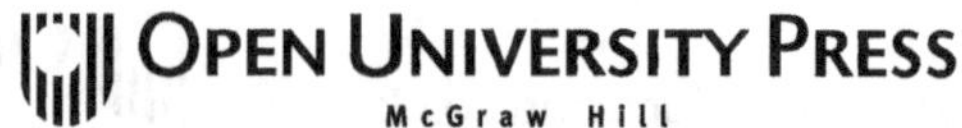

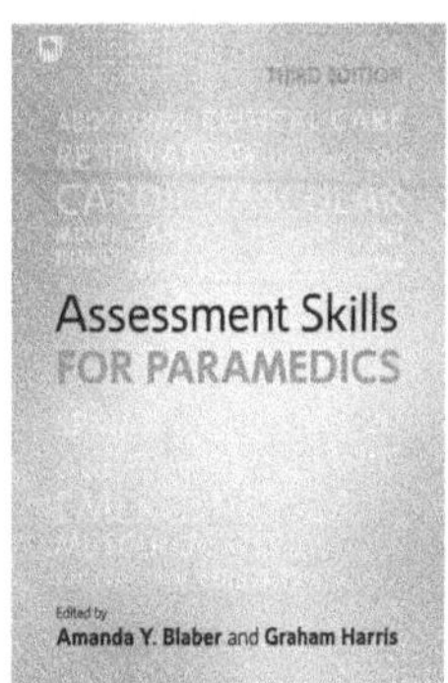

Assessment Skills for Paramedics

Amanda Blaber, Graham Harris

3rd edition

ISBN: **9780335249954** (Paperback)
eISBN: 9780335249961

2021

Now in its third edition, this highly acclaimed resource is the ideal guide for student and practicing paramedics looking to refresh and consolidate their assessment skills. Assessment Skills for Paramedics has been thoroughly revised with fresh, up-to-date knowledge and national guidance. Divided into body systems and presented in a clear, accessible format the book takes the reader through the considerations and actions required for each type of emergency presentation.

New to this edition:

- **Histories, assessments and scenarios across multiple chapters.**
- **Content covering the well-being of the paramedic.**
- **Chapters including the review of systems (RoS) approach.**
- **A systematic format of primary and secondary survey in each chapter that relates to current practice.**
- **Reflects updates to Ambulance Clinical Guidelines, and the National Institute for Health and Care Excellence Guidelines, and The Joint Royal Colleges Ambulance Liaison Committee guidelines.**

Written by experienced paramedics, specialist health care professionals and doctors, this book will enable readers to enhance their practical knowledge and to make accurate, timely and thorough assessment of patients across the lifespan.

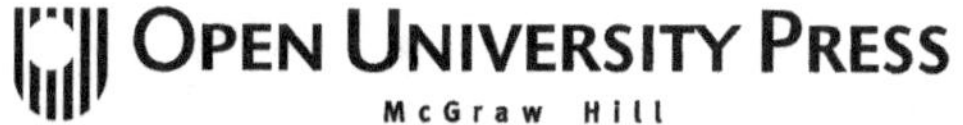

www.mheducation.co.uk

OPEN UNIVERSITY PRESS

McGraw Hill